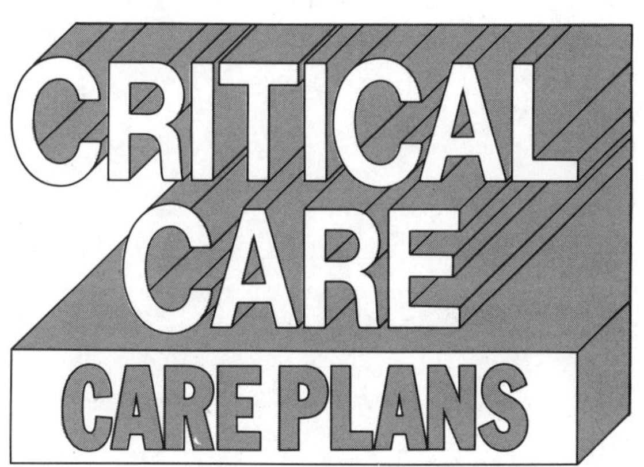

NANCY M. HOLLOWAY, RN, MSN, CCRN, CEN

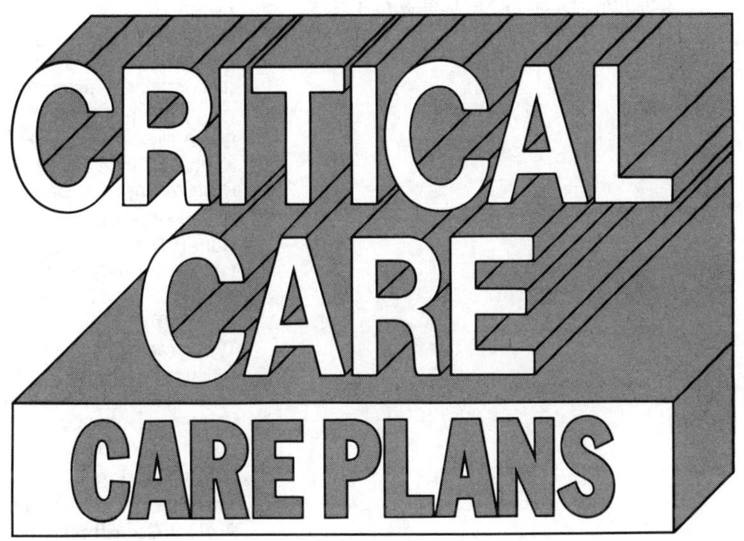

NANCY M. HOLLOWAY, RN, MSN, CCRN, CEN

Springhouse Corporation
Springhouse, Pennsylvania

Staff For This Volume

CLINICAL STAFF

Clinical Director
Barbara McVan, RN

Clinical Editor
Diane Schweisguth, RN, BSN, CCRN, CEN

Consulting Editor
Ruth E. Malone, RN, CEN
Staff Nurse, Emergency Department
Children's Hospital Medical Center
Oakland, Calif.

PUBLICATION STAFF

Executive Director, Editorial
Stanley Loeb

Executive Director, Creative Services
Jean Robinson

Design
John Hubbard (art director), Stephanie Peters (associate art director), Elaine K. Ezrow

Editing
Susan L. Taddei (senior acquisitions editor), David Prout, Bernadette M. Glenn (acquisitions assistant)

Copy Editing
David Prout (supervisor), Nick Anastasio, Keith de Pinho, Elizabeth B. Kiselev, Doris Weinstock, Debra Young

Art Production
Robert Perry (manager), Mark Marcin, Loretta Caruso, Anna Brindisi, Donald Knauss, Robert Wieder, Christina McKinley

Typography
David Kosten (manager), Diane Paluba (assistant manager), Brenda Mayer, Valeria L. Rosenberger, Joyce Rossi Biletz, Robin Rantz, Brent Rinedoller

Manufacturing
Deborah Meiris (manager), T.A. Landis

Project Coordination
Aline S. Miller (supervisor), Laurie J. Sander

The clinical procedures described and recommended in this publication are based on research and consultation with nursing, medical, and legal authorities. To the best of our knowledge, these procedures reflect currently accepted practice; nevertheless, they can't be considered absolute and universal recommendations. For individual application, all recommendations must be considered in light of the patient's clinical condition and, before administration of new or infrequently used drugs, in light of latest package-insert information. The authors and the publisher disclaim responsibility for any adverse effects resulting directly or indirectly from the suggested procedures, from any undetected errors, or from the reader's misunderstanding of the text.

Printed in the United States of America. For information write Springhouse Corporation, 1111 Bethlehem Pike, Springhouse, Pa. 19477.

CCCP-020189

Library of Congress Cataloging-in-Publication Data
Holloway, Nancy Meyer, 1947-
Critical-care care plans/ Nancy M. Holloway.
p. cm.
Includes bibliographies and index.
1. Intensive care nursing. I. Title.
[DNLM: 1. Critical Care—nurses' instruction.
2. Nursing Assessment. 3. Patient Care Planning—nurses' instruction. WY 154 H745c]
RT120.I5H63 1988
610.73'61—dc19
DNLM/DLC
for Library of Congress
ISBN 0-87434-168-X 88-24813
CIP

Contents

Contributors and Consultants

CONSULTING EDITOR

Ruth E. Malone, RN, CEN
Staff Nurse, Emergency Department
Children's Hospital Medical Center
Oakland, California

Contributors

Nancy Newell Bell, RN, MN, CCRN, CEN
Critical Care/Trauma Clinical Nurse Specialist
Eden Hospital Medical Center
Assistant Clinical Professor
School of Physiological Nursing
University of California at San Francisco
(Multiple Trauma)

Phyllis R. Easterling, RN, MS, CEN
Assistant Professor, Department Chairperson
Medical-Surgical Nursing
Samuel Merritt College of Nursing
Oakland, California
(Acute Renal Failure, Major Burns, Thoracotomy)

Patricia C. Hanson, RN
President
Healthcare Management Services
Eagan, Minnesota
(Delivering Quality Care in a Cost-Conscious Environment, DRG Information, Nursing Transfer Criteria)

Ruth E. Malone, RN, CEN
Staff Nurse, Emergency Department
Children's Hospital Medical Center
Oakland, California
(Grieving and Dying, Ineffective Coping, Impaired Physical Mobility, Sensory-Perceptual Alteration, Guillain-Barré Syndrome, Seizures, Gastrointestinal Hemorrhage, Pancreatitis, Acquired Immunodeficiency Syndrome, Drug Overdose, Organ Donation appendix, Pediatric Considerations appendix, Postoperative Considerations appendix)

Cecilia E. Shaw, RN, C, OCN, BSN
Clinical Supervisor
Cancer Care Associates
Tulsa, Oklahoma
(Pulmonary Embolism)

Susan A. VanDeVelde-Coke, RN, MA, MBA
Director of Nursing, Medical/Surgical, General Hospital
Health Sciences Center
Winnipeg, Manitoba, Canada
(Liver Failure)

Patricia Harvey Webb, RN, BSN, MS
Assistant Professor
Samuel Merritt College of Nursing
Oakland, California, and
Staff Nurse, Critical Care Units
Mt. Diablo Hospital Medical Center
Concord, California
(Craniotomy, Increased Intracranial Pressure)

Consultants

C. Russell Baker, BSN, CRNA
Maryland Institute for Emergency Medical Services Systems
Baltimore, Maryland
(Mechanical Ventilation)

Diane Sadler Benson, RN, MEd, MS
Nurse Specialist/Educator
Private Practice
Eureka, California
(Acute Pain, Appendices, Cardiac Surgery, Diabetic Ketoacidosis, Grieving and Dying, Guillain-Barré Syndrome, Hyperglycemic Hyperosmolar Nonketostis, Knowledge Deficit, Liver Failure, Nutritional Deficit, Pulmonary Embolism, Shock, Thoracotomy)

Carolyn Childs, RN, MSN
Head Nurse
Orthopedic and Neurosurgical Operating Rooms
Johns Hopkins Hospital
Baltimore, Maryland
(Acquired Immunodeficiency Syndrome)

Michelle Gilmore, RN
Children's Hospital Medical Center of Northern California
Oakland, California
(Pediatric Appendix)

Michael J. Groves, RN, BSN
Nurse Clinician I, Admitting Area
Maryland Institute for Emergency
Medical Services Systems
Baltimore, Maryland
(Drug Overdose, Ineffective Coping)

Deana Lee Holler, RN, BSN
Nurse Clinician II
Trauma Resuscitation Area
Shock Trauma Clinical Center
Maryland Institute for Emergency
Medical Services Systems
Baltimore, Maryland
(Disseminated Intravascular Coagulation)

Susie C. Mull, RN, BSN
Staff Nurse
Telemetry Unit
Prince George's Hospital
Prince George's County, Maryland
(Acute Heart Failure, Acute Myocardial
Infarction)

Paula Sallese, RN
Primary Nurse I, Trauma Center
Maryland Institute for Emergency
Medical Services Systems
Baltimore, Maryland
(Acute Renal Failure)

William L. Shopp, RN, BSN
Head Nurse
Neurosurgical Intensive Care Unit
Cleveland Clinic Hospital
Cleveland, Ohio
(Guillain-Barré Syndrome)

Julie Mull Strange, RN, CCRN
Trauma Program Coordinator
Temple University Hospital
Philadelphia, Pennsylvania
(Adult Respiratory Distress Syndrome,
Gastrointestinal Hemorrhage, Impaired
Physical Mobility, Increased Intracranial
Pressure, Major Burns, Multiple Trauma,
Pancreatitis, Seizures, Sensory-
Perceptual Alteration)

Theresa Supik Wilson, BSN, MSN
Nurse Clinician I
Operating Room
Maryland Institute for Emergency
Medical Services Systems
Baltimore, Maryland
(Craniotomy)

Acknowledgments

Many talented people contributed to this book's genesis. I extend a special thank you to our contributors and consultants, acknowledged by name on a separate page. In addition, I thank the following people for their extraordinary contributions:

Ruth Malone, consulting editor. A gifted writer, Ruth's perception, sensitivity, and commitment to this project played a major role in this book's quality.

Camden Rutter, administrative assistant, whose computer wizardry and willingness to work within seemingly impossible deadlines eased project management immeasurably.

Julie Strange and Diane Sadler Benson, clinical reviewers. Julie's thoughtful feedback helped clarify the plans, while Diane's perceptive comments both strengthened individual plans and crystallized the book's mission.

Patricia Hanson, consultant, whose expertise in DRGs and discharge planning added a unique flavor to this book.

The talented publishing team at Springhouse Publishing Company, particularly Susan Taddei, senior acquisitions editor. Susan, your editorial guidance, loyalty to this project, and sponsorship were major factors in this book's publication. I will always be grateful to you for helping to turn the vision into reality.

Dedication

This book is dedicated to Hazel Pye Meyer, my mother, for her strength and inspiration; D. Michael Holloway, my husband, for championing my dreams; and Jason Holloway, my son, for making it all worthwhile.

Preface

This book is essential. Why? Because it integrates three major trends in nursing: care planning, nursing diagnosis, and diagnosis-related groups (DRGs). Written by American and Canadian clinical experts with the "front-line" nurse in mind, these practical plans help the nurse resolve three challenges in planning patient care: distinguishing nursing from medical care, balancing standardized versus individualized care, and reconciling cost containment versus quality care.

Focusing on the critical care patient, this is the first book to:

- distinguish clearly between nursing's collaborative functions (those shared with medicine) and its independent functions (those uniquely nursing's)
- offer the less-experienced bedside nurse, nursing student, and nursing instructor comprehensive, realistic clinical plans
- offer the experienced bedside nurse condensed plans concise enough to be used easily in today's hectic, cost-conscious environment.

This book provides a comprehensive—yet concise—data bank for the clinical nurse to use daily in planning quality nursing care. The 30 comprehensive care plans are straightforward and easily individualized. The book also contains selected condensed care plans in a special section designed for fast access. These fill a long-existing need for a clinically relevant reference that meets different requirements in developing effective, professional care plans.

Distinguishing features

The blend of standardized and individualized features provides the advantages of standardized care plans but also surmounts their limitations. This approach will help you save time and avoid repetition in preparing plans while promoting personalized care.

Plans cover major clinical disorders, such as acute myocardial infarction, as well as important general conditions nurses encounter daily, such as grieving and dying. Other care plan books may contain one or the other but not both.

Plans for clinical disorders include both collaborative problems and nursing diagnoses. This dual focus is unique. Collaborative problems are named with familiar medical terminology, for example, shock. Nursing diagnoses are named with selected terminology from NANDA's Seventh Conference on the Classification of Nursing Diagnoses. This refreshing approach helps you:

- see the complete picture of patient care
- differentiate clearly between areas of collaborative and independent nursing responsibility
- apply the latest official information on nursing diagnoses
- avoid force-fitting all patient care under nursing diagnosis terminology. Used in other care plan books, that process only renames medical diagnoses and fosters confusion between nursing and medicine.

Each plan contains the latest clinically relevant DRG information, including DRG numbers, principal diagnoses, and mean length of stay, which helps you:

- understand the reimbursement system that is the primary cause of today's cost-conscious environment
- know the mean length of stay of patients with this disorder, which is a benchmark for judging speed of recovery and in planning patient teaching.

Common historical and subjective findings for a clinical disorder are presented according to Gordon's Functional Health Patterns, a widely known nursing assessment format that blends both traditional and contemporary areas of nursing assessment. Objective findings are presented in a body systems format. This approach helps you:

- recognize pertinent data reported or displayed by the patient
- understand the basis on which the collaborative problems and nursing diagnoses were identified.

Why are care plans important?
Clinically, care plans offer a way to plan for and communicate appropriate patient care. Legally, they offer a framework for establishing the standard of care in a given situation. Financially, they can validate appropriateness of care given and justify staffing levels and patient-care charges.

If care plans are so important, why don't more nurses use them?
Most nurses are first exposed to care plans as students. They learn rapidly that writing care plans can be frustrating and time-consuming. As graduates, many nurses view care plans as irrelevant or too cumbersome to use; this is particularly true in critical care.

Even nurses who would like to use written care plans may find themselves at a loss about how to integrate the concepts of nursing diagnosis and DRGs. Overwhelmed, they may turn to previously published books for guidance, only to encounter frustration there, too. You'll hear them say, for instance:

"These care plans won't work for me—they're too general. I'd have to rewrite everything for a 'real' patient."

"This is great information on nursing diagnosis, but I can't figure out quickly which ones go with which medical disorder!"

"This information's too theoretical—it doesn't fit the real world."

"This is amazing! Everything's written as a nursing diagnosis. Why rename problems we already have names for?"

And yet, it's obvious that nurses would welcome the guidance that could be provided by clinically relevant care plans. If you listen closely to their questions about patient care, you hear concerns like these:

- Problems nurses face on admission:

  "What's really important to note when doing a physical assessment? I haven't got time to check everything!"

  "What laboratory tests and diagnostic procedures should I anticipate? What do they usually show?"

  "What are the nursing priorities for this patient?"

- Problems nurses face in providing care:

  "What are the usual problems encountered with this type of patient?"

  "Why are certain interventions important?"

  "What are the complications that can occur with this disorder?"

- Problems nurses face in discharge planning

  "How long is this patient likely to be in the hospital?"

  "Realistically, what patient teaching can I accomplish?"

  "From a nursing standpoint, how do I know when a patient's ready for discharge?"

The solution: This book

This book provides clinically relevant answers to these questions because they are targeted to the needs of the "hands-on" nurse clinician.

Standardized vs. individualized care

The most common and important question nurses raise about written care plans is: "How can I write care plans? Who has the time?" Their concern about time is valid because most nurses practice in a hectic, complex environment that allows little time for thoughtful care planning.

To cope with this problem, some nurses have turned to published standard care plans. Nurses like standard care plans because they decrease the repetition involved in writing individual care plans, help inexperienced staff learn about patient care, and remind experienced staff about aspects of care they may have overlooked. But standard care plans have some disadvantages, too. They may be misused as the *only* care plan—promoting standardized rather than individualized care—or they may be ignored altogether.

Major differences of opinion exist in nursing concerning standardized versus individualized care plans. Opponents of standardization argue that it equals depersonalization in delivering care. Advocates argue that standardization is efficient because it limits care planning time without sacrificing quality and that it fosters quality assurance. This disagreement cannot be resolved easily; however, this book combines the advantages of standard care plans with unusual features that help to overcome their disadvantages:

• The plans blend standardized and individualized aspects of care. Standardization works better in some areas of care planning than others: problems, priorities, and interventions can usually be standardized, but outcome criteria, timing of interventions, and discharge criteria require a significant amount of individualization. This book takes both sets of factors into account and encourages flexibility in areas that vary significantly among patients.
• Space is provided at the end of each problem to append "additional individualized interventions."

These unusual features challenge the nurse to think creatively. Because the resulting plan is pertinent and individualized, its clinical usefulness is assured. *These* care plans won't be dismissed—they'll be used every day.

The most important point to remember in the debate over standardized versus individualized care plans is this: *it is not a care plan that causes depersonalized care; it is the nurse's attitude.* The nurse who appreciates patients as individuals will use a standardized care plan as a basis from which to work creatively, staying attuned to individual patient responses while applying the art and science of nursing.

Because of its unusual focus, this book helps resolve three major issues nurses struggle with: medical versus nursing care, standardized versus individualized care, and cost containment versus quality care. These stances need not be adversarial; in fact, the nurse as well as the patient can benefit from the best aspects of all these approaches to patient care. Ultimately, any care plan is only as good as the nurse who provides the care. Conscientious nurses find care plans a resource for learning new information quickly, refreshing their knowledge, and focusing their energy on the most important problems their patients may encounter. The contributors have based these care plans on a blend of clinical expertise, nursing diagnosis, and care planning—and always kept the nurse on the front line in mind. Recognizing that most nurse clinicians welcome help in dealing with these problems, the contributors provided expert assistance in this unique book.

—Nancy Meyer Holloway

Section I

With sicker patients, shorter stays, and burgeoning technology, the critical care nurse faces three professional challenges, which are covered here: differentiating nursing from medical care, balancing standardized and individualized care, and reconciling cost-containment and quality care.

Delivering Quality Care in a Cost-Conscious Environment

The advent of Medicare's prospective payment system (PPS) in 1983 dramatically altered the U.S. health care system in ways that nurses are only now beginning to understand. Faced with new restrictions and regulations affecting delivery of care, nurses are confronted by twin challenges: sicker patients and shorter hospitalizations. Nurses also play a key role in maintaining a hospital's financial viability in this competitive, market-driven health care environment. So, to maintain quality patient care under PPS, they must become increasingly sophisticated and innovative.

Evolution of PPS

Before 1983, charges for hospital care were based on a retrospective method of payment. Hospital charges reflected what the market would bear and often were arbitrary, unrelated to the actual costs of delivering services. Nursing, for the most part, was a nonbillable direct service that was "bundled" under room and board charges in the hospital bill. But since 1983, third-party payers have demanded more explicit accounting for all services and appropriate charges for every area of health care delivery. In response, hospitals have begun to "unbundle" all units of service, including nursing.

Medicare, as one of the nation's primary insurers, was the first to change its reimbursement method. PPS was a desperate attempt to conserve the rapidly dwindling dollars available in the Medicare trust fund set up in the 1960s to ensure that America's elderly would have access to health care.

Under Medicare's PPS, diagnosis-related groups (DRGs) were developed to identify clinically homogeneous groups of diagnoses that use similar tests, treatments, and services and therefore could be reimbursed at similar rates. This federal system is now mandatory for Medicare recipients at all acute-care hospitals. Besides standardizing payment, the purpose of this classification system was to put acute hospitalized patients into groups that could be used to predict resource consumption.

At present, 475 DRGs are grouped into 23 Major Diagnostic Categories (MDCs) based on anatomical organ systems such as the respiratory system. The predetermined rate of reimbursement for each DRG is based on numerous factors, including the principal diagnosis, the patient's age, the presence of complications or comorbidities, and the occurrence of an operating room procedure. All these factors are taken into account upon patient discharge to determine which of the 475 DRGs will be assigned.

The DRG system is incongruous in many ways, the most important of which for critical care is that it does not take into account the severity of the patient's illness. Thus, a patient who is severely ill and needs more services and a longer length of stay has hospitalization paid for at the same rate as a patient with the same illness and assigned DRG who is not severely ill. DRGs are, in effect, an averaging system: a hospital will lose money on cases whose cost of care will be more than the amount paid for the assigned DRG, and will make money on cases whose costs are less than the DRG payment. Many patients who would have been hospitalized in the past, however, now receive treatment in outpatient settings; since only patients who meet strict criteria may be admitted to acute-care facilities, hospitals have, overall, sicker patients to care for than in the past. Thus, patient care must be managed as efficiently as possible for a hospital to maintain financial viability.

TEN FREQUENTLY OCCURRING DRGs

127 Heart Failure and Shock
89 Simple Pneumonia and Pleurisy
182 Esophagitis, Gastroenteritis, Digestive Disorders
140 Angina Pectoris
14 Cerebrovascular Disorders
96 Bronchitis and Asthma
138 Cardiac Arrhythmia
296 Nutritional and Metabolic Disorders
88 Chronic Obstructive Pulmonary Disease
121 Circulation Disorders and Acute Myocardial Infarction

How DRGs are assigned

After discharge, a patient is assigned a DRG based on the following factors:

- principal diagnosis—the diagnosis that necessitated admission to the hospital
- secondary diagnosis—all secondary conditions that exist at the time of admission or that develop during hospitalization and affect the treatment or length of stay (LOS)
- operative procedures—any surgical procedures performed for definitive treatment rather than for diagnostic or exploratory purposes
- age—for some conditions, a different reimbursement rate applies for patients under and over age 17
- discharge status—for example, discharged home or transferred to another hospital

• complications—any conditions arising during hospitalization that may prolong LOS at least 1 day in 75% of patients (diabetes is an example)
• comorbidity—a preexisting condition that will increase LOS at least 1 day in 75% of cases.

All these factors need to be considered and the presence or absence of each factor determined to identify the correct DRG.

How DRGs are used

Once the correct DRG has been determined, further statistical measures affecting reimbursement can be identified:

• geometric mean LOS—each DRG has an assigned geometric mean LOS. The terms "geometric mean LOS" or "mean LOS" in this book refer to specific DRG statistical data for *groups* of patients. (The unqualified term "LOS" is a general abbreviation referring to an *individual* patient's length of stay.) The geometric mean LOS usually is thought of as the average LOS for all patients within a specified DRG; however, this is a misconception. Actually, the geometric mean LOS is a statistical measure used in cost accounting for the sole purpose of determining when a patient becomes a "day outlier," a status discussed in the second bullet below.

The geometric mean LOS is an average derived from 1986 data that indicated the mean LOS for patients with specific diagnoses or procedures at the time the DRG system was updated. This fact has four important implications:

□ The geometric mean LOS should be understood as an indicator of when most patients within each DRG *were* discharged in 1986. It was never intended as a guide to determine when a specific patient *should* be discharged.

□ Current hospital stays are significantly shorter than the geometric mean LOS. Since 1984, the actual LOS across the country for nearly every DRG has decreased dramatically as doctors have learned to treat in outpatient facilities, in their offices, and within a much shorter length of time in the hospital.

□ The geometric mean LOS has nothing to do with the point after which a hospital loses money on a case. That point can be determined only after studying each case.

□ In most cases, a hospital begins losing money before the geometric mean LOS is reached because actual costs of caring for the patient usually exceed designated costs before this point. This is partially because hospital costs have continued to increase as actual LOS has continued to decrease.

• relative weight—a statistical term used in DRG reimbursement that determines the actual dollars a particular hospital is paid for a given DRG. Among other factors, it is based on categorizing the hospital as acute or chronic, teaching or nonteaching, urban or rural. The weight assigned each DRG has been reevaluated and revised at regular intervals. Because relative weights vary greatly from hospital to hospital and area to area, and because of their periodic revision, they are not specified in the care plans in this book.

• outlier—a case that uses more than the assigned resources. Two types of outliers exist: day outliers and cost outliers. A day outlier is a case that remains hospitalized, on average, at least 17 days beyond the geometric mean LOS. Although hospitals receive an additional payment for cases that reach day outlier status, payment is never enough to cover the costs or charges incurred during an extended LOS.

Day outliers were predicted to be 5% of all Medicare discharges when PPS was begun. The latest data suggest only 1.5% of discharges are reaching outlier status. In nearly every instance, day outliers are those patients that have multisystem failure and are severely ill. Preventing a patient from becoming a day outlier is rarely under the control of the nurse.

A cost outlier is a case that does not exceed the allowed number of days but does exceed the expected cost. Cost outliers are even rarer than day outliers. This book does not include information on cost outliers.

Keys to success under DRGs

Several major factors affect financial success under DRGs:

• accurate coding of all medical record data upon patient discharge. This is achieved by choosing the diagnosis that was chiefly responsible for the admission and taking into account all of the factors that will place the diagnosis in the highest-paying category, for example, complications and comorbidities. Medical record professionals, responsible for coding, depend on the documentation in the medical record when assigning the DRG.

• effective and efficient management of the "products" of hospitals—that is, hours of nursing care, laboratory tests, medications, supplies, and other services. The more efficiently care is delivered, the greater the hospital's profit.

• an appropriate "case mix" (a hospital's mixture of patients, defined by severity of illness and by assigned DRGs). A hospital must maintain a mixture of patients with various DRGs to plan and manage resource allocation within defined reimbursement parameters.

• utilization of the appropriate site of care and LOS. Care will be reimbursed only if it is provided in the appropriate setting; for example, hospitals will not be reimbursed for care that could have been appropriately provided in an outpatient setting. LOS also must be appropriate. Patients must not be discharged before they are medically stable, yet the hospital must ensure that unnecessary costs will not be incurred.

• prevention of complications. Because development of complications increases the likelihood that care costs will exceed reimbursement, their prevention is a key factor in maintaining fiscal control.

The nurse's role in a PPS

The increasing impact of government regulations and third-party payers on the health care delivery system presents the nurse with challenges and opportunities. The nurse is instrumental in assuring both the quality of care and the hospital's financial success under any PPS. Some of the ways the nurse can maintain quality care and yet dramatically affect a hospital's reimbursement include:

- care planning. The nurse must be able to prioritize and deliver care that realistically correlates with the projected LOS—which means establishing and following an explicit plan of care. Care planning provides an essential means of determining goals and desired outcomes of care delivery. Only by this means can care be managed effectively and efficiently. This book is designed to help the nurse provide quality care in the age of cost containment.

  Caring for a patient without a care plan can be likened to starting out on an unfamiliar trip without a road map. You may end up getting to the desired destination, but most certainly it will involve many unnecessary detours and take more time, effort, and money. This book identifies the "destination" of care—the target outcome criteria—as well as the best "roads" for getting there.
- early discharge planning. Besides developing and using care plans, the nurse must become involved in the discharge planning process from the moment of patient admission, whenever possible. By beginning the process early, the nurse can help ensure appropriate posthospital care. For example, the nurse can emphasize patient and family education, maximize self-care abilities, and arrange for continued care by other professionals when indicated, such as home care nursing or nursing home placement.
- patient education. Patient and family education is a key element in preventing readmissions. The patient's perception of quality care is also enhanced by the nurse's promoting self-care and teaching about posthospital management of health problems.
- documentation. Accurate documentation promotes communication among caregivers that maximizes the benefits of hospitalization while minimizing LOS. Also, documentation is crucial for assigning appropriate reimbursement for services.
- quality assurance. This mandatory element should include both specific nursing standards and monitoring of adherence to those standards.

The nurse also needs to become aware of the impact of the new economics on the professional status of nursing. This is an opportune time to advance the function and image of nursing as an independent health care practice that can be judged not only on its benefits for patients but also on its contribution to hospitals' economic viability. Nursing services now can be costed out and charged for separately, based on their use by patients.

Advent of retrospective review

Besides DRGs, other changes occurring in health care are increasing the pressure to deliver care in the most efficient manner possible. Particularly important is the advent of health maintenance organizations (HMOs) and other competitive medical plans.

The nurse should be aware of the complexity of reimbursement methods now used in health care. Most third-party payers (not just Medicare) are using some form of prospective payment mechanism to reimburse hospitals. For example, many HMOs currently pay hospitals on a negotiated rate not unlike DRGs. Also, all third-party payers are negotiating discounted rates for services provided in acute-care facilities in return for guaranteeing that their subscribers will use those specific facilities for their acute-care needs. Such arrangements are important for hospitals because they ensure a constant volume of patients. With LOSs much shorter than they were before PPS, hospitals must count on a stable census to ensure maximum efficiency and a constant cash flow.

For patients, the hospital incentives in every PPS mean shorter stays and potential decreases in hospital services. Some patients who have been accustomed to remaining in the hospital until they perceive themselves as ready for discharge believe that they are being discharged prematurely; nurses, doctors, and other health care providers have expressed the same concern. Because of these perceptions of premature patient discharges and underutilization of necessary services, state peer review organizations (PROs) have been mandated to increase review of care provided in acute-care facilities.

This mandate has led PROs to establish explicit review criteria specific to the provision of medical care. Within the DRG system, however, information is evolving that could be useful to nurses and may become mandatory—specifically, the screening criteria being developed and used by the Health Care Financing Administration (HCFA) and state PROs. The PROs are using generic and disease-specific criteria retrospectively to identify the appropriateness of admission and discharge and the quality of care.

Although PROs are reviewing only Medicare cases now, in the near future all hospital admissions, outpatient procedures, home care services, and care in doctors' offices and long-term settings will be reviewed in much the same manner.

The nursing challenge

Today, the nurse faces greater challenges than ever: sicker patients, more complex care, and shorter patient stays. This book offers the nurse the expertise of professional colleagues who understand the complexities of those challenges and who offer powerful help in meeting them.

Nursing Diagnosis

The American Nurses Association Social Policy Statement (1980) defines nursing as "the diagnosis and treatment of human responses to actual or potential health problems." Gordon (1987) defines a nursing diagnosis as "an actual or potential health problem amenable to nursing intervention." Although nurses have been diagnosing patient problems for years, the term "nursing diagnosis" is relatively new.

Past diagnostic efforts have been hampered by the lack of a common language for labeling nursing problems. To remove this barrier, the National Conference Group on the Classification of Nursing Diagnoses began identifying and classifying health problems that nurses treat. That organization, formed at the first National Conference on Classification of Nursing Diagnoses in 1973, is now the North American Nursing Diagnosis Association (NANDA).

This book identifies nursing diagnoses using the terminology recommended by NANDA whenever possible. The NANDA list represents those diagnoses that the organization has accepted for study and clinical testing. The current list appears in the Appendix.

Two major issues relate to the NANDA diagnoses: clinical usefulness of the terminology and the renaming of medical diagnoses.

Because the nursing diagnosis movement is evolving, nurses have encountered significant difficulty in using the list. Gordon (1986a) has reported that some authors have criticized the categories' complexity, esoteric language, lack of specificity, and differing levels of abstraction. Others have described the terminology as wordy, vague, confusing, and inconsistent (Iyer et al., 1986). These responses highlight an important problem: some NANDA diagnostic labels are not yet useful. Because the clinical experts who wrote the care plans in this book found some of the NANDA diagnoses functional and others not, the editor has made the following decisions reflected in the care plans:

- Some of the NANDA diagnosis labels contain a general classification and a specific diagnosis (Gordon, 1986b). In these situations, we have dropped the categorical labels and used the most precise term.
- We used alternate terminology for one diagnosis because of its wordiness. In place of "Alteration in nutrition: less than body requirements," we used "nutritional deficit."
- Because people do not speak in the language of nursing diagnoses (for example, "airway clearance, ineffective"), we have modified the wording slightly to reflect usual conversational sequences and phrasing.

As noted, the NANDA list is incomplete. So, if an author could not find a diagnosis on the list to fit a patient problem, a new diagnosis was generated. In that case, the diagnosis is followed by an asterisk and a footnote identifying it as a non-NANDA diagnosis.

Another issue has provoked substantial controversy and major differences of opinion within the nursing diagnosis community: the renaming of medical diagnoses. Many nurses believe that several of the accepted nursing diagnoses rename medical diagnoses; examples are decreased cardiac output, decreased tissue perfusion, and impaired tissue integrity. In part, this controversy stems from the continued difficulty nurses face in articulating the dimensions of their practice and, particularly, in differentiating it from medical practice.

Because the editor believes that renaming problems already defined by other disciplines simply perpetuates the confusion between nursing and medicine, these diagnoses have not been used as identified nursing diagnoses. Instead, such problems are clearly identified as *collaborative* problems requiring both medical and nursing interventions and named with familiar terminology; for example, shock is used instead of decreased cardiac output, and ischemia instead of impaired tissue perfusion. In some cases, a nursing diagnosis fits a nonacute problem but not a related acute problem, such as fluid volume deficit. In a nonacute fluid volume deficit, independent nursing interventions, such as providing preferred fluids and encouraging fluid intake, are paramount. In an acute fluid volume deficit, however, medical interventions, such as ordering the insertion of an intravenous catheter and prescribing specific intravenous solutions, are paramount. For diagnostic clarity, fluid volume deficit was used in the first situation and hypovolemia in the second. The distinction between acute and nonacute gives new direction to the use of NANDA diagnoses and may prove a fruitful path for exploration in further attempts to increase their clinical usefulness.

References

American Nurses Association, Congress for Nursing Practice. *Nursing: A Social Policy Statement.* Kansas City, Mo.: American Nurses Association, 1980.

Gordon, Marjory. "Nursing Diagnosis and the Diagnostic Process," *American Journal of Nursing* 76(6):1298-1300, 1986a.

Gordon, Marjory. "Structure of Diagnostic Categories," in *Classification of Nursing Diagnoses: Proceedings of the Sixth NANDA Conference.* Edited by Hurley, M. St. Louis: C.V. Mosby Co., 1986b.

Gordon, Marjory. *Nursing Diagnosis: Process and Application*, 2nd ed. New York: McGraw-Hill Book Co., 1987.

Iyer, Patricia, et al. *Nursing Process and Nursing Diagnosis.* Philadelphia: W.B. Saunders Co., 1986.

McLane, Audrey, ed. *Classification of Nursing Diagnoses: Proceedings of the Seventh NANDA Conference.* St. Louis: C.V. Mosby Co., 1987.

Using the Care Plans

These care plans are designed to give the practicing nurse a maximal amount of clinically relevant information within a minimal number of pages. This book is intended not as a substitute for the broad clinical knowledge base found in more exhaustive nursing references, but as a guide for providing quality "hands-on" nursing care to patients in the critical care setting.

Every care plan is subdivided into sections, each presenting the nurse with a different type of information. Becoming familiar with the basic format will enhance their practical value for the clinical nurse. Explanations of each section follow, along with specific recommendations for using the care plans in practice.

DRG information

Immediately after the name of the clinical plan, abbreviated *DRG information* appears, including:

• relevant DRG number(s). Some clinical disorders always have the same DRG, such as myasthenia gravis. Others, such as circulatory disorders, are subdivided into several DRGs. Where appropriate in the care plans, relevant DRGs are indicated.
• mean geometric LOS for each DRG
• comments, if any, designed to provide a perspective on the DRG.

Ideally, each care plan would include the usual LOS for the patient's particular disorder to guide patient and family teaching and to provide a benchmark against which the nurse could assess the patient's progress toward discharge. Unfortunately, such information is not available. However, this book provides the best substitute: the mean LOS, previously defined. The mean LOS gives you an idea of the average LOS for patients with this diagnosis. You could use this information to anticipate when teaching and discharge planning should be well under way and when maximum hospital benefit usually has been reached. Do not use the mean LOS as a target for discharge; doing so will almost certainly ensure that the hospital loses money. Instead, plan for a LOS shorter than the mean LOS, when possible, yet appropriate for the patient's needs. Remember that the mean LOS relates to discharge from the hospital, not transfer from the critical care unit. Mean LOSs are updated periodically; the nurse should consult the *Federal Register* if updates are desired.

Introduction

In *Definition and Time Focus,* the disease process, surgical procedure, or patient problem that forms the focus of the care plan is briefly discussed within a specific time frame. Surgical care plans generally cover the immediate preoperative and postoperative phases of care. Medical care plans focus on the most acute phase of the illness, the period in which the patient is most likely to be hospitalized in the critical care unit.

Listed next in *Etiology and Precipitating Factors* are factors that directly or indirectly contribute to the condition's development, grouped according to pathophysiologic mechanism when possible.

Focused assessment guidelines

This section is further subdivided into *Nursing History, Physical Findings, Diagnostic Studies,* and *Potential Complications.*

The assessment guidelines delineate specific findings common to most patients with the identified condition. The intent is to give the clinician a vivid picture of the typical patient presentation in a given condition.

The first assessment section, *Nursing History (Functional health pattern findings),* presents subjective and historical data organized by Gordon's *Functional Health Patterns* framework. The health patterns represent 11 broad categories within the holistic wellness-illness system. Each of the health patterns provides useful parameters for assessment of any given patient. Because the emphasis here is on definitive or common findings, only those patterns with data relevant to the condition are included. If the patient presenting with a specified condition does not typically give information about a particular health pattern, the pattern is not listed.

The second assessment section, *Physical Findings,* presents typical objective findings in a patient who presents with the identified condition. The physical findings are organized in the body systems format familiar to most nurses.

Diagnostic Studies, the next section of the care plan, provides the nurse with information regarding laboratory and diagnostic tests usually performed for the diagnosis and treatment of a patient with the specified condition. Not all the tests listed may be performed on a particular patient; what actually is ordered depends on individual factors. However, the astute nurse is aware of the significance of studies and tests that may pertain to the patient's condition and, when indicated, offers collaborative input to the doctor regarding selection of such studies.

Finally, *Potential Complications* are listed for the identified condition. The complications listed are those most common for patients with the condition. Activities that promote wellness and preventive health care practices now constitute a significant focus in nursing practice. Nurses must be aware of associated complications to take preventive action on the patient's behalf.

Collaborative problems and nursing diagnoses

This section contains the main body of the care plan: the major problems specific to the condition. They are the predictable patient health responses usually caused by the pathophysiology of the disorder.

Problems may be actual or potential. An actual problem is one that usually is present and presents identifiable signs and symptoms. A potential problem is one the patient is at high risk of developing; although signs and symptoms are not present, risk factors are.

Because nursing practice is based on both medical and nursing diagnoses, a patient problem is identified as either a *Collaborative Problem* or *Nursing Diagnosis,* represented by two distinctive logos. Care plans that focus only on nursing diagnoses are shown with a circle in a box, which symbolizes independent action. Disease-related care plans are shown with two boxes joined together forming a plus sign, which symbolizes collaboration.

Collaborative problems are those that fall within the domain of both medicine and nursing; their etiologies are amenable primarily to medical interventions. The nurse does not treat them independently but may initiate monitoring for them. Nursing diagnoses are those problems that fall within nursing's expertise. They are responses that the nurse can identify and treat independently; etiologies are primarily amenable to independent nursing interventions.

Some problems identified here as nursing diagnoses have the potential to become collaborative problems; for example, the nurse may have primary responsibility for airway clearance, but if complications necessitate endotracheal intubation, the problem becomes a collaborative one. The intent in this book is not to split hairs over functional terminology but to increase nursing awareness of the diagnostic activities that are currently a part of nursing practice.

In most plans, the patient problems are presented in order of descending importance. Exceptions may be found in some surgical-procedure care plans, where preoperative problems are presented first to provide logical continuity.

After problem identification, the *Nursing Priority* in dealing with the problem is specified. The nursing priority indicates the focus for the nursing interventions that follow. *Interventions* and *Rationales* are presented in a two-column format. Interventions are based on clinical experience and the nursing literature and thus represent a blend of practice and theory.

Interventions usually are ranked in order of decreasing priority. Interventions may be interdependent or independent in nature: for interdependent functions, initiation is the responsibility of another health care provider, typically a doctor. However, whether performed under direct or indirect supervision or under

FUNCTIONAL HEALTH PATTERNS

1. Health Perception–Health Management Pattern
- perceived pattern of health and well-being
- general level of health care behavior (how health is managed)
- health status related to future planning

2. Nutritional-Metabolic Pattern
- food and fluid consumption relative to metabolic need
- pattern, types, quantity, and preferences of food and fluids
- skin lesions and healing ability
- indicators of nutritional status (such as skin, hair, and nail condition)

3. Elimination Pattern
- patterns of excretory function
- routines and devices used

4. Activity-Exercise Pattern
- exercise, activity, leisure, recreation
- activities of daily living
- sports
- factors interfering with activity

5. Sleep-Rest Pattern
- pattern of sleep, rest, and relaxation
- perception of quantity and quality of rest
- energy level
- sleep aids and problems

6. Cognitive-Perceptual Pattern
- adequacy of sensory modes
- pain perception and management
- cognitive functional ability

7. Self-Perception–Self-Concept Pattern
- attitudes about self
- perception of abilities
- body image, identity, and general emotional pattern
- pattern of body posture and speech

8. Role-Relationship Pattern
- role engagements—family, work, social
- perception of responsibilities

9. Sexuality-Reproductive Pattern
- satisfaction or disturbances in sexuality
- reproductive stage
- reproductive pattern

10. Coping–Stress Tolerance Pattern
- general coping pattern and effectiveness
- perceived ability to manage situations
- reserve capacity and resources

11. Value-Belief Pattern
- values, goals, or beliefs that guide choices
- conflicts related to health status

Adapted from: Gordon, Marjory. *Nursing Diagnosis: Process and Application,* 2nd ed. New York: McGraw-Hill Book Co., 1987.

protocol, they always require the application of nursing judgment. Independent functions do not require initiation by another health care provider; they are initiated by the nurse under his or her professional license. The rationales, although purposely brief, incorporate relevant physiologic mechanisms whenever possible, along with other helpful data.

Nurses have long recognized that patients respond best to care that takes personal characteristics and preferences into consideration. Space is provided at the end of each problem section for notation of additional individualized interventions.

Each problem is followed by specific *Target outcome criteria,* defined as ideal expected patient responses to the interventions. These criteria, based on the clinical expertise of the nurses who contributed to this book, focus on specific, measurable patient responses that provide the nurse with guidance in evaluating the results of care provided. Outcome criteria are grouped according to ideal time periods for achievement. These criteria are intended only as a guide; individual variation is to be expected, and professional judgment must be used because outcomes obviously depend on many factors.

Transfer planning and documentation

The final section of the care plan includes three guides for the nurse to use in planning for transfer and in documenting care. *Nursing Transfer Criteria* provides the nurse with specific guidelines for assessing the patient's readiness for transfer from the critical care unit. These guidelines were developed by clinical experts and a discharge planning expert. Criteria listed in this section help alert the nurse to factors that must be considered before the doctor makes the decision to transfer the patient. They are particularly helpful in situations where a rapid transfer decision must be made, for example, when the unit is full and a critically ill patient still must be admitted from the emergency department. The criteria in this section are in addition to the general transfer criteria contained in Appendix H, "Transfer Criteria Guidelines." Again, these criteria are intended only as a guide; some patients may not meet them, but if not, it is imperative that appropriate special planning be accomplished to avert any lapse in needed care.

The *Patient-Family Teaching Checklist* ensures that needed patient and family teaching related to the specified condition has been considered. Teaching should begin on admission, when appropriate, and continue throughout hospitalization. Therefore, teaching interventions in the plan reflect only what may be reasonable to accomplish in the critical care unit. Interventions related to teaching are interwoven throughout the plan or included in a special "Knowledge deficit" problem. (General teaching information is contained in the comprehensive "Knowledge Deficit" care plan.) Such teaching can be, and usually is, done by various health professionals besides the nurse. It can be expected that dietitians, physicians, clinical specialists, social workers, and others will be responsible for various aspects of patient education during hospitalization.

Finally, the *Documentation Checklist* provides a summary of items that should be documented in the patient record. As has been previously noted, recent changes in health care payment systems make thorough documentation more essential than ever. Accurate documentation also helps protect the nurse in the event of case-related litigation, although now, as always, the best way to avoid legal problems is to maintain high standards of care, impeccable professionalism, and warm, caring relationships with patients.

Concluding each care plan is a list of *Associated Care Plans* found elsewhere in this book and *References,* which may be helpful to the nurse seeking further information.

In using these care plans in clinical practice, the nurse may benefit from closely reading the applicable care plan first. Thereafter, the care plan should be referred to on a shift-by-shift basis, with problems addressed and interventions documented in the nurse's notes. Before the patient is transferred, the nurse should review the appropriate sections and evaluate all teaching and documentation, using the checklists as a guide.

Organization of the book

The comprehensive clinical care plans contain the depth of detail appropriate for education and reference, but nurses already familiar with the care appropriate for a particular condition may prefer an abbreviated version. So this book includes a special section containing condensed care plans (arranged alphabetically) for selected conditions nurses encounter most frequently.

This book contains two types of care plans: those pertaining to a specific medical diagnosis or surgical procedure, which constitute the main portion of the book, and those referred to as "general" care plans, which are presented in a separate section. The general care plans provide the nurse with detailed interventions for dealing with common patient problems (for example, pain, knowledge deficit, and grieving and dying) that may be encountered in caring for any patient. They are designed to be used with the diagnosis- or procedure-based clinical plans.

References

Health Care Financing Administration. "Changes to the In-Patient Hospital and Prospective Payment System and Fiscal Year 1988 Rates; Final Rule," *Federal Register* 52:33-34, September 1, 1987.

Health Systems International. *Diagnosis Related Groups,* 4th revision. New Haven, Conn.: Health System International, 1987.

Prospective Payment: Laws, Regulations, Guidelines and Decisions. Owings Mills, Md.: National Health Publishing, 1984.

Section II

Comprehensive care plans cover general nursing problems or major medical diagnoses, arranged by body systems. These plans incorporate functional health patterns, nursing diagnoses, collaborative problems, prioritized interventions, target outcome criteria, nursing transfer criteria, and DRGs.

Acute Pain

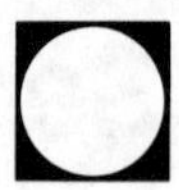

Introduction

DEFINITION AND TIME FOCUS

Acute pain represents neurologic or emotional suffering of brief duration in response to a noxious stimulus. Commonly encountered in critical care nursing, pain is best prevented and relieved when the nurse continuously maintains an anticipatory attitude toward it. Although individuals experience pain differently, pain's symbolic meaning as a danger and threat commonly heightens a person's perceptions of it. Sophisticated pain management demands patient sensitivity, compassion, and a repertoire of pain-control techniques. Because of individual factors and various pain-control techniques, selecting the best strategy for a particular patient at a particular time represents an important area of nursing judgment.

This clinical plan focuses on the care of a patient experiencing pain lasting minutes to days, rather than chronic pain, because acute pain is more common in the critical care setting.

ETIOLOGY AND PRECIPITATING FACTORS

- surgical or accidental trauma
- inflammation
- musculoskeletal disorders, such as muscle spasm
- neuropathies, such as multiple sclerosis
- visceral disorders, such as myocardial infarction
- vascular disorders, such as sickle cell anemia
- invasive diagnostic procedures
- excessive pressure, such as with immobility
- cancer

Focused assessment guidelines

NURSING HISTORY (Functional health pattern findings)

Health perception–health management pattern

- reports acute physical discomfort, typically described as pain, pressure, tightness, soreness, or a crushing or burning sensation

Nutritional-metabolic pattern

- may describe anorexia, nausea, or vomiting

Activity-exercise pattern

- commonly reports intense fatigue

Sleep-rest pattern

- may report inability to rest or sleep

Cognitive-perceptual pattern

- commonly reports inability to concentrate

Self-perception–self-concept pattern

- may report anxiety or depression

Role-relationship pattern

- may express concern that others discount presence of pain
- may describe decreased desire to interact with others

Coping-stress tolerance pattern

- may report increased stress level
- may report decreased ability to deal with frustration or other stress

PHYSICAL FINDINGS

General appearance

- tense, guarded posture
- facial grimacing
- crying
- moaning

Musculoskeletal

- writhing
- muscle spasms
- unnatural stillness
- increased physical activity (uncommon)

Integumentary

- diaphoresis
- pallor

Neurologic

- impaired concentration
- irritability
- restlessness

Cardiovascular

- hypertension and tachycardia
- hypotension and bradycardia (uncommon)

Respiratory

- tachypnea
- gasping

DIAGNOSTIC STUDIES

No specific studies indicate the presence or degree of pain. Various procedures may be indicated in the differential diagnosis of pain. For example, for chest pain, the patient may undergo a 12-lead EKG, chest X-ray, creatine phosphokinase (CPK) level measurements, and pulmonary ventilation scan to differentiate acute myocardial infarction from pulmonary embolism. See care plans on specific disorders for details.

Nursing diagnosis: *Acute pain from tissue injury, ischemia, infarction, inflammation, edema, tension, or spasm*

NURSING PRIORITY: Prevent or ameliorate pain.

Interventions	Rationales
1. Monitor continuously for possible indicators of pain, including verbalization, grimacing, diaphoresis, tense posture, splinting, restlessness, irritability, emotional withdrawal, and vital sign changes.	1. The critically ill patient may not be fully conscious because of the underlying disease process or medications that blunt perception. As a result, verbal reports alone may not adequately indicate the presence and degree of pain. Astute observation may provide ongoing protection against unreported or underreported pain.
2. Analyze and document pain characteristics systematically; for example, use the PQRST mnemonic: P = precipitators Q = quality R = region and radiation S = severity T = time Report promptly to the doctor any new or increased pain.	2. Careful analysis of pain characteristics aids in the differential diagnosis of pain. Systematic analysis prevents hasty and possibly inaccurate conclusions about the quality or probable cause of pain. New or increased pain requires prompt medical evaluation.
3. Prepare the patient for brief, unavoidably painful experiences, such as percutaneous skin puncture for arterial blood gas sampling. State clear expectations for behavior, such as, "If it hurts, squeeze my hand but hold your other arm still."	3. The psychological assault of unexpected pain can unnerve even the most stoic person and make coping with the pain needlessly stressful. Brief explanations decrease fear of the unknown and assist the patient to prepare for the experience. Positive suggestions provide an appropriate way to cope with the pain.
4. When preparing the patient for a painful experience, try to find out how much the patient wants to know. If possible, tailor the degree of detail to the patient's preference for information and the procedure's extensiveness.	4. Recent research suggests that patient teaching does not necessarily reduce anxiety; people vary in the degree of detail they find helpful. According to Watkins and Odegaard (1986), "blunters," who tend to avoid threatening aspects of situations to lessen their psychological impact, usually want to know relatively little about impending experiences, whereas "monitors," who tend to seek information about stressful events to lessen their psychological impact, want to know a great deal. Providing a "blunter" with detailed information increases anxiety, whereas withholding it from a "monitor" worsens stress. When possible, appropriate matching of preference and preparation honors individual differences and supports the patient's preferred coping style.
5. During painful procedures, provide ongoing support and positive reinforcement:	5. Providing support and encouragement during the experience increases the patient's sense of security and control.
• Use brief, simple directions, as needed. Use therapeutic touch, if accepted by the patient.	• Brief, simple directions are necessary because pain reduces comprehension and retention of information. Touch may convey comfort more profoundly than words.

(continued)

Interventions	Rationales
• When the experience is over, encourage the patient to ventilate feelings, if desired. Convey acceptance for the way the patient handled pain, using praise generously when appropriate.	• Discussing the pain experience afterward provides an opportunity for psychological integration and closure of the experience, which is necessary to "let go" of it. Conveying acceptance is particularly important for patients who scream or otherwise lose control because it reassures them and may relieve any residual feelings of shame.
6. For patients with ongoing pain, explicitly convey the goal of aggressive pain management. State the intent to prevent or "stay on top" of the pain and to work with the patient to identify the most effective methods. Explain the rationale for and importance of reporting a painful episode as soon as possible.	6. A sense of isolation can increase pain. Explicit goals imply that the situation is manageable, which is reassuring. The power of suggestion may reduce anxiety. Involving the patient promotes a sense of mastery that reduces fears of helplessness or loss of control. Pain can be more easily brought under control in its early stages.
7. Use a repertoire of nonpharmacologic pain-control strategies:	7. Because various factors may cause or exacerbate pain, various techniques may bring relief. A multifaceted approach is more likely to be successful than a single strategy.
• Positioning—Cushion and elevate the painful area, if possible. Avoid pressure or tension on it. Encourage the patient to rest in a comfortable position, but also to change position every hour, while awake. Explain the rationale for position changes, provide gentle reminders, and assist with movement, as necessary.	• Cushioning increases comfort, whereas elevation reduces edema. Avoiding pressure or tension eliminates additional painful stimuli to an already sensitive area. Rest increases pain tolerance. Position changes improve perfusion, helping remove chemical mediators of inflammation and bringing oxygen and other nutrients to healing tissue. Position changes also help prevent complications of immobility. Because moving the painful area may temporarily increase pain, patient education, gentle but firm reminders, and active assistance may be necessary to ensure attention to this important need.
• Cutaneous stimulation from massage or applications of heat, cold, or mentholated ointments	• Pain impulses are believed to be transmitted to the brain along peripheral nerve fibers to ascending pathways in the spinal cord. Sharp, acute pain is transmitted along small-diameter, type A fibers, whereas dull, chronic pain is transmitted along type C fibers. Stimulation of nearby sensory fibers inhibits these ascending pain pathways. In addition, massage increases perfusion and reduces muscle tension. Cold-induced vasoconstriction reduces edema, and is especially helpful in the first 24 hours after injury. Heat increases circulation, mobility, and muscle relaxation, which is particularly helpful in decreasing painful reflex muscle spasms.
• Contralateral stimulation, such as scratching or massage, when the injured area is not directly accessible (for example, under a cast).	• Stimulation of the area opposite the painful one may provide relief, probably by triggering release of endorphins, opiate-like substances that relieve pain.
8. Explore various behavioral pain-control strategies, including:	8. Behavioral strategies divert attention away from the pain, promote a sense of self-control, help increase muscle relaxation, and may stimulate endorphin release.
• Distraction techniques, such as talking or listening to lively music	• Distraction is especially helpful for brief episodes of pain, but may increase pain perception and fatigue after the distracting stimulus is removed.
• Relaxation techniques, such as rhythmic breathing, progressive muscle relaxation, listening to relaxation tapes or soothing music, or meditation.	• These techniques reduce muscle tension, enhance rest, and promote a sense of well-being.

Interventions

9. If the above methods are inappropriate or ineffective, collaborate with the doctor and clinical pharmacist, as needed, to determine an effective analgesic regimen. Administer and document analgesics, as ordered, which may include:

- potent narcotics, such as morphine and meperidine (Demerol)
- mild narcotics, such as codeine, and narcotic agonists or antagonists, such as butorphanol (Stadol)
- nonnarcotic analgesics, such as aspirin, acetaminophen (Tylenol), and ibuprofen (Motrin)
- analgesic adjuncts, such as diazepam (Valium).

Rationales

9. The above methods require a certain amount of emotional energy and ability to concentrate, which the patient may lack, or pain may be too severe for them to be effective. Personalizing the analgesic regimen recognizes individual differences in pain perception and provides the most effective control for a particular patient.

- Narcotics act centrally to blunt pain perception. Potent narcotics, although effective in relieving severe pain, may cause sedation, respiratory depression, nausea, vomiting, and other adverse effects.
- Used for moderate pain, these agents are less likely to cause respiratory depression.
- Appropriate for mild pain, these agents block synthesis of prostaglandins (inflammatory mediators that increase pain).
- Adjuncts increase the analgesic's effects, lessen muscle spasm, cause sedation, and may diminish pain recall.

10. Involve the family in pain-relief strategies. Help them understand the patient's behavior in the context of the pain. Explain the rationale for pain-control techniques. Correct misconceptions, if present. When possible, have family members participate in providing the pain relief, such as massage. Explicitly acknowledge the difficulty in observing a loved one's pain, and provide emotional support.

10. Capitalizing on family bonds can provide a level of interpersonal comfort that exceeds what concerned, supportive staff can provide. Understanding pain behaviors may help the family be more patient, and correcting misconceptions (such as the danger of addiction) may relieve unwarranted anxiety. Acknowledgment of family members' emotional suffering conveys respect and concern for them, and nurturing family members increases their coping skills and ability to support the patient.

11. If chronic pain is present, collaborate with the patient, family, doctor, and pharmacist to optimize pain relief, through such measures as:

- transcutaneous electrical nerve stimulation (TENS) or acupuncture
- epidural or intrathecal narcotic administration
- continuous I.V. or subcutaneous infusion or patient-controlled analgesic devices
- hypnosis, guided imagery, and biofeedback
- tricyclic antidepressants.

11. Persistent pain (for example, from bone cancer) may demoralize the patient and make suffering seem unbearable. A collaborative approach using several options increases the likelihood of finding the optimal pain-control regimen for a given patient.

- TENS transmits an electrical stimulus to the painful area, whereas acupuncture uses needles to stimulate sensitive areas. The techniques are thought to stimulate endorphin and enkephalin release, thus providing analgesia, and to block ascending pain transmission pathways.
- These techniques deliver small doses of narcotics directly to endorphin receptor sites, allowing powerful pain control without the usual systemic effects of narcotics.
- Continuous infusions allow for more effective control by maintaining constant analgesic blood levels. Patient-controlled analgesic devices allow for immediate pain relief, increasing the patient's sense of control over pain.
- These techniques alter pain perception but require motivation and training, so they may not be appropriate for some patients.
- Tricyclic antidepressants block the synaptic removal of serotonin. Serotonin stimulates the production of enkephalins, chemical mediators that inhibit pain impulses.

12. Additional individualized interventions: ____________

12. Rationales: ____________

Target outcome criteria
Within 1 hour after the onset of pain, the patient will:
• verbalize increased comfort
• have a relaxed posture and facial expression
• have vital signs within normal limits.

Transfer planning

NURSING TRANSFER CRITERIA
Upon transfer, documentation shows evidence of:
• pain-relief measures effective in reducing pain to tolerable level
• vital signs within normal limits.

PATIENT-FAMILY TEACHING CHECKLIST
Document evidence that the patient and family demonstrate understanding of:
__ anticipated course of pain in relation to the medical condition
__ importance of prompt reporting of pain
__ effective analgesics
__ nonpharmacologic relief strategies.

DOCUMENTATION CHECKLIST
Using outcome criteria as a guide, document:
__ clinical status on admission
__ significant changes in status
__ pertinent laboratory and diagnostic test findings
__ pain characteristics
__ analgesic administration
__ nonpharmacologic strategies
__ behavioral strategies
__ effectiveness of measures
__ patient's and family's response to pain
__ patient-family teaching
__ transfer planning.

ASSOCIATED CARE PLANS
Grieving and Dying
Impaired Physical Mobility
Ineffective Coping
Sensory-Perceptual Alteration

REFERENCES

Carpenito, L. *Nursing Diagnosis: Application to Clinical Practice*. Philadelphia: J.B. Lippincott Co., 1983.

Gregory, C., and Holloway, N. "Pain," in *Nursing the Critically Ill Adult*, 3rd ed. Edited by Holloway, N. Menlo Park, Calif.: Addison-Wesley Publishing Co., 1988.

Guyton, A. *Textbook of Medical Physiology*, 7th ed. Philadelphia: W.B. Saunders Co., 1986.

Hinton-Walker, P. "Pain," in *Medical-Surgical Care Plans.* Edited by Holloway, N. Springhouse, Pa.: Springhouse Corp., 1988.

McCaffery, M. "Patients Shouldn't Have to Suffer: How to Relieve Pain with Injectable Narcotics," *Nursing80* 10(10):34-39, October 1980.

McCaffery, M. "Relieving Pain with Noninvasive Techniques," *Nursing80* 10(12):55-57, December 1980.

Watkins, L., Weaver, L., and Odegaard, V. "Preparation for Cardiac Catheterization: Tailoring the Content of Instruction to Coping Style," *Heart & Lung* 15(4):382-89, 1986.

Grieving and Dying

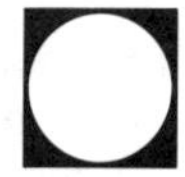

Introduction

DEFINITION AND TIME FOCUS

Loss is a fundamental, universal human experience repeated throughout the life span, beginning with the infant's first temporary separation from the mother and ending with death. The grieving process, a natural response to loss, involves acknowledging, accepting, mourning, and integrating the reality of the loss into new life patterns. Grieving is an essential part of effectively coping with loss, and serious emotional, social, and even physical problems may result if normal grieving does not take place.

Death represents an immediate threat to every patient admitted to the critical care unit. Dr. Elisabeth Kübler-Ross has described death as "the key to the door of life," and the critical care nurse can help patients and families use this key. Awareness of death's inevitability, and the unflinching contemplation of our own fears and feelings about it, can lead to a heightened appreciation for life and a more courageous and thoughtful response to the challenges life provides.

As a critical care nurse, you will deal with loss and death on a day-to-day basis and, thus, will have an opportunity to make a profoundly meaningful contribution to patients and families who are grieving. More than any other professional, you have the kind of close and continuing contact with patients, the direct experience with those who have faced such losses, and the concern for both emotional and physiologic problems needed to help patients and families cope. Although death remains a "great unknown," patients and their loved ones have the right to continue sharing life until until the end, and you can facilitate this process.

Because issues of death are so immediate for critical care patients, this care plan focuses on the needs of dying patients and of families who are facing the loss of a loved one. Normal grieving, however, may also follow many other kinds of losses; the same care principles apply to both.

ETIOLOGY AND PRECIPITATING FACTORS

Grieving occurs as a response to loss:
- of body image (such as amputation) or self-image (such as different social role)
- of loved one or significant other (such as through separation, divorce, or death)
- of material possessions (such as home, income, or pets)
- through a maturational or developmental process (such as weaning, graduation, retirement, death).

Death may result from:
- disease (or, occasionally, complications of treatment)
- injury or accident
- aging or debilitation
- suicide or homicide.

Focused assessment guidelines

NURSING HISTORY (Functional health pattern findings)

Because dying patients present with many different etiologic factors, no typical findings exist. Instead, this section presents an assessment guide to assist in planning care for patients facing death. No guide is appropriate for all patients. You must use professional judgment in deciding when and how much to ask patients, but the answers to the following questions may help determine how to intervene most effectively on behalf of the dying and the grieving.

Health perception–health management pattern

- Is the patient aware of the prognosis? If so, for how long?
- If the patient is not aware of the prognosis, why not? What does he believe is the reason for hospitalization?
- What measures have been taken to help the patient's physical or mental condition before this hospitalization? Does the patient believe they have helped? If so, how? If not, why not?
- What are the patient's expectations about admission to and treatment in the critical care unit?

Nutritional-metabolic pattern

- Does the patient have any particular dietary preferences, intolerances, or restrictions?
- Has the patient been anorectic, vomiting, or dysphagic?

Elimination pattern

- What is the patient's present elimination status and pattern?
- Are any elimination aids presently used?

Activity-exercise pattern

- What is the patient's current activity level and tolerance?

Sleep-rest pattern

- What are the patient's sleeping habits? Does the patient feel he has been getting enough sleep? If not, why not?

Cognitive-perceptual pattern

- Is the patient's pain, if present, controlled? By what?
- Does the patient display any perceptual deficits?

Self-perception–self-concept pattern

- What events or achievements in life have brought the patient most satisfaction?
- What does the patient want most to accomplish before he dies?

Role-relationship pattern
• Who are the patient's significant others?
• Among these, are there any with whom the patient has long-standing, unresolved conflicts or other "unfinished business"?
• Has the patient been able to talk about the subject of dying and death with significant others?
• How are significant others handling the situation?

Coping-stress tolerance pattern
• Have the patient and family suffered other recent losses?
• If the patient is aware of the prognosis, how is he coping?
• What resources are available to help the patient cope?
• What resources are available to the family?

Value-belief pattern
• What are the patient's religious or spiritual beliefs?
• How does the patient conceptualize death?

PHYSICAL FINDINGS
Physical findings in critically ill patients vary widely depending on the medical condition; refer to the care plan in this book on the patient's specific disorder.

DIAGNOSTIC STUDIES
See the care plan on the patient's specific disorder.

POTENTIAL COMPLICATIONS
• ineffective coping
• dysfunctional grieving
• crisis state

Nursing diagnosis: *Grieving related to actual or impending loss*

NURSING PRIORITY: Facilitate the grieving process.

Interventions	Rationales
1. Assess patient and family members for features of normal grieving, including emotional numbness and denial of the loss; anxiety and somatic signs or symptoms (such as sighing, hyperventilation, restlessness, or weakness); transient confusion and disorientation; crying and pining; anger toward self or others; guilt; expression of a sense of "internal mutilation" (for example, "My job was a big part of me" or "Her dying left a hole in my life"); or identification with the loss (for example, behavior that tries to recreate a sense of the world as it was before the loss). Display acceptance of such behaviors, if observed.	1. Any patient who is hospitalized in the critical care setting and his family have suffered a significant loss. Grieving is an appropriate and necessary response. The characteristics of normal grieving commonly prove alarming to others. Even experienced professionals may find it difficult to watch suffering and may be uncomfortable with expressions of loss. Identifying the features of grief and displaying acceptance are the first steps in helping the patient and family cope with loss.
2. Listen actively. Express concern, but avoid trying to smooth over difficult topics or distract the grieving person from the loss. Encourage him to express feelings. When possible, meet with the patient or family in a private area.	2. Listening helps the grieving person feel that his sense of loss is recognized and validated. Attempts to redirect the flow of expression may interfere with the grieving process and contribute to delayed, prolonged, or pathologic grieving. Encouraging verbalization decreases the sudden sense of isolation that loss can bring. Grieving persons may need privacy to express themselves freely.
3. Help the grieving person to identify the loss, and try to determine the meaning of the loss in the context of the individual's current and previous life circumstances.	3. Helping the person identify the specific loss can focus the grief process and may reduce the sense of being overwhelmed by it. Understanding the significance of the loss in relationship to other events or circumstances in the person's life is essential because other stressors can affect coping ability.
4. Allow time for adaptation to loss. Prepare the grieving person to expect and accept feelings, which may surface months or even years after the loss.	4. The grieving process is a nonlinear struggle to integrate a significant loss into daily life; steps often do not follow each other in a smooth, logical progression. Eventually, time softens the impact and immediacy of the loss, but grieving may continue in some form long after the individual has resumed normal activities and relationships. Being prepared for such feelings helps the individual cope effectively when they occur.

Interventions

5. Observe for evidence of unhealthy coping behaviors, such as drug or alcohol abuse, persistent self-recrimination or aggression toward others, or suicidal behaviors. Report and intervene as needed to prevent injury. See the "Ineffective Coping" care plan, page 26.

Rationales

5. Early identification of unhealthy coping behaviors allows intervention to avert further losses that may result from such destructive behaviors. The "Ineffective Coping" care plan contains interventions helpful in refocusing the individual's coping strategy toward a more healthful one.

6. Additional individualized interventions: ____________

6. Rationales: ____________

Target outcome criteria

According to individual readiness, the grieving person will:

- express feelings regarding loss freely, as desired
- identify the specific loss and contextual meaning for the individual
- use effective coping behaviors.

Nursing diagnosis: *Fear related to potential pain, loss, emotional upheaval, and "unknowns" of the dying process*

NURSING PRIORITY: Promote identification and confrontation of specific, realistic fears.

Interventions

1. Examine your personal fears and feelings about death before becoming involved with the critical patient and his family. Identify previous experiences with death, and be aware of personal emotions, spiritual or religious beliefs, and fears that may influence your perceptions. If talking about death seems too uncomfortable for you, refer the patient and family to another professional with the necessary skills.

Rationales

1. The clinician's personal feelings and experiences with death affect the ability to promote healthy emotional responses. A nurse who has not faced the death of a loved one may be less able to empathize with the patient and family. Appropriate referral allows the emotional needs of others to be addressed.

Interventions

2. Assess the patient's coping style and stage of acceptance. Assess his previous experience with death. Observe the patient's behaviors, and confer with the family and other caregivers as needed.

Rationales

2. Each person responds differently to mortality. When threatened, most people initially revert to familiar coping mechanisms, which caregivers must be aware of in establishing therapeutic communication. Recognizing the stage of acceptance helps determine appropriate interventions. Previous experiences with death strongly influence behavioral responses and may contribute significantly to the patient's or family's overall ability to achieve acceptance. Conferring with the family or other caregivers may provide insights into the patient's behavior and feelings.

Interventions

3. Use role modeling, as appropriate, to encourage the expression of feelings, for example, "If I were facing your situation, I think I might feel scared or angry or depressed."

Rationales

3. The patient and family members may need "permission" to discuss their fears. Opening the discussion by stating your feelings allows the person to express their feelings, if they want to, and reassures them that such feelings are normal, expected, and acceptable.

Interventions

4. Support coping mechanisms. Avoid forcing the patient or family member to confront emotional issues.

Rationales

4. Each person moves through various stages at different times in coping with the ultimate loss of individuality. Forcing issues is counterproductive and may damage the therapeutic relationship. Recognizing individual readiness conveys respect for the individual, which promotes trust.

(continued)

Interventions	Rationales
5. As indicated by the patient's responsiveness to role modeling, help him identify specific fears and prioritize them. Acknowledge the unknowns.	5. Identifying explicit fears, such as pain, loss of control, or being a burden to others, helps reduce the sense of being overwhelmed and encourages the patient to plan for specific problems that may arise. Acknowledging the unknown reassures the patient or family member that caregivers recognize the enormity of the questions faced.
6. Identify the patient's support system and resource base. Coordinate involvement of patient, family, and caregivers in planning for anticipated problems and needs.	6. Coordinating resources and support for the patient is essential in reducing isolation, which contributes to fear.
7. Arrange for appropriate referrals, as needed, such as psychiatric liaison nurse, social worker, chaplain, hospice, or peer support group, for the specific disorder.	7. The patient and family may be unaware of resources available. Even if referrals are not used, knowledge of their availability may be comforting.
8. Provide companionship, when possible.	8. Simply sitting quietly beside the patient communicates concern and decreases the sense of aloneness.
9. If patient is confronting imminent, unexpected death (for example, in a sudden worsening of condition or in trauma), provide brief, clear explanations, even if the patient appears unresponsive. Offer to call a spiritual advisor. Provide a support person to be with the family, and—if at all possible—allow a family member to see the patient before death.	9. Even in an emergency, the patient has the right to caring communication, which may help reduce fear. Survivors of near-death experiences report hearing conversation and being aware of activities around them even when they appeared unresponsive. Surviving spouses have remarked that the inability to see their husband or wife during resuscitation or before death caused the most anguish for them.
10. Additional individualized interventions: ______	10. Rationales: ______

Target outcome criteria

According to individual readiness, the patient or family member will:

- identify specific fears
- express feelings, as desired
- use appropriate resources.

Nursing diagnosis: *Powerlessness related to inevitability of death, lack of control over body functions, and/or dependence on others for care*

NURSING PRIORITY: Increase the patient's sense of personal power while promoting acceptance of his condition.

Interventions	Rationales
1. Encourage personal decision-making whenever possible. Allow maximum flexibility for scheduling of activities, treatments, or visitors. Include the patient as a participant in making decisions about care, as condition permits.	1. The hospitalized patient relinquishes many freedoms, regardless of the reason for his hospitalization. Allowing as many choices as possible promotes a sense of control and increases the patient's coping ability. Taking-over behavior by caregivers (for example, arbitrarily making decisions the patient could make) has a devaluing effect on the patient's self-esteem and should be avoided unless absolutely necessary.
2. Recognize and support courageous attitudes.	2. Regardless of external circumstances, people maintain the freedom to choose their attitude and approach to life. Acknowledging courageous attitudes in adverse situations reinforces feelings of self-worth.

Interventions	Rationales
3. Accept personal powerlessness to alter many aspects of the patient's critical condition.	3. Health care professionals commonly find it difficult to be unable to "make it better" for the patient. Realistic self-assessment is essential to prevent caregiver burnout and maintain the potential for effective intervention in areas that can be altered.
4. Help the patient identify inner strengths. Ask the patient to recall past losses: How were they dealt with? What was learned from them?	4. Recalling other losses may help the patient build on previously learned coping skills. Losses throughout life may have uniquely prepared that individual with qualities that can be used in facing death.
5. Encourage the patient to establish realistic goals for the remainder of his life.	5. Establishing goals provides a focus for energy and reduces the patient's sense of helplessness. Realistic evaluation of capabilities helps in the process of acceptance.
6. Assist the patient, as needed, to put affairs in order by, among other things, determining resuscitation status and preferences, planning the funeral and memorials, making a will, and settling economic affairs.	6. Putting affairs in order increases the patient's sense of control and may help soften the effect on loved ones.
7. Additional individualized interventions: ____________	7. Rationales: ____________

Target outcome criteria

According to individual readiness, the patient will:

- participate in decisions about care
- verbalize inner strengths
- set realistic goals
- initiate activity to put affairs in order.

Nursing diagnosis: *Disturbed self-concept: personal identity related to imminent threat of loss of self*

NURSING PRIORITY: Help patient maintain and enrich personal identity throughout remainder of life.

Interventions	Rationales
1. Use active listening skills, paying special attention to nonverbal or symbolic communication. Use reflective statements and open-ended observations to provide an opportunity to discuss difficult issues. Accept and respect the patient's need for denial or avoidance behavior. Whatever the patient's response, try to communicate understanding and acceptance.	1. The patient facing death commonly uses nonverbal or symbolic communication to describe his experience and to test others' willingness to talk about it. Rushed or distracted behavior from caregivers may distance the patient and contribute to feelings of alienation. Active listening and sharing show concern and respect for the patient as an individual. Some patients choose denial or avoidance to the end, and their right to make this choice should be respected as a reflection of their unique selfhood.
2. Be honest with the patient in answering questions, but do not force discussion of issues the patient has not introduced or has not responded to in discussion.	2. Honesty, even when painful, reflects respect for the person. The patient has the right, however, to choose which issues shall be discussed.
3. Encourage reminiscence and review of life experiences.	3. Life experiences have helped shape the patient's unique identity. Reminiscence helps the patient remain connected to important core experiences (that is, experiences central to the patient's self-concept) and provides the caregiver with a greater understanding of the patient's behavior.

(continued)

Interventions	Rationales
4. Promote creative expression. Encourage family and friends to provide, or obtain from the occupational therapy department, materials for drawing, painting, writing, or other creative pursuits, as the patient's condition permits.	4. Creative activities encourage individual expression, helping the patient maintain a sense of uniqueness. Drawings, music, and other artistic expressions may also provide clues to the patient's stage of acceptance.
5. Explore the option of preparing audiotaped or videotaped messages or mementos for family and friends to share after the patient's death, or earlier, if the patient wishes.	5. Some patients may feel more comfortable expressing feelings in this way. The process of recording helps in accepting an impending death. Such mementos may offer the patient comfort in knowing that some record of his life will endure. Families also value recordings that preserve the loved one's memory.
6. Use touch generously when providing care, unless it makes the patient uncomfortable. Encourage family affection, including holding, rocking, even lying next to the patient. If equipment and tubing are not likely to have life-sustaining value, consult with the doctor about discontinuing their use.	6. Illness and hospitalization reduce the frequency of physical contact with others that normally helps provide self-definition of body image. Touch also provides comfort and communicates genuine caring more effectively than almost any other single measure. High-technology equipment and tubes can be a barrier to personal contact and may increase anxiety for the patient and family.
7. Additional individualized interventions: ______	7. Rationales: ______

Target outcome criteria

According to individual readiness, the patient will:
- maintain preferred coping behaviors
- reminisce about life experiences
- participate in creative activity, as able
- touch family members freely.

Nursing diagnosis: *Potential spiritual distress related to confronting the unknown*

NURSING PRIORITY: Help the patient savor the remaining period of life and identify meaning in impending death.

Interventions	Rationales
1. Support the patient's personal spiritual beliefs, even if they seem unusual or unfamiliar.	1. Spiritual beliefs are extremely varied and provide comfort depending on their meaningfulness to the patient. Attempting to alter such beliefs or supplant them with others shows disrespect and may precipitate undue conflict and distress.
2. Maintain a positive attitude. Promote activities that provide at least some enjoyment. Avoid generalizations that attempt to provide pat explanations for suffering.	2. The caregiver's positive attitude may help the patient maintain hope and find pleasure in living, even while facing death. Small gestures may be extremely meaningful when the patient's world view is narrowed by illness. Generalizations or facile explanations (such as "It may actually be a blessing") indicate a shallow appreciation of the patient's situation and may be interpreted as dismissal of real concerns.
3. Recognize that facing death is a developmental task for all humans, as is separation. Promote a focus on growth and learning rather than disease or injury.	3. Because our culture places such emphasis on youth, we lack the societal integration of death as part of life that many primitive cultures take for granted. To help the patient accept his impending death, caregivers must acknowledge it as a stage of development and validate its importance. Interventions not related to the disease process (discussed throughout this plan) help redirect coping efforts toward positive life closure.

Interventions	Rationales
4. Acknowledge what the dying patient has to teach others, and express this to the patient and family, when appropriate.	4. Nurses can learn much from the dying patient that may help them care for others. In such ways, the patient may touch the lives of others he will never meet. Recognizing this can help both the nurse and the patient find meaning in death.
5. Provide privacy, according to the patient's wishes.	5. The hospital environment may allow the patient minimal time to be alone. A patient struggling with spiritual issues may need uninterrupted time for prayer or meditation.
6. Offer to call the spiritual advisor, counselor, or friend of the patient's choice. Obtain and provide religious texts or other inspirational readings, if requested.	6. A spiritual advisor may provide guidance or perform essential rituals for the patient. Many patients find religious readings comforting, while others prefer poetry or literature that has a special personal significance.
7. Explore the possibility of organ donation, if appropriate, with the patient and family. Be familiar with your hospital's policy and procedure for arranging organ donation. Consider the underlying disorder before discussing donation of specific organs.	7. Many patients and families can find meaning and consolation in knowing others may benefit from organ donation. Many transplant programs now have a broad interlinking system for identification of donors and the harvest and transplantation of donated organs. Underlying disease (such as cancer) may make some organs unsatisfactory for donation, but others (such as corneas or skin) are usually still useful and do not always require immediate transplantation.
8. Address the patient while providing care, even if the patient has apparently become unresponsive or comatose. Encourage family members to continue talking to the patient.	8. Persons who recover from deep or prolonged coma commonly report remembering conversation around them while they were apparently unconscious.
9. Worry less about saying the "wrong thing" than about being afraid to communicate caring. In this way, set an example family members may follow.	9. Because of prolonged close contact with dying patients and interaction with their families, nurses are uniquely suited to help encourage dialogue between a dying patient and the family. Usually, the patient and family avoid raising the issue with each other directly, concerned they may cause pain or emotional upset. No cultural prescriptions exist to guide families, but the nurse may be able to act as a liaison to help communication, thereby reducing guilt and anxiety and further preparing both the patient and family for separation.
10. Additional individualized interventions: ______	10. Rationales: ______

Target outcome criteria
Throughout remainder of life, the patient will:

- maintain personally meaningful spiritual or religious practices
- express pleasure periodically in meaningful activity.

Nursing diagnosis: *Alteration in family processes related to imminent death of family member*

NURSING PRIORITY: Minimize disruption in family integrity by facilitating healthy coping, mutual support, and communication with the dying person.

Interventions	Rationales
1. Assess the family's level of acceptance and coping by observing behaviors and interactions of family members with the patient and providing time for private discussions with them, as needed. Be alert to differences among individual family members and clues to the family's previous experience with death, if any.	1. Effective intervention must be appropriately correlated to the stage of acceptance. Each member of the family may respond differently to impending loss. Previous family deaths may affect family members' ability to cope in a mutually supportive way.
2. Liberalize visiting policies, as needed. Allow private time for the family to be with the patient. Encourage family members to participate in care, remaining alert for signs of possible anxiety or discomfort. Avoid giving the impression of dismissing or neglecting the patient.	2. Family integrity is more likely to be maintained when members can continue their usual level of contact with one another. Helping with care reduces the family's sense of helplessness and provides a special comfort to the patient. However, this is not a substitute for the nurse's close involvement with the patient and family.
3. When possible, facilitate family dialogue, remaining cognizant of established family roles and expectations. Offer to introduce topics as needed; strive to promote face-to-face communication when possible.	3. Discussing issues surrounding death is difficult for most families and may be compounded by unresolved conflicts, guilt, or role demands. The nurse may be able to act as a liaison to help open communication about sensitive issues. Family stability is related to long-standing family patterns of behavior, so interventions that are at odds with these patterns may be unsuccessful. Direct communication promotes maximum understanding and helps minimize later guilt over things left unsaid.
4. Be aware of cultural attitudes that may affect family response.	4. Different cultures view death in different ways. Some observe specific rituals around the occasion, and others withdraw or avoid contact with others. Being aware of cultural differences helps the nurse plan appropriate interventions.
5. Help the family identify and mobilize external resources, such as friends, clergy, counselors, and financial support. Provide referrals to a pastoral care person, psychiatrist, or social worker, as needed.	5. Families coping with death, especially a prolonged death, commonly require added support to deal with stresses caused by a family member's illness. Other professionals may offer spiritual or psychological counseling, temporary housing placement, and financial aid programs.
6. Encourage family members to care for their own physical and emotional needs. Emphasize importance of adequate rest, food, and exercise. Suggest that family members take turns at the bedside, if they seem reluctant to leave the patient unattended.	6. Maintenance of physical well-being is essential if family members are to continue providing support for the patient and each other. Taking breaks helps the family maintain contact with external resources and reduces the emotional drain of constantly attending to the patient's needs.
7. If the patient is to be transferred or discharged before impending death, take time to prepare the patient and family for the transition. If possible, orient them to the new unit staff and environment. Discuss the patient's wishes regarding resuscitation status. If the patient is going home, ensure that the family has adequate support and knows what to do when death is imminent and after death occurs.	7. The stress of transfer or discharge of a dying patient can be emotionally traumatizing, because both patient and family members are already coping with difficult issues. Careful preparation is essential to reduce fear and ensure that the patient's wishes are identified and carried out in the new setting.

Interventions	Rationales
8. Additional individualized interventions: ________	8. Rationales: ________

Target outcome criteria
Throughout hospitalization, family members will:
- participate in care, as condition permits
- share concerns with the patient and each other
- appear well-rested most of the time
- use external resources, as appropriate
- display healthful coping behaviors.

Nursing diagnosis: *Family coping: potential for growth related to bereavement and mourning*

NURSING PRIORITY: Facilitate initiation of healthy grieving after death occurs.

Interventions	Rationales
1. If not already acquainted with the family, introduce yourself, identify your relationship as the patient's nurse, and express sympathy.	1. If the family arrives after death has occurred, or if the family does not know caregivers from previous contact, such an introduction serves to reassure them that the patient died with concerned caregivers at hand.
2. Allow the family members to see and touch the body. If death was sudden and unexpected, prepare them for the appearance of the body in advance, explaining that all measures were tried in the attempt to restore life. Ensure that the body is respectfully covered but not inaccessible. Do *not* clean up all indications of emergency intervention before allowing the family into the room.	2. Seeing and touching the body of the loved one helps the family accept the reality of death. If death was sudden and resuscitation efforts altered the body's appearance, advance preparation for viewing the body may help reduce distress for the family. Gross blood or other secretions should be cleaned up before the family enters, but putting away all supplies and cleaning the room before the family sees the body may leave the family with doubts that "everything possible" was done for the patient.
3. Use direct, simple sentences, avoiding use of euphemisms to describe death. Provide comforting observations, when possible, for example, "He died quietly and appeared to have no pain" or "She told me last night about the good times you used to have and she seemed very happy."	3. Most family members are too anxious at this time to comprehend complex explanations. Euphemisms, such as "passed on," may offend some family members and can potentially interfere with reality orientation. Sharing selected, specific observations with family members may help minimize guilt and promote healthy grieving.
4. Acknowledge the family's loss by gently reorienting them to the reality of death: "It must be hard to realize he's really dead." Avoid oversentimental responses, especially if you are unfamiliar with the family (for example, "God must have wanted her for an angel.").	4. Shock and disbelief are normal initial responses to sudden death and, to a certain degree, even to expected death. Gentle reorientation aids in the process of integrating death into reality. Oversentimental responses may be inappropriate to the family's actual relationship with the deceased or offensive to their beliefs.
5. Avoid recommending the sedation of a family member, unless severely dysfunctional behavior is present.	5. Sedation may delay initiation of the normal grieving process.
6. Offer to call a friend, clergy member, or counselor of choice to help with immediate arrangements. If the family does not designate such a person, offer the services of hospital chaplain, liaison nurse, or other in-house professional skilled in dealing with grief.	6. During the initial stages of the grieving process, decision-making becomes difficult and disorganization and disorientation are common. Providing an advocate helps reduce family members' distress while they are making necessary arrangements, such as for disposition of the body.

(continued)

Interventions	Rationales
7. Prepare the family for the work of grieving. Emphasize the normalcy of a wide range of emotional responses (such as anger, guilt, sadness, frustration, resentment, fear, and depression) and behaviors (such as crying, laughing, withdrawal, and confusion) in response to the loss of a loved one.	7. Family members are sometimes unprepared for the various feelings experienced in the grieving process. Some may feel they're "going crazy" when unexpected feelings occur. Understanding that such emotional disorganization is a normal (and healthy) response to loss can help families deal with these feelings.
8. Listen patiently to retelling of the story of death, especially if it was unexpected. Avoid responses that might be interpreted as judgmental or disinterested.	8. Retelling of events by survivors is an essential part of reality acceptance and coping. Judgmental responses may provoke severe guilt reactions in family members, whereas disinterested ones may provoke alienation.
9. Reemphasize the need for health-promoting behavior during the grieving period.	9. Grief work places additional stress on survivors, who are at increased risk for developing physical illness during mourning. Health-promoting behavior, such as exercise, can help release emotional energy and reduce the effects of stress.
10. Ensure that someone will be available to be with survivors before they leave the hospital.	10. The grieving process is facilitated by sharing feelings with others. Few instances of loneliness are as profound as that of a bereaved person, newly alone.
11. If possible, provide a follow-up call to surviving family members 1 to 3 months after bereavement. Keeping a callback calendar on the unit will help in organizing this task.	11. Follow-up from caregivers to survivors is the final step in the care of a dying patient and provides family members with added assurance that their loved one was special and received care accordingly. This call also provides an opportunity to identify dysfunctional grieving and make appropriate referrals, if needed.
12. Additional individualized interventions: ________	12. Rationales: ________

Target outcome criteria

Before the survivors leave the hospital, they will:
• view and touch the body, if desired
• express initial grief and disbelief
• establish contact with advocacy and support persons.

One to 3 months after death, the family members will verbalize coping effectively, with adequate support.

Transfer planning

NURSING TRANSFER CRITERIA

If the patient is to be transferred from the unit before death, documentation should show evidence of:
• discussion of transfer with patient and family
• resuscitation status.

PATIENT-FAMILY TEACHING CHECKLIST

During hospitalization, document evidence that the patient and family demonstrate understanding of:
__ common reactions to grief
__ positive coping mechanisms
__ resources available
__ organ donation procedure, if desired.

If the patient is discharged home before anticipated death, document evidence that patient and family demonstrate understanding of:
__ support and resources available
__ what to do when death is imminent
__ what to do after death occurs
__ normal mourning and grieving and what to expect.

DOCUMENTATION CHECKLIST

Using outcome criteria as a guide, document:
__ fears
__ feelings expressed
__ goals identified
__ preferred coping behaviors
__ spiritual or religious practices
__ pain-control measures
__ family members' behaviors
__ referrals.

After the patient's death, document:
__ time and circumstances of death
__ disposition of body and effects
__ family support measures implemented

ASSOCIATED CARE PLANS

Acute Pain
Ineffective Coping
(See also care plans for specific disorders.)

REFERENCES

Fanslow, J. "Needs of Grieving Spouses in Sudden Death Situations: A Pilot Study," *Journal of Emergency Nursing* 9(4):213-16, 1983.

Frankl, V.E. *Man's Search for Meaning.* New York: Washington Square Press, 1969.

Hoff, L.A. *People in Crisis: Understanding and Helping,* 2nd ed. Menlo Park, Calif.: Addison-Wesley Publishing Co., 1984.

Hudak, C., et al. *Critical Care Nursing: A Holistic Approach,* 4th ed. Philadelphia: J.B. Lippincott Co., 1986.

Jung, C. *Modern Man in Search of a Soul.* New York: Harcourt, Brace and Co., 1934.

Kneisl, C., and Ames, S.A. *Adult Health Nursing: A Biopsychosocial Approach.* Menlo Park, Calif.: Addison-Wesley Publishing Co., 1986.

Kübler-Ross, E. *Death, The Final Stage of Growth.* Englewood Cliffs, N.J.: Prentice-Hall, 1975.

Kübler-Ross, E. *Living With Death and Dying.* New York: Macmillan Publishing Co., 1981.

Mueller, S. "Grief and Grieving," in *Medical-Surgical Care Plans.* Edited by Holloway, N. Springhouse, Pa.: Springhouse Corp., 1988.

Tatelbaum, J. *The Courage to Grieve.* New York: Harper & Row Publishers, 1980.

Note: Portions of this care plan previously appeared in Malone, R. "Death and Dying," in *Medical-Surgical Care Plans.* Edited by Holloway, N. Springhouse, Pa.: Springhouse Corp., 1988.

Ineffective Coping

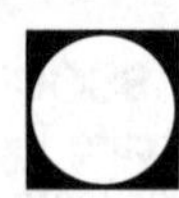

Introduction

DEFINITION AND TIME FOCUS

The stress of critical illness or injury places an enormous burden on the coping resources of the patient and his family. Besides the physiologic stress of the disorder itself, the patient and family face significant emotional, financial, physical, and social effects on their lives related to the hospitalization. Sometimes the illness itself may be indirectly caused by stress, as in myocardial infarction, and the patient may have a history of dysfunctional or unhealthy coping behaviors before hospitalization. Or the disorder may represent a sudden, catastrophic disruption in normal coping patterns, as in multiple trauma or major burns. Regardless of the reason for the patient's hospitalization, a stay in the critical care unit is threatening and disorganizing, taxing the resources of patient and family on many levels. Ineffective coping results when the patient and family are unable to adapt behaviors effectively to cope with the hospitalization, the illness, and its attendant problems. This care plan focuses on interventions to increase the coping abilities of critical care patients and their families throughout the critical care experience.

ETIOLOGY AND PRECIPITATING FACTORS

- disruption in routines
- pain and physical discomfort
- financial stress
- unanticipated changes
- knowledge deficit
- sleep deprivation
- sensory overload or deprivation
- isolation from others
- excessive anxiety
- fear
- loss of control
- effects of medications
- lack of resources

Focused assessment guidelines

NURSING HISTORY (Functional health pattern findings)

Health perception–health management pattern

- usually perceives condition leading to hospitalization as a threat to life

Nutritional-metabolic pattern

- may display reduced appetite or forget to eat
- may report nausea or vomiting
- may indulge in excessive eating or drinking

Elimination pattern

- may report diarrhea or constipation in response to physiologic or emotional stress

Activity-exercise pattern

- likely to report fatigue

Sleep-rest pattern

- commonly reports insomnia (difficulty falling asleep or early awakening)
- may report feeling constantly tired or sleeping excessively

Cognitive-perceptual pattern

- may display reduced ability to follow instructions, make decisions, perform complex motor tasks, or remember teaching
- may report headaches, neck pain, or abdominal discomfort
- may report pain uncontrolled by medication

Self-perception–self-concept pattern

- likely to report feeling overwhelmed
- may view self as victim
- may neglect personal grooming

Role-relationship pattern

- may display emotional lability
- may withdraw from others
- may report few social contacts or limited local support network
- may express unresolved guilt
- may exhibit aggressive or suicidal behavior

Sexuality-reproductive pattern

- may report loss of libido

Coping-stress tolerance pattern

- may minimize severity of condition
- may have postponed seeking medical help until condition became severe
- may exhibit inappropriate or exaggerated emotional responses
- may have history of unhealthy coping behaviors, such as drug or alcohol dependency

Value-belief pattern

- may express belief that illness is punishment or is otherwise linked to previous behavior

PHYSICAL FINDINGS

The following are common physiologic effects of stress that may be observed in patients or family members. In addition, the patient's physical findings vary according to the underlying disorder.

General appearance

- anxious facial expression
- reduced eye contact
- tense posture
- flat affect
- unkempt appearance

Cardiovascular

- tachycardia
- elevated blood pressure
- occasionally, increased ventricular or atrial dysrhythmias

Respiratory

- hyperventilation
- sighing

Gastrointestinal

- vomiting
- diarrhea
- abdominal pain
- air swallowing
- dry mouth
- yawning

Neurologic

- dilated pupils (if sympathetic nervous system response)

Musculoskeletal

- tremorous extremities
- fidgeting
- increased muscle tension

Integumentary

- flushing
- occasionally, diaphoresis

DIAGNOSTIC STUDIES

No laboratory or diagnostic tests specifically assess ineffective coping. However, remember that physiologic responses to stress often mimic or exacerbate disease, so carefully review appropriate laboratory tests, such as the following:

- white blood cell (WBC) count—may be increased
- arterial blood gas measurements—respiratory alkalosis may be present in stress-induced hyperventilation.

POTENTIAL COMPLICATIONS

- crisis state
- suicide or homicide
- disintegration of family unit
- major depression
- psychosis

Nursing diagnosis: *Ineffective coping related to overwhelming threat*

NURSING PRIORITIES: (a) Establish therapeutic communication and (b) minimize or reduce threatening stimuli.

Interventions	Rationales
1. Establish rapport. Introduce yourself to the patient and family, and provide a clear explanation of your role. Emphasize the staff's availability, for example, "I'll be your nurse today until 11 o'clock, but four other nurses are also here. We will be in and out of your room frequently checking on you, but here is your call bell if you need us sooner. I'll be glad to answer any questions you may have." Try to provide consistency in staffing on a day-to-day basis.	1. Establishing a therapeutic relationship reduces the threat of hospitalization by decreasing the strangeness of the environment and providing the patient and family with a source of information, comfort, and familiarity. Consistency in staffing encourages development of trust and promotes a sense of "surrogate family," which can be particularly reassuring in the intimidating environment of the critical care unit. Predictability reduces stress.
2. Communicate nonverbally to reinforce what you're saying: maintain eye contact, be aware of body language, and use touch generously unless the patient and family appear uncomfortable with physical contact.	2. Nonverbal communication is extremely effective when anxiety is high and cognitive abilities are compromised.

(continued)

Interventions	Rationales
3. Provide orientation to the unit, explaining routines and equipment in simple, direct lay terms. Avoid using technical jargon or unfamiliar medical terminology. Provide accurate information.	3. Orientation to the unit reduces the threat of unfamiliarity. Explaining routines provides structure and promotes a sense of security, helping the patient and family to define the altered reality of critical illness. In the anxiety-provoking setting of a critical care unit, simple and direct terms are most readily understood. Complex explanations or technical jargon may confuse or alienate, adding to the perceived threat.
4. Interpret stimuli, such as sounds, which may contribute to tension or anxiety.	4. The high-technology environment of the critical care unit is filled with unfamiliar and sometimes distressing sounds. Understanding their source may help minimize such effects.
5. Repeat explanations, as necessary.	5. Anxiety interferes with the ability to comprehend and retain new information.
6. Allow and encourage verbalization of feelings. Ask direct questions, such as "How do you feel about what has happened?" Use open-ended questions that cannot be answered by a simple yes or no. Avoid asking "why" questions.	6. Verbalization of feelings is the first step in accepting and dealing with the perceived threat. Direct, open-ended questions help the person explore emotional issues. "Why" questions may be considered threatening or blaming.
7. Recognize the patient's and family's need to share or repeat details of events leading to hospitalization. Provide positive feedback when possible, such as "It was good you called the ambulance when you did," or "You were a big help in bringing in the list of medicines your father has been taking." Avoid making recriminating or judgmental statements.	7. Repeating the details of the events helps the person accept the reality of the situation. Reliving the events through verbalization also allows for ventilation of anxiety-producing feelings and provides the nurse with an opportunity to correct misconceptions the patient or family may have about their responsibility for the problem. Families may feel guilty or anxious that something they did or did not do has caused the problem. Providing reassurance that they acted wisely, even in small ways, promotes competence and reinforces coping skills.
8. Help the patient and family define the components of a perceived threat, encouraging them to separate and prioritize problems. Ask questions that help in defining boundaries, for example, "What is the scariest thing about this situation? What is the least scary?" Focus discussion on modifiable factors, emphasizing and allowing choices wherever possible.	8. Ineffective coping is commonly linked with feeling overwhelmed by all-encompassing problems. When the problems are broken down into separate parts, the patient and family may feel better able to deal with smaller issues on a step-by-step basis. Defining the perceived parameters of the problem helps reduce free-floating anxiety and provides the nurse with information about the personal perspectives and values of the patient and family. Focusing discussion on factors about which something can be done promotes a sense of self-control and reduces panic.
9. Additional individualized interventions: ____________	9. Rationales: ____________

Target outcome criteria

Within the first 24 hours, the patient (depending on level of responsiveness) or family will:

- know the names of primary caregivers
- ask appropriate questions
- identify immediate problems.

Nursing diagnosis: *Ineffective coping related to inadequate resources*

NURSING PRIORITY: Help the patient and family identify and practice appropriate coping behaviors.

Interventions	Rationales
1. Assess previous health history, noting similar situations the patient and family have previously experienced. Ask the patient and family how they have handled problems before.	1. Previous coping behaviors provide the best clues for evaluating the adequacy of the patient's and family's support system and understanding current coping styles. Reviewing past coping strategies links the patient and family with previously learned lessons in coping with stress and may help the nurse identify beliefs about health or illness that impact coping ability.
2. Share specific observations of positive family interactions or personal strengths, such as "You really know how to talk to your Dad. He always relaxes after you visit," or "You have a great sense of humor. I can imagine that gets you over a lot of humps." Identify and support strengths, such as "It sounds like your family really sticks together when things get tough."	2. Sharing observations of the behavior of patients and families can illumine and reinforce strengths they may not realize they possess. Such sharing also provides reassurance that their caregiver takes a personal interest in them, reducing fear and isolation.
3. Assess patient's and family's external resource base, including evaluation of the following: • financial needs • transportation problems • housing and home care arrangements • other ill family members • preexisting problems • social and family support • language and cultural barriers. Arrange appropriate referrals to social service staff or other agencies and caregivers as indicated.	3. Coping ability is reduced if multiple stressors are present, a common circumstance when critical illness occurs. Providing referrals to link the patient and family with appropriate resources can enhance the ability to utilize adaptive behaviors most effectively.
4. Explore, with the patient and family, new ways of looking at identified problems. Use "reframing" when possible; for example, a patient who considers his myocardial infarction (MI) as "Just one more thing to show I'm really a loser," may be encouraged to identify how the MI may have positively affected his life (time for reflection, closer ties with family, and reevaluation of life goals may be potentially positive outcomes).	4. Emphasizing that one's attitude toward a problem remains a choice even when external restrictions allow only limited decision-making can restore a sense of self-control and shore up the patient's and family's ability to deal with difficulties constructively. Positive "self-talk" reduces anxiety.
5. Consider organizing an ongoing family support group for family members of critical care patients. Even without a formally organized group, try to facilitate supportive interactions among families when possible, providing introductions and a space away from the unit for conversation. Enlist the help of the hospital chaplain, psychiatric liaison nurse, or family guidance professional, as needed.	5. Families may derive mutual support from sharing feelings with others in similar circumstances. Such support may also decrease the sense of isolation and helplessness felt by family members of a critically ill patient. "Older" families may help in orienting "new" families to unit and hospital routines and resources.
6. Encourage family members to participate in patient care, even if only in small ways. For example, the family may be able to help with mouth care or back rubs, or assist the patient with meals. Provide supervision and guidance, teaching as necessary.	6. Family participation in care may help decrease the anxiety associated with "waiting for something to happen," a common phenomenon among families of critically ill patients. Having something useful to do enhances coping ability and promotes supportive interactions between patient and family. Supervision and guidance help minimize anxiety over unfamiliar tubes and equipment on or around the patient.
7. Additional individualized interventions: ____________ ____________	7. Rationales: ____________ ____________

Target outcome criteria
Within 48 hours, the patient or family will:
• review family coping strategies
• identify one internal resource
• identify external stressors and contact referral as needed
• participate in care, to extent possible.

Nursing diagnosis: *Ineffective coping related to inability to mobilize existing resources*

NURSING PRIORITY: Facilitate mobilization of coping behaviors.

Interventions	Rationales
1. Allow time for adaptation. Anticipate and accept the normally varied emotional plumage associated with reaction to loss, including shock and denial, anger, withdrawal, and depression. Avoid forcing issues; respect the communication implicit in periods of silence, but ask for clarification as needed. Be especially alert to nonverbal cues and avoided topics.	1. Successful adaptation to change requires time for grieving before reorganization can begin. Patients' coping styles vary widely, and the nurse must be supportive of the individual's defense mechanisms in order to facilitate adjustment. Forcing emotional issues before the person is ready can interfere with the therapeutic relationship and become counterproductive. Avoided topics and nonverbal cues may indicate anxiety-producing issues.
2. Consider and evaluate for possible organic causes of altered behavior patterns.	2. Behavioral changes that sometimes indicate ineffective coping may actually be caused by physiologic disturbances, such as fluid or electrolyte imbalances, disease, drug reactions, or hypoxia.
3. Wherever possible, reduce or eliminate environmental factors that decrease coping ability. Control pain, noise, temperature, and unpleasant stimuli. Group procedures to allow maximum sleep-rest cycles. Encourage adequate dietary intake. Provide privacy, as possible. Establish routines.	3. Pain, tension, inadequate rest and nutrition, and disturbing environmental factors can all contribute to decreased ability to cope with illness. Lack of privacy contributes to a sense of helplessness and dependency. Routines increase security and promote trust.
4. If maladaptive behavior is present, reexamine your own personal biases and values in relationship to the behavior. Consider altering your response to the behavior. Attempt to understand behavior in terms of the threat to the individual; try to convey acceptance.	4. Recognizing personal biases is the first step in avoiding judgmental responses. Difficult patients are often simply those with different cultural value systems. The ability to mobilize effective coping skills depends, at least in part, on sensing others' acceptance. Even inadvertently judgmental responses may reduce the individual's already precarious confidence level.
5. Teach the patient and family about effective relaxation techniques, such as massage, guided imagery, and progressive relaxation response.	5. Such techniques decrease tension and anxiety and may permit the individual to mobilize coping skills.
6. Help the patient and family develop specific plans for dealing with individual, identified problems. Encourage them to identify goals and to break them down into small, specific, and measurable components. For example, a family member whose health is suffering from lack of sleep may be unwilling to leave the hospital for fear something will happen. A goal for this person may simply be arranging for a trusted friend to stay with the patient for an hour or two while the family member goes home for a nap. Encourage all affected persons to participate in developing plans. Consider their functional level, developmental level, dependency needs, cultural factors, and medical condition when developing plans. Make all plans time-limited and include arrangements for follow-up and renegotiation of further goals.	6. When problems have been identified, addressing each individually helps reduce the threat to a manageable level. Likewise, goal-setting may seem overwhelming initially, but setting realistic, measurable subgoals promotes restoration of self-control. Including all affected persons in planning is essential because "taking over" by others devalues a person's self-esteem. Individual considerations are essential to success-oriented interventions. Follow-up provides an opportunity for reinforcement of positive adaptive skills.

ASSESSING SUICIDE POTENTIAL

The alert nurse is aware of suicide risk factors and assesses patients at risk specifically by asking direct questions.

MAJOR RISK FACTORS	SAMPLE QUESTIONS
Intent Contrary to popular myth, asking patients directly about suicide does not precipitate attempts. Patients tend to answer truthfully and are often relieved that someone has acknowledged their distress.	"Are you thinking about killing yourself?" or "Are you considering suicide?"
Plan Patients who verbalize clearly defined, detailed plans for suicide are at greater risk than those who express vaguely that they want to die.	"Do you have a plan to do it?"
Lethality of method Highly lethal methods (such as shooting, hanging, jumping from a height) greatly increase risk.	"How would you do it?"
Availability of means Patients who have the means readily available are at greater risk.	"Do you have a gun at home?"
Personal/family history A majority of people who succeed at suicide have made previous attempts. If previous attempts used highly lethal means or were unsuccessful only by accident (that is, if the plan did not allow for rescue), risk is increased. Those who have lost loved ones to suicide are at greater risk.	"Have you tried to kill yourself before?" "How? What happened?" "Has anyone in your family committed suicide?"
Goals Patients unable to envision or articulate goals or plans are at increased risk.	"Where do you see yourself next month? In 1 year? In 5 years?"

These factors associated with serious suicide risk also should be assessed by questioning the patient's family or other health care providers.

ADDITIONAL RISK FACTORS

Resources
Lack of social and personal resources to deal with external or internal crises, or a perception by the patient that such resources are unavailable, increases the likelihood of suicide.

Recent loss or life changes
Loss or the threat of loss increases suicide risk. Even other kinds of change (a promotion, a household move, or changes in roles or responsibilities) can increase stress and overwhelm the individual's coping abilities.

Physical illness
Physical illness may increase suicide risk, particularly if the illness involves major life changes or a threat to essentials of self-image.

Alcohol or drug abuse
Substance abuse may increase impulsive behavior and contribute to depression, thus increasing suicide risk. Additionally, alcohol or drugs may increase lethality by potentiating other drugs or decreasing overall level of awareness.

Sudden behavior change
Abrupt changes in behavior, of any kind, may signal suicidal intent.

Isolation
Physical or emotional isolation from others greatly increases suicide risk.

Age, sex, marital status
Older men have a higher rate of successful suicide, possibly because they tend to choose more lethal means. Risk of suicide may be increased for separated, widowed, or divorced persons. These parameters, however, are less reliable predictors than those above.

Mueller, S., and Malone, R. "Grief and Grieving," in *Medical-Surgical Care Plans.* Edited by Holloway, N. Springhouse, Pa.: Springhouse Corp., 1988.

Interventions

7. Assess suicide potential by asking direct questions, and intervene as indicated (see *Assessing Suicide Potential).* Recognize that issues of death and dying underlie all experiences with critical illness, and provide opportunities for frank, realistic discussion of death. See the "Grieving and Dying" care plan for details.

Rationales

7. The individual who feels unable to cope may contemplate suicide as a release from an apparently insoluble problem. Direct questioning is the best way to ascertain suicide risk. Discussing the underlying (and often unspoken) issues of death and dying may relieve tension and allow healthy coping to begin.

(continued)

Interventions	Rationales
8. As much as possible, prepare the patient and family in advance for eventual and possibly abrupt transfer out of the critical care unit. Explain how care routines will be different and how, as condition improves, care needs will be reduced. Anticipate increased anxiety as transfer nears. Make efforts to introduce the patient and family to post–critical care unit staff before transfer.	8. Transfer from the unit can precipitate a crisis if the patient and family are unprepared. Transfer may be misinterpreted as "giving up on" the patient. Addressing concerns in advance, and preparing the patient and family for the possibility that, as the condition improves, the patient may be considered for transfer if more critical patients need unit placement, can reduce anxiety and promote a smooth transition.
9. Additional individualized interventions: ____________	9. Rationales: ____________

Target outcome criteria
Within 48 hours, the patient or family will develop a specific plan for coping with at least one identified problem.

Transfer planning

NURSING TRANSFER CRITERIA

Upon transfer, documentation shows evidence of use of adaptive coping behaviors.

PATIENT-FAMILY TEACHING CHECKLIST

Document evidence that the patient and family demonstrate understanding of:

__ diagnosis, treatment plan, and prognosis
__ expected psychological responses
__ resources available for help
__ effective coping strategies.

DOCUMENTATION CHECKLIST

Using outcome criteria as a guide, document:

__ clinical status on admission
__ significant stress-related physiologic responses
__ patient's and family's subjective perception of threat
__ identified problems
__ response to staff members
__ patient-family support and interaction
__ coping history
__ pain-control measures
__ sleep patterns
__ nutritional intake
__ relaxation techniques
__ other interventions to increase coping ability
__ suicide assessment
__ referrals made
__ teaching.

ASSOCIATED CARE PLANS

Acute Pain
Grieving and Dying
Knowledge Deficit
Sensory-Perceptual Alteration

REFERENCES

Burgess, A.W., and Hartman, C.R. "Patient's Perceptions of the Cardiac Crisis: Key to Recovery," *American Journal of Nursing* 86(5):568-71, 1986.

Clark, S. "Ineffective Individual Coping," in *Medical-Surgical Care Plans.* Edited by Holloway, N. Springhouse, Pa.: Springhouse Corp., 1988.

Daley, L. "The Perceived Immediate Needs of Families with Relatives in the Intensive Care Setting," *Heart & Lung* 13:231-37, 1984.

Hoff, L.A. *People in Crisis: Understanding and Helping,* 2nd ed. Menlo Park, Calif.: Addison-Wesley Publishing Co., 1984.

Hudak, C., et al. *Critical Care Nursing: A Holistic Approach,* 4th ed. Philadelphia: J.B. Lippincott Co., 1986.

King, S., and Gregor, F. "Stress and Coping in Families of the Critically Ill," *Critical Care Nurse* 5:48-51, 1985.

McGovern, W.N., and Rodgers, J.A. "Change Theory," *American Journal of Nursing* 86(5):566-67, 1986.

Whittaker, A. "Ineffective Family Coping," in *Medical-Surgical Care Plans.* Edited by Holloway, N. Springhouse, Pa.: Springhouse Corp., 1988.

Impaired Physical Mobility

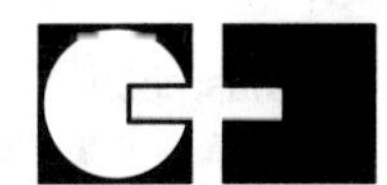

Introduction

DEFINITION AND TIME FOCUS

Impaired physical mobility is a problem for almost every patient in the critical care unit. Critically ill or injured patients are physically unable to engage in normal activities; often activity limitations also comprise part of the therapeutic regimen. Rest is essential for healing and should be encouraged; however, prolonged bed rest results in well-documented physical and emotional disabilities that can create even more problems for the patient. The effects of decreased mobility must be addressed early in care planning and reviewed frequently throughout the patient's hospitalization. This care plan focuses on the care of the critical patient whose condition causes or necessitates impaired physical mobility.

ETIOLOGY AND PRECIPITATING FACTORS

- injury that prevents weight bearing (such as trauma)
- illness that causes activity intolerance (such as cardiopulmonary disorders)
- chronic or acute disabling conditions (such as severe arthritis or Guillain-Barré syndrome)
- sensory-perceptual alterations (as in cerebrovascular accident)
- therapeutic restrictions
- reluctance to attempt movement

Focused assessment guidelines

NURSING HISTORY (Functional health pattern findings)

Because the patient's subjective responses to immobility vary widely, depending on the underlying condition, this section presents a guide to assessing the patient with a mobility impairment.

Health perception–health management pattern

- Is the patient's mobility problem of new onset, or does it reflect long-standing disability?
- What is the extent of the patient's activity limitation?
- Does the patient normally use any mobility aids at home (such as a walker, cane, or wheelchair)?
- Does the patient have a cast, splint, traction, or other immobilization device?
- Does the patient have equipment that interferes with normal mobility, such as a ventilator or multiple I.V. lines?
- Does the patient have previously existing conditions that affect mobility, such as a stroke or amputation?
- Does the patient have a history of blood disorders, integumentary problems, pulmonary disease, or cardiac disease?

Nutritional-metabolic pattern

- What is the patient's baseline nutritional status? (See the "Nutritional Deficit" care plan, page 53.)
- Is the patient able or permitted to take oral nourishment?

Elimination pattern

- When was the patient's last bowel movement?
- Does the patient normally use elimination aids, such as laxatives or enemas?
- Does the patient have a history of calculi, renal disease, or recurrent urinary tract infections?
- If the patient has a urinary catheter, when was it placed?

Activity-exercise pattern

- Is the patient able to perform any self-care activity?
- What was the patient's baseline activity tolerance before hospitalization?
- Are all joints capable of full range of motion?

Cognitive-perceptual pattern

- Is the patient conscious and alert?
- Does the patient have any sensory deficits (such as blindness, deafness, or hemiparesis)?

Self-perception–self-concept pattern

- What is the patient's attitude toward resuming physical activity?

Role-relationship pattern

- Does the patient's occupation require full mobility?

Sexuality-reproductive pattern

- Does the patient's mobility impairment potentially affect sexual function?

Coping-stress tolerance pattern

- Has the patient utilized physical activity as a primary coping behavior or stress-relieving measure?

PHYSICAL FINDINGS

Because physical findings vary widely in patients with reduced mobility, depending on their underlying condition, this section has been refocused to outline some of the major physiologic effects of immobility on body systems.

Cardiovascular

- orthostatic hypotension (related to reduced autonomic neurovascular reflex response)
- reduced stroke volume
- gradually increasing tachycardia (related to deconditioning effects)
- decreased oxygen uptake

- venous pooling (related to lack of muscle activity)
- plasma volume loss
- blood volume loss
- reduced cardiac reserve

Respiratory
- restricted diaphragmatic and costal excursion
- reduced ciliary activity
- reduced vital capacity
- reduced gas exchange (related to gravitational effects)
- reduced production of surfactant

Gastrointestinal
- decreased peristalsis
- increased sphincter tone
- abdominal distention
- anorexia

Neurologic
- decreased sensorium

Integumentary
- reduced skin turgor (related to fluid shifts and volume loss)
- impaired wound healing
- dependent edema

Musculoskeletal
- reduced muscle mass
- decreased strength and endurance
- bone demineralization (at increased rate)
- fibrosis or ankylosis
- calcium deposition in soft tissue

Renal
- hypercalciuria and precipitation of calcium salts (related to bone demineralization)
- increased renal blood flow
- initial diuresis (related to decreased antidiuretic hormone [ADH] release)
- bladder distention
- urinary stasis

Metabolic
- increased rate of catabolism
- decreased basal metabolic rate
- increased excretion of electrolytes

DIAGNOSTIC STUDIES

Because no diagnostic studies are specifically applicable to all patients with impaired mobility, only the usual laboratory test findings related to the physiologic changes described in the preceding section are presented here. Laboratory tests include:
- serum protein level—usually decreased from accelerated catabolism
- serum and urine calcium and phosphate levels—increased from bone demineralization
- arterial blood gas (ABG) measurements—may show reduced PaO_2 and increased $PaCO_2$, indicating hypoventilation and impaired gas exchange
- blood urea nitrogen level—may be elevated from catabolic activity
- urine pH—may be elevated from decreased levels of acid end products released by muscle activity
- hematocrit—may be increased from plasma and blood volume losses and diuresis.

POTENTIAL COMPLICATIONS
- thromboembolic phenomena
- atelectasis
- pneumonia
- infections
- skin breakdown
- constipation
- contractures
- osteoporosis
- muscle wasting
- urinary calculi
- ineffective coping

Nursing diagnosis: *Potential ineffective airway clearance related to reduced diaphragmatic and costal excursion, stasis of secretions, decreased ciliary activity, weakness, and underlying disease process*

NURSING PRIORITIES: (a) Maintain a clear airway and (b) prevent or promptly treat pulmonary complications.

Interventions	Rationales
1. Assess pulmonary capabilities at least every 2 hours while awake. Evaluate the patient's level of alertness, ability to cough and deep breathe, respiratory rate and effort, and lung sounds.	1. Initial and ongoing assessments provide direction for care planning. The factors listed are crucial determinants of the patient's capability to counteract the effects of bed rest on pulmonary function.

Interventions	Rationales
2. Evaluate for risk factors that affect pulmonary status, such as obesity, lung disease, incisions, abdominal distention, neuromuscular dysfunction, chest wall pathology, and medications that depress respirations.	2. The risk factors listed are associated with increased incidence of serious pulmonary complications.
3. Monitor vital signs, intake and output, hemodynamic pressures, and EKG findings according to Appendix A, "Monitoring Standards," or unit protocol. Report changes or abnormal findings promptly.	3. Bed rest has significant effects on cardiovascular function, including a reduction in stroke volume (which may be compensated by tachycardia), redistribution of blood flow (which may contribute to orthostatic hypotension), and decreased cardiovascular reserve (resulting in reduced exercise tolerance and general deconditioning). Careful monitoring of cardiovascular parameters aids in early detection of preventable complications.
4. Obtain and monitor arterial blood gas (ABG) measurements as ordered. Monitor vital capacity and other pulmonary function studies, as ordered, and report any abnormal findings promptly.	4. ABG measurements provide direct evaluation of ventilatory status. Pulmonary function studies aid further in classifying and evaluating the effects of bed rest on lungs, since bed rest is associated with decreased ventilatory capacity.
5. Initiate measures to promote effective breathing:	5. Maintaining an effective breathing pattern reduces the risk of developing pulmonary complications.
• Place the patient in Fowler's or semi-Fowler's position, as permitted by condition, and change position at least every 1 to 2 hours.	• Patients on bed rest commonly assume a slumped position, decreasing the adequacy of chest expansion. Frequent repositioning helps facilitate gravity drainage of secretions.
• Encourage deep breathing at least every hour while awake, and assist the patient using an incentive spirometer, as ordered.	• Deep breathing and incentive spirometry may increase inspiratory reserve volume, promote maximum alveolar inflation, and improve ventilation-perfusion ratios. Deep breathing may actually reverse microatelectasis related to hypoventilation. The incentive spirometer also provides a "goal" for the patient.
• Teach or assist the patient to splint incisions, if present.	• Splinting may decrease the fear of pain and promote deeper breathing and fuller chest wall expansion.
• Reduce abdominal distention, when possible, through use of gastric suction, return-flow enema, or other measures, as ordered.	• Abdominal distention exerts upward pressure on the diaphragm, reducing chest excursion.
6. Initiate measures to promote airway clearance:	6. Pulmonary hygiene measures help reduce the risk of developing pulmonary complications.
• Encourage deep breathing at least every 2 hours, and check with the doctor about including coughing with deep breathing.	• The effectiveness and desirability of coughing as an airway clearance measure are controversial because its direct effects on small airways have not been shown, and in fact, coughing may increase intrathoracic pressure and lead to alveolar microatelectasis. Some clinicians believe coughing may result in a "milking" effect from smaller to larger airways. If coughing is used, it should always be followed by several deep breaths to help reinflate alveoli.
• Provide humidification of inspired air.	• Humidification may help decrease the viscosity of secretions and helps minimize upper airway irritation if constant oxygen is required.
• Encourage an adequate fluid intake, typically 2,000 to 3,000 ml/day as condition allows.	• Rehydration of dehydrated patients has been shown to promote increased mucociliary clearance.
• Suction, as needed, providing supplemental oxygen before and after the procedure.	• Suctioning may be necessary for airway clearance, especially in persons with weak or absent cough or artificial airways. Supplemental oxygen is essential because suctioning has been shown to cause significant reduction in PaO_2 without it.

(continued)

Interventions	Rationales
• Perform chest physiotherapy every 4 hours while awake (or more frequently, as indicated by patient's condition).	• Chest physiotherapy may be helpful in preventing pooling of secretions and in loosening mucus plugs. When used in combination with postural drainage, it can help bring secretions into larger airways where they are more easily expectorated.
7. Monitor for evidence of pulmonary complications associated with bed rest, as follows:	7. Pulmonary insult complicates treatment of underlying conditions and increases mortality in the critically ill.
• pneumonia—crackles, rhonchi, chest pain, fever, productive cough, tachypnea, tachycardia, whispered pectoriloquy, consolidation or effusion on chest X-ray.	• Prompt detection and treatment of pulmonary infections is essential because their presence exacerbates ventilatory compromise related to bed rest. Purulent sputum is more tenacious because it contains viscous leukocyte deoxyribonucleic acid. In addition, proteolytic enzymes released from destroyed leukocytes can increase inflammation, resulting in bronchoconstriction.
• atelectasis—bronchial breath sounds or decreased breath sounds, dull percussion note over affected side, tachypnea, tachycardia, restlessness, tracheal shift toward affected side on chest X-ray, or cyanosis (if advanced macroatelectasis)	• Bed rest contributes to the development of atelectasis because of reduced chest expansion, ventilatory capacity, and secretion clearance. Microatelectasis is common and may be undetectable on chest X-ray. When atelectasis occurs, ventilatory capacity is reduced because inspired air cannot reach the affected areas.
• pulmonary embolus. (See the "Potential thromboembolic phenomena" problem below.)	• Pulmonary embolus is the most immediately life-threatening complication associated with bed rest, with a mortality of approximately 38%.
8. Additional individualized interventions: ____________	8. Rationales: ____________

Target outcome criteria

Throughout the critical care unit stay, the patient will:

• exhibit effective breathing pattern
• change position (or be turned) every 1 to 2 hours
• perform pulmonary hygiene measures at least every 2 hours, as condition permits
• exhibit no evidence of pneumonia, atelectasis, or pulmonary embolus.

Collaborative problem: *Potential thromboembolic phenomena related to venous pooling, loss of vasomotor tone, lack of skeletal muscle contraction, and increased blood viscosity*

NURSING PRIORITY: Prevent or promptly detect and treat thromboembolic complications.

Interventions	Rationales
1. Evaluate the patient for factors that increase the risk of thromboembolism, including: • previous history of deep vein thrombosis • abdominal, pelvic, or orthopedic surgery • trauma • history of varicosities, cancer, smoking, stroke, or bleeding disorders • use of oral contraceptives or other medications that affect clotting • dehydration • obesity • hypertension, diabetes mellitus, or renal disease • paralysis • decreased alertness • age (>40 years).	1. Any factor that contributes to venous stasis, hypercoagulability, trauma, or degeneration of blood vessels increases the risk of thromboembolism. Because bed rest alone increases the incidence of thromboembolic complications, noting any additional contributing factors will help identify the highest-risk patients for individual care planning.

Interventions

2. Initiate measures to promote venous return and decrease venous pooling:

• Teach the patient to perform leg exercises every 1 to 2 hours while awake, such as dorsiplantar flexion and quadriceps sets. Elevate legs 15 degrees.

• Avoid use of the knee gatch, leg crossing, or pillows placed directly under the popliteal area.

• Apply graded antiembolic hose, taking care to remove them at least three times daily for 30 to 60 minutes, or according to unit protocol. Discuss use of pneumatic devices such as special boots with doctor.

• Increase activity to permit ambulation as soon as the patient's condition permits. Use caution when first getting patient out of bed.

3. For high-risk patients, administer prophylactic anticoagulants, if ordered (typically low-dose heparin or warfarin sodium). Monitor clotting studies (prothrombin time [PT] or partial thromboplastin time [PTT]) daily for these patients, as ordered. Question anticoagulant orders for trauma patients or others with possible cardiovascular instability or bleeding problems.

4. Monitor for evidence of thromboembolic complications, including:

• pulmonary embolus—tachypnea, sudden dyspnea, pleuritic chest pain, restlessness, feelings of impending doom, diaphoresis, hypotension, pallor, or cyanosis. If these signs and symptoms occur, elevate the head of the bed, administer oxygen, obtain a specimen for ABG study, and notify the doctor immediately.

• thrombophlebitis—erythema, edema, tenderness, venous patterning or engorgement, positive Homans' sign, cording, or calf pain. Avoid deep palpation of affected area. If swelling is suspected, initiate daily measurements of leg circumference at a designated reference point. If these signs and symptoms occur, notify the doctor immediately and elevate the affected extremity.

5. Additional individualized interventions: ______________

____

Rationales

2. Venous stasis is associated with increased incidence of thromboembolic complications.

• Leg exercises cause muscle contraction, promoting venous return toward the heart. Elevation of the extremities promotes gravity drainage from peripheral vessels.

• These measures may cause venous compression or occlusion, increasing the risk of thromboembolic complications.

• Antiembolic hose "squeeze" superficial vessels and are thought to promote venous return. Removal permits examination of the skin and allows for drying if moisture has accumulated. Pneumatic devices may also promote venous return, and their use is particularly desirable if heparin is contraindicated by the patient's condition.

• Weight bearing increases muscle contraction and also decreases bone demineralization associated with immobility. Clots that have formed during periods of immobility are most likely to embolize when the patient first resumes activity.

3. Heparin inactivates fibrin, thus preventing formation of a fibrin clot and reducing the risk of enlargement of existing clots. Warfarin interferes with vitamin K production, thus decreasing production of clotting factors. Monitoring PT and PTT permits dosage adjustment as needed. Anticoagulants may precipitate bleeding in susceptible patients.

4. Early detection and treatment of thromboembolic phenomena may minimize their effects.

• Pulmonary embolus is the blockage of a pulmonary artery by a thrombus. As a result, alveoli are ventilated but not perfused, resulting in increased alveolar dead space in the affected areas of lung tissue. A large embolus may cause significant increases in pulmonary vascular resistance, which may contribute to the development of right-sided heart failure. Pulmonary infarction may also occur if the embolus is large. ABG findings guide intervention.

• Thrombophlebitis may occur in superficial or deep veins; the leg veins are most frequently affected. Superficial thrombophlebitis, although not dangerous, can cause significant discomfort; deep vein thrombophlebitis, however, may lead to life-threatening embolization to the lung. Initial erythema, swelling, and tenderness are related to inflammatory changes, while later signs (such as cording and a positive Homans' sign) represent actual thrombus formation. Deep palpation may cause dislodgment of clots. Circumferential measuring of the leg provides an objective means of evaluating swelling. Elevating the affected extremity helps minimize venous stasis, which may contribute to enlargement of the thrombus.

5. Rationales: ______________________________

____

Target outcome criteria
Throughout the critical care unit stay, the patient will:
- perform leg exercises at least every 2 hours as instructed or receive range-of-motion exercises
- increase activity to maximum level permitted
- display no signs of pulmonary embolus or thrombophlebitis.

Nursing diagnosis: *Potential impaired skin integrity related to impeded capillary flow, possible altered sensation, and/or venous stasis*

NURSING PRIORITY: Prevent skin breakdown.

Interventions	Rationales
1. On admission to the unit, and at least daily thereafter, inspect the skin carefully, evaluating color, texture, turgor, dryness, sensation, and capillary refill.	1. Initial and ongoing assessment is the first step in providing individualized care. Abnormal findings may provide clues to problem areas and can be used to guide care planning.
2. Evaluate for factors that increase the risk of skin breakdown, such as nutritional deficit, obesity, diabetes mellitus (or other conditions affecting vascular status), incontinence, decreased sensation, infection, excessive moisture, old age, decreased alertness, and paralysis.	2. Bed rest alone places any patient at increased risk for skin problems because pressure areas may develop rapidly if motion is restricted or impossible. The patient who presents with one or more of the conditions listed should be considered at extremely high risk. Early evaluation of such factors allows for institution of preventive measures.
3. Initiate measures to prevent skin breakdown, including:	3. Preventing skin breakdown is much easier than treating a problem after it develops.
• turning and repositioning every 1 to 2 hours, massaging areas of pressure or bony prominences	• Repositioning allows redistribution of pressure. Massage stimulates circulation and promotes comfort; bony prominences are the most common sites of skin breakdown.
• careful turning technique	• Rapid or overly vigorous turning may cause delicate skin to shear.
• judicious use of lotion, avoidance of harsh soaps, and careful cleansing, especially if incontinence is present, followed by gentle but thorough drying	• Dry skin is more prone to cracking and peeling, but excessive moisture provides a medium for bacterial growth and may lead to maceration. Soaps may be irritating. Urine or fecal material, if left in contact with skin, may cause chemical irritation and contribute to rapid breakdown of tissue.
• egg-crate mattress, flotation pad or water bed, sheepskins, air mattress, air-fluidized bead systems, low-air-loss bed or kinetic bed, as available and indicated	• Special bedding or beds may help improve patient comfort, distribute pressure more evenly, and reduce the deleterious effects of impaired mobility.
• adequate nutrition.	• Immobility contributes to increased catabolism and tissue breakdown; also, using stored fats as an energy source may cause reduction in cushioning provided by adipose tissue. Protein is essential for maintenance and rebuilding of tissue.
4. Monitor for evidence of impending skin breakdown: edema, blanching, coldness, tenderness, redness, or blistering. Brief reactive hyperemia of the skin is normal following relief from pressure. If reactive hyperemia does not resolve after 15 minutes, institute additional protective measures for the affected area.	4. Early detection of impending problems permits treatment before actual breakdown occurs. The signs and symptoms listed result when pressure and immobility diminish perfusion. Pressure ulcers can result from as little as 1 hour of pressure and immobility, if the pressure is high enough to impede capillary flow. Additionally, subcutaneous tissue and muscle have usually suffered ischemia before the ulcer becomes apparent on the skin surface, so early detection and treatment are vital.

Interventions	Rationales
5. If a pressure sore develops, institute a therapeutic regimen immediately, according to the doctor's orders or unit protocol.	5. Treatment of pressure sores varies among practitioners and institutions. Prompt treatment is essential to avert development of additional complications, such as osteomyelitis.
6. Additional individualized interventions: ____________	6. Rationales: ____________

Target outcome criteria
Throughout the critical care unit stay, the patient will:
- maintain clean, intact skin
- exhibit no evidence of skin breakdown
- maintain adequate nutritional intake.

Nursing diagnosis: *Potential altered urinary elimination pattern related to diuresis, stasis of urine, positioning, and/or bone demineralization*

NURSING PRIORITIES: (a) Promote normal urinary elimination and (b) prevent urinary system complications.

Interventions	Rationales
1. Assess the patient's normal urinary elimination pattern, if possible, by noting the following: • frequency, times, and amounts of voidings • any change in the usual pattern • continence • special measures used to initiate or control voiding.	1. Assessment of the patient's normal elimination status is the first step in planning individualized care.
2. Evaluate factors that may increase the risk of urinary complications, such as: • dehydration • incontinence • indwelling catheters • narcotics, sedatives, diuretics, or other medications that affect renal function or alertness • diabetes • neurogenic bladder dysfunction • pregnancy • immunosuppression • shock • altered acid-base or electrolyte status.	2. Immobility has several effects on urinary elimination. Bed rest increases the solute load of the kidneys because tissue breakdown and bone demineralization both occur at an increased rate. The increased thoracic blood volume associated with the supine position triggers decreased ADH release, resulting in diuresis. The supine position also contributes to urinary stasis, because downward urinary flow is normally enhanced by gravity. Additionally, complete bladder emptying may be harder to achieve in the supine position. Any additional factors, such as those listed, contribute further to the risk of complications and must be considered in care planning.
3. Initiate measures to promote normal urinary elimination:	3. Measures to promote normal elimination may help reduce the risk of developing urinary system complications.
• Get the patient up to a bedside commode or allow a male to stand to urinate, if his condition permits.	• The upright position facilitates improved urinary flow from the ureters and bladder and is usually more comfortable for patients. In addition, studies report no significant differences in oxygen consumption and cardiovascular response between in-bed and out-of-bed toileting. Weight-bearing exercise of any kind, including the effort to stand at the bedside, may also help reduce deleterious orthostasis and bone demineralization.
• Encourage adequate fluid intake, unless contraindicated by underlying condition, to between 2,000 and 3,000 ml/day.	• Calcium precipitation, and resultant calculi formation, is less likely to occur in dilute urine. In addition, an adequate quantity of dilute urine increases frequency of micturition, reducing the likelihood of infection from stasis.

(continued)

Interventions	Rationales
• Promote as much activity as condition permits—turning, sitting, dangling, standing, walking, or range-of-motion exercise.	• Position changes promote urinary drainage, minimize stasis, and reduce protein breakdown associated with immobilization.
• Provide privacy during attempts to void.	• The sphincter relaxation necessary for voiding may be difficult to achieve unless privacy is ensured.
• Use measures to promote full emptying of the bladder, as needed, such as running water nearby, pouring warm water over the perineum, and applying manual pressure over the bladder.	• Bladder distention may cause back pressure and eventual nephron damage. Incomplete bladder emptying is also associated with increased risk of infection.
• Use urinary catheterization only as needed to prevent distention and stasis. Exercise impeccable aseptic technique in insertion and care of catheters, if used.	• Urinary catheterization is associated with a high incidence of nosocomial infections. Entry into the normally sterile urinary tract exposes the patient to pathogens that may result in infection.
4. Measure urine output hourly and report values <60 ml/hour for 2 hours. Assess for bladder distention at least every 8 hours. Measure urine pH every 8 hours and report levels >6. Monitor routine urine cultures, as ordered.	4. Urine output of <60 ml/hour may indicate impending renal failure or other complications. Bladder distention and resultant urinary stasis may occur even in a catheterized patient, if the tube becomes obstructed by sediment, blood clots, or calculi. Alkaline urine contributes to the formation of calcium calculi. Routine urine cultures allow early detection of infection.
5. Monitor for indications of urinary tract complications, as follows:	5. Urinary tract complications usually are the result of several interrelated factors.
• infection—burning, frequency, and urgency (if voiding voluntarily); cloudy, foul-smelling urine; hematuria; fever; or low back pain	• Urinary tract infection may be related to stasis, dehydration, bladder distention, or any factor that damages the protective mucosal lining of the bladder, such as calculi or catheterization.
• calculi—severe flank pain, lower abdominal pain, hematuria, nausea, or altered urinary stream (if a calculus lodges in the bladder neck or urethra)	• Calcium excretion is increased in patients on prolonged bed rest because of increased bone breakdown. Most calculi are composed of calcium salts. Such factors as stasis, infection, and decreased urine volume contribute to the precipitation of calculi. Also, because of low levels of muscle contraction, a smaller-than-normal quantity of acid end products is excreted, and the urine becomes increasingly alkaline, a condition that favors calculus formation.
6. If indications of urinary complications are detected, notify the doctor promptly and collaborate in treatment.	6. Treatment of urinary pathology in critically ill patients must be carefully coordinated with treatment of the patient's primary condition to avert development of further complications.
7. Additional individualized interventions: ____________	7. Rationales: ____________

Target outcome criteria

Throughout the critical care unit stay, the patient will:
- maintain urine output of at least 60 ml/hour
- maintain fluid intake of at least 2,000 ml/day, unless contraindicated
- exhibit no signs of urinary tract infection or calculi.

Nursing diagnosis: *Potential altered bowel elimination related to lack of contraction of abdominal muscles, weakness, loss of defecation reflex, slowed peristalsis, altered nutritional intake, and/or psychological inhibition*

NURSING PRIORITY: Promote normal bowel elimination.

Interventions	Rationales
1. Assess the patient's normal bowel elimination pattern, if possible, noting the frequency, times, color, and consistency of stools; any change in the usual pattern; continence; use of laxatives or enemas; date and time of last bowel movement; and bowel sounds. Monitor bowel status on a daily basis.	1. Assessment of the patient's normal elimination status is the first step in planning individualized care. Daily monitoring helps in early identification of potential problems.
2. Evaluate the patient for factors that may increase the risk of constipation, including dehydration; narcotics, iron, anticholinergics, or other medications affecting peristaltic function; paralysis; age (because of reduced colonic tone); cachexia; emphysema (because of reduced ability to increase intra-abdominal pressure); abdominal surgery; abdominal tumors; pregnancy; ascites; hemorrhoids; NPO status; and trauma.	2. Because normal bowel motility depends in part upon abdominal muscle contraction and physical activity, immobility predisposes patients to constipation. Any additional factors, such as those listed, contribute further to the risk of complications and must be considered in care planning.
3. Initiate measures to promote normal bowel elimination:	3. Maintaining normal bowel elimination reduces the risk of developing bowel complications.
• Allow the use of a bedside commode or toilet, if condition permits. Encourage the patient to attempt defecation at usual times, or whenever he experiences the urge.	• The normal defecation position facilitates evacuation. If defecation is suppressed despite impulses from rectal distention, colonic motility eventually may be inhibited.
• Encourage the patient to contract abdominal muscles while exhaling during defecation attempts. Instruct the patient to avoid Valsalva's maneuver.	• Contraction of abdominal muscles increases intra-abdominal pressure and aids in evacuation. Valsalva's maneuver causes a vagal response and, in susceptible patients, may result in undesirable bradycardia, heart block, or other cardiovascular complications.
• As the patient's condition permits, teach exercises to maintain or strengthen abdominal musculature, such as contracting and relaxing abdominal muscles several times per hour and performing leg lifts.	• Bed rest results in generalized muscle atrophy. Weakness of the abdominal muscles may render the patient unable to voluntarily assist with evacuation.
• Encourage an adequate fluid intake, unless contraindicated.	• Inadequate fluid intake may form dry, hard stools that are more difficult to expel.
• If the patient can tolerate oral food intake, encourage natural laxatives and high-fiber foods, as permitted.	• Whole-grain cereals, fruits and vegetables, and prune juice help promote natural elimination.
• Provide privacy and comfort measures during toileting, such as ensuring warmth and providing air freshener.	• Bowel activity may be inhibited if the patient is anxious, embarrassed, or uncomfortable.
4. Assess for indications of constipation, such as absence of bowel movements; hard, dry, small stools; rectal pressure sensation; abdominal distention or mass; headache; decreased appetite; hard stool felt in rectal vault on digital examination; or ribbonlike diarrhea.	4. In the absence of normal bowel elimination, water continues to be reabsorbed from the stool that remains in the bowel, and the stool becomes harder, dryer, and more compacted. As softer stool collects behind it, increasing peristaltic pressure may result in a forceful expulsion of diarrhea past the hard mass of stool.
5. As necessary, collaborate with the doctor to select appropriate elimination aids, such as laxatives, suppositories, enemas, or stool softeners.	5. Laxatives, suppositories, and enemas may be necessary occasionally, but their frequent use may disrupt normal bowel functioning. Stool softeners may help in the natural expulsion of stool and are nonhabit-forming.
6. Additional individualized interventions: __________	6. Rationales: __________

Target outcome criteria

Throughout the critical care unit stay, the patient will:
- maintain normal bowel elimination
- perform abdominal exercises as taught, if condition permits
- exhibit no signs of constipation.

Collaborative problem: *Potential muscle atrophy and/or joint contractures related to disuse, nonfunctional positioning, and/or reduced muscle tone*

NURSING PRIORITY: Maintain maximum functional integrity of bone and muscle.

Interventions

1. Evaluate the patient for factors that increase the risk of significant muscle, bone, and joint complications, including preexisting conditions that reduce mobility (arthritis, paralysis, paresis, or debilitation), decreased level of alertness, spinal injury or surgery, major burns, and trauma.

2. Initiate measures to preserve motor function and strength:
- weight bearing, as condition permits, even if only standing at the bedside or on a tilt table several times daily
- active exercise, as condition permits, including hourly ankle rotation, dorsiplantar flexion, and quadriceps setting
- complete range of motion to all joints at least four times daily, as condition permits
- careful positioning to maintain functional alignment, using such measures as trochanter rolls, hand rolls, splints, footboards, and padding between thighs (if hip adduction is a problem). Alternate flexion and extension of extremities when turning and repositioning at least every 1 to 2 hours.

3. Additional individualized interventions: ____________

Rationales

1. Normal bone and muscle function are dependent on activity, which maintains and increases muscle strength, maintains balanced muscle tone, and promotes normal bone formation. When a muscle is immobilized, 10% to 15% of its strength may be lost in as little as 1 week, and it may atrophy to half its size within a month. Disuse atrophy leads to shortening of muscle fibers and reduces joint motion. Immobilization decreases osteoblastic deposition of bone matrix, but normal osteoclastic destruction continues, depleting calcium and other minerals essential for bone stability. The other factors listed may add further to the risk of significant bone- and muscle-related complications.

2. Maintaining healthy bone and muscle function is easier than restoring function once disability occurs.
- Weight-bearing exercise stimulates osteoblastic activity by providing normal stress to bones. Lack of weight bearing is the primary contributor to development of osteoporosis, a condition in which the bones are so weakened that the patient is prone to fractures.
- Active exercises promote maximum muscle contraction and help maintain strength and endurance.
- Putting the joint through its full range of motion stretches the surrounding muscle fibers and maintains the coordinated function of joint structures.
- Serious joint contractures requiring surgical intervention or prolonged corrective physical therapy may result if functional alignment is not maintained.

3. Rationales: ____________

Target outcome criteria

Throughout the critical care unit stay, the patient will:
- perform exercises as taught, if condition permits
- maintain functional alignment of all joints.

Nursing diagnosis: *Disturbed self-concept: body image, role performance related to dependent patient role*

NURSING PRIORITY: Promote positive self-image.

Interventions	Rationales
1. Assess the effects of reduced mobility on self-concept. Encourage ventilation of feelings and identification of primary losses.	1. Identifying what the loss of normal mobility means to the individual is the first step in care planning. A patient's reaction to immobility can vary enormously, depending on his baseline activity level and the importance of physical function to his identity.
2. Encourage the patient's participation in his own care and decision-making, to the extent permitted by condition.	2. Participating in his own care, even in small ways, preserves a patient's sense of identity and integrity.
3. Anticipate such behaviors as regression, withdrawal, aggression, apathy, and crying. Try to help the patient interpret these normal responses to loss.	3. Immobility may cause disorganization of the psyche as the individual attempts to cope with the profound losses of usual roles, stimulation, and independence. Helping the patient to understand the normalcy of his reactions may reduce psychic disequilibrium and facilitate initiation of healthy coping strategies.
4. See the "Sensory-Perceptual Alteration" care plan, page 60.	4. Immobility results in significant reduction in normal sensory stimulation. This can contribute to decreased motivation, reduced ability to learn and problem-solve, sleep disturbances, and other problems that may compound the patient's distress. The "Sensory-Perceptual Alteration" care plan contains detailed information on preventing, detecting, and treating this problem.
5. See the "Ineffective Coping" care plan, page 26.	5. The "Ineffective Coping" care plan contains further interventions that may be helpful in caring for the patient with a disturbed self-concept.
6. Additional individualized interventions: ______	6. Rationales: ______

Target outcome criteria
Throughout the critical care unit stay, the patient will:
- express feelings related to losses
- participate in decision-making related to care
- exercise healthy coping behaviors.

Transfer planning

NURSING TRANSFER CRITERIA
Upon transfer, documentation shows evidence of no life-threatening or disabling complications of immobility.

PATIENT-FAMILY TEACHING CHECKLIST
Document evidence that patient and family demonstrate understanding of:
__ activity recommendations, restrictions, and limitations
__ measures to avert orthostatic hypotension and activity intolerance
__ indicators of clinically significant activity intolerance
__ signs of complications related to impaired mobility
__ use of any mobility aids.

DOCUMENTATION CHECKLIST
Using outcome criteria as a guide, document:
__ clinical status on admission
__ significant changes in status
__ pertinent laboratory and diagnostic test findings
__ protective measures initiated
__ response to resumption of activity
__ complications of immobility, if any
__ patient-family teaching
__ transfer planning.

ASSOCIATED CARE PLANS

Acute Pain
Ineffective Coping
Nutritional Deficit
Sensory-Perceptual Alteration

REFERENCES

Cosenza, J., and Norton, L. "Secretion Clearance: State of the Art From a Nursing Perspective," *Critical Care Nurse* 6(4):23-36, 1986.

Holloway, N. *Nursing the Critically Ill Adult,* 3rd ed. Menlo Park, Calif.: Addison-Wesley Publishing Co., 1988.

Kozier, B., and Erb, G. *Fundamentals of Nursing: Concepts and Procedures,* 3rd ed. Menlo Park, Calif.: Addison-Wesley Publishing Co., 1987.

Luckmann, J., and Sorensen, K. *Medical-Surgical Nursing: A Psychophysiologic Approach,* 3rd ed. Philadelphia: W.B. Saunders Co., 1987.

Olson, E.V., et al. "The Hazards of Immobility," *American Journal of Nursing* 67:781-96, 1967.

Rubin, M. "The Physiology of Bed Rest," *American Journal of Nursing* 88:50-55, 1988.

Traver, G.A. "Ineffective Airway Clearance: Physiology and Clinical Application," *Dimensions of Critical Care Nursing* 4(4):198-207, 1985.

Westra, B. "When Your Patient Says 'I Can't Breathe,'" *Nursing84* 14(5):34-39, May 1984.

Winslow, E., et al. "Oxygen Uptake and Cardiovascular Responses in Patients and Normal Adults During In-Bed and Out-of-Bed Toileting," *Journal of Cardiac Rehabilitation* 4:348-54, 1984.

Knowledge Deficit

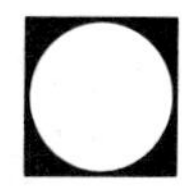

Introduction

DEFINITION AND TIME FOCUS

A lack of knowledge or skills necessary for health recovery or maintenance comprises a knowledge deficit. This teaching plan, adapted from a similar care plan that originally appeared in the author's *Medical-Surgical Care Plans,* focuses on the critically ill patient and family. Although the teaching and learning principles for medical-surgical and critical care patients have many similarities, the emphasis is different. In critical care, the patient is usually too ill for formal teaching; physiologic needs take precedence, and extensive teaching may be deferred until after the patient stabilizes. Although a major teaching program during this period is inappropriate for most patients, you can capitalize on serendipitous teaching opportunities to meet immediate learning needs as well as to identify long-range learning needs. The latter are usually addressed after the patient has been transferred to a more conducive environment than the often hectic critical care unit.

Although teaching usually cannot be completed during the unit stay, it can begin there. Through expert teaching, you can provide a context for the patient and family to understand the rationale for immediate therapeutic interventions and lay a foundation for further teaching by colleagues on step-down units and general medical-surgical units. Teaching is most effective when an awareness of its importance pervades all phases of patient care.

ETIOLOGY AND PRECIPITATING FACTORS

- unfamiliar diagnostic procedure
- new diagnosis
- alteration in preexisting health problem
- unfamiliar or altered treatment plan
- complex treatment regimen
- denial
- anxiety

Focused assessment guidelines

NURSING HISTORY (Functional health pattern findings)

Note: Because no typical presentation of a patient with a knowledge deficit exists, this section presents an assessment guide for teaching and learning factors.

Health perception–health management pattern

- Did the patient delay seeking needed medical attention?
- Does the patient lack knowledge about the disorder?
- Does the patient express lack of confidence in his ability to manage the condition?
- Does the patient express misconceptions about health status?
- Has the patient failed to comply with recommended health practices?
- Does the patient fail to carry out self-care, even though physically able?

Nutritional-metabolic pattern

- Does the patient express concerns about the effects of the disorder on nutrition and eating habits?
- Has the patient had difficulty staying on a prescribed dietary regimen?

Activity-exercise pattern

- Does the patient express concerns about life-changing limitation of activity because of the disorder?

Cognitive-perceptual pattern

- Does the patient have concerns about the specific details of a diagnostic or therapeutic procedure?
- Does the patient have sensory deficits, such as visual or hearing impairments?
- Does the patient lack psychomotor skills needed to maintain a home treatment regimen?
- Has the patient experienced confusion or changes in thought processes from the disorder?
- Has the patient shown signs of misinterpreting information, for example, by asking inappropriate questions?

Self-perception–self-concept pattern

- Does the patient express concerns about an inability to maintain treatment regimen?
- Does the patient report anxiety about changes in body image from the disorder?

Role-relationship pattern

- Does the patient want a significant other present or available during procedures?
- Does the patient express concerns about job, income, or family responsibilities because of the disorder?
- Does the patient express concerns about family's response to life style changes because of the disorder?

Sexuality-reproductive pattern

- Does the patient report concern about the impact of the disorder on sexual activity?
- Does the patient express concern about the impact of changes in sexual activity on a spouse or partner?

Coping-stress tolerance pattern

- Does the patient display an unusual amount of anxiety?
- Does the patient display denial of his disorder?
- Does the patient report depression because of lifestyle changes caused by his disorder?
- Does the patient express concerns about coping behaviors and motivation?

PHYSICAL FINDINGS
Not applicable

DIAGNOSTIC STUDIES
Not applicable

POTENTIAL COMPLICATIONS
- Exacerbation of disorder

Nursing diagnosis: *Potential knowledge deficit related to lack of readiness to learn**

NURSING PRIORITY: Determine readiness to learn.

Intervention	Rationales
1. Assess the impact of the patient's disorder on lifestyle.	1. The degree of impact determines the extent of teaching necessary. Areas of impact provide foci around which learning experiences should be structured.
2. Determine the patient's stage of adaptation to the disorder: shock and disbelief; developing awareness; or resolution and reorganization. Dovetail teaching objectives and content with psychological issues during each phase.	2. Different psychological work occurs in each of these phases. Attempting to provide teaching inappropriate for a particular phase results in increased learner anxiety or irritation and inability to absorb information.
3. Assess the patient's physical readiness to learn: Is he physiologically stable, rested, and pain-free? If not, defer participation in a formal teaching program.	3. Teaching is most effective when the patient is ready to learn. Readiness to learn depends on physical as well as psychological factors. Determining readiness to learn requires weighing the interaction of numerous variables. Learning requires energy that will not be available if the patient is unstable, tired, or in pain. Because of shortened critical care unit (CCU) stays, very few CCU patients reach physical readiness to learn much before transfer, except stable acute myocardial infarction patients.
4. Determine the patient's motivation to learn. For example, are appropriate questions asked about status or care? Is the patient preoccupied, distracted, or emotionally labile?	4. Motivation is the crucial variable in learning and may be absent initially because of anxiety or preoccupation with other needs. Prolonged absence of interest in learning about the condition may be a clue to an underlying emotional disorder requiring treatment before the patient assumes independent self-care responsibility. Motivation may be developed through teaching by linking relevant learning to the patient's particular concerns.
5. Determine the general pattern of health maintenance; for example, has the patient sought regular medical checkups, followed previous health recommendations, eaten a balanced diet, and exercised regularly?	5. The general pattern can provide clues to overall acceptance of responsibility for self-care and likelihood of receptivity to teaching.
6. Assess the patient's current knowledge of the disorder and its implications, the likelihood of complications, and the likelihood of cure or disease control. Specifically ask about the doctor's explanations, the patient's past experiences, and information received from family, friends, and the media.	6. Adults learn best when teaching builds on previous knowledge or experience. Assessing recall of the doctor's explanations as well as the patient's past experiences and exposure to health information provides an opportunity for assessing attitudes and the accuracy and completeness of knowledge.

*Because of the importance of knowledge deficit as a patient problem and because of the large number of possible interventions, problems in this plan are subdivided by etiology.

Interventions	Rationales
7. Ask the patient how much he wants to know, if possible. Consider the patient's preference for information in planning teaching.	7. Recent research suggests that the common assumption that teaching reduces anxiety or otherwise helps the patient is not always true; people vary in the degree of detail they find helpful. According to Watkins and Odegaard (1986), learners fall into two groups: those who cope with a threatening experience by avoiding its aspects ("blunters") and those who cope by learning as much as possible about its aspects ("monitors"). Blunters generally want to know relatively little about impending experiences, whereas monitors want to know a great deal. Providing a blunter with detailed information increases anxiety, whereas withholding it from a monitor worsens stress. When possible, match preference and teaching appropriately to respect individual differences and support the patient's preferred learning style.
8. Determine learning needs. Consider needs expressed by the patient and family; predictable disorder-related concerns and responses; and activities necessary to monitor health status, prevent disease, implement prescribed therapy, and prevent complications or recurrence.	8. Learning needs determine appropriate content. Learning occurs most rapidly when it is relevant to current needs and past experiences. Responding to expressed needs displays sensitivity to the patient's and family's concerns. Predictable concerns and responses and necessary self-care activities help the nurse identify learning needs of which the patient and family may be unaware.
9. Estimate learning capacity. Assess the patient's age; language skills; ability to read, write, and reason; and educational, religious, and cultural background.	9. Sociocultural factors affect the speed and degree of learning. Awareness of the patient's age, background, and general ability to think logically and express himself helps you present material at an appropriate intellectual level.
10. Additional individualized interventions: ____________	10. Rationales: ____________

Target outcome criteria

Before initiation of teaching, the patient will:
- be physiologically stable
- discuss current knowledge of disorder
- identify primary perceived learning needs
- display motivation to learn; for example, by asking appropriate questions.

Nursing diagnosis: *Potential knowledge deficit related to a teaching program that is inappropriate for the patient's current needs*

NURSING PRIORITY: Plan an individualized teaching strategy.

Interventions	Rationales
1. Determine realistic goals for learning while the patient is in the CCU. Work with the patient and family to ensure that goals are mutually acceptable.	1. Goals determine content. Goal-directed learning is more efficient than fragmented, unfocused learning. Active participation in goal-setting increases the likelihood that the patient and family will understand goals and support them.
2. Determine what to teach by assessing what is essential from the patient's viewpoint. Set priorities for content by dividing it into "need to know now" and "need to know later" categories.	2. Because the patient's attention span may be limited and the patient's hospitalization may be short, priorities for content must be set. Content largely determines the choice of teaching method.

(continued)

TEACHING STRATEGIES

Method	Characteristics	Most appropriate for	Disadvantages
Individual bedside instruction	One-on-one interaction between teacher and learner Immediate feedback Informal	Acute phase Sensitive topics "Private" person Emotionally labile person Persons with language difficulties Persons with limited education	Time-consuming
Group session	Small or large number of people Informal Interchange of ideas	General content Persons with similar readiness-to-learn levels	Lack of individualization
Lecture	Highly structured Efficient	Large amount of factual content Rehabilitation program	Lack of opportunity for teacher-learner interaction Possible failure to engage learner's interest (Disadvantages may be overcome by alternating lectures with interactive learning opportunities, such as question-and-answer periods or skill demonstrations.)
Discussion	Interchange of ideas More informal than lecture More opportunity to adapt content and evaluate learner comprehension	Acute phase Sensitive topics When attitudinal change is desired Highly verbal patients	Time-consuming May be uncomfortable for some patients because of their cultural norms against expression
Demonstration/return demonstration	Observation and supervised practice Immediate feedback	Teaching psychomotor skills	Requires realistic equipment

Interventions	Rationales
3. Provide an appropriate sequence to the information presented. In general, in the CCU teach only:	3. Proper sequencing allows the patient to build upon current knowledge and experience.
• information about expressed concerns	• Learning is strongest when it occurs in response to perceived needs. Dealing with initial concerns displays sensitivity to the patient, helps establish rapport and trust, and frees the patient's energy to focus on further learning. In general, only crucial questions are answered in the CCU and the remainder deferred.
• high-priority information—specific teaching without which the patient's condition may be seriously jeopardized.	• Presenting essential information early in the teaching period helps ensure that all the critical information will have been covered by the time of hospital discharge.

Interventions	Rationales
4. Select appropriate teaching methods: • individual bedside instruction • discussions • demonstrations.	4. Although various teaching methods exist (see *Teaching Strategies*), individual instruction, discussion, and demonstration are most appropriate in the CCU because of constraints imposed by the patient's condition and the environment.
5. Be creative in choosing appropriate teaching materials, such as booklets, instruction sheets, films, videotapes, models or dolls, slides, and audiotapes. In choosing, consider the advantages, availability, patient's learning style, and the learning environment.	5. The more senses involved in learning, the more likely the patient will retain the material. Printed materials provide consistency, reinforce orally presented information, and provide a source to which the patient can refer as needed. Models (for example, of the heart and a pacemaker) help the patient visualize how something works. Dolls may be useful adjuncts for teaching children. Slides, audiotapes, films, and videotapes can vividly present an experience—for example, by showing a diagnostic procedure from the patient's viewpoint. These audiovisuals may not be suitable, however, unless the patient is stable enough to focus his attention on them and the learning environment is conducive to using them. If used, they should be supplemented by a one-on-one follow-up discussion.
6. Determine how best to teach the content to an individual patient at a particular time. Consider the advantages and disadvantages of various teaching methods, the appropriateness and availability of educational materials, and the patient's personality.	6. In many cases, several combinations of content, teaching methods, and educational materials can achieve a desired goal. Selecting the combination most appropriate to this patient makes learning "come alive."
7. Decide who should teach what: Consider the primary nurse, a nurse with special related expertise, and other health care professionals. Mention the availability of visitors from community or self-help groups when the patient is more stable physiologically.	7. Depending on the content and patient preferences, different teachers may be necessary or appropriate to reinforce learning. Support groups may provide especially relevant information based on personal experience with the patient's disorder. In many cases, their credibility makes them invaluable in helping the patient accept the need for long-term education and rehabilitation. Their visits may need to be deferred until after patient transfer from the unit, when he can benefit more from their insight and competencies. Knowing that others have coped productively with similar experiences may provide a sense of rapport and trust that facilitates the necessary learning.
8. Decide when to teach.	8. Choosing appropriate times to teach capitalizes on learning readiness. Appropriate sequencing builds upon previously presented material and enhances integration of learning.
9. Plan evaluation strategies, such as observation, questions, and having the patient demonstrate new skills, that are based on goals and objectives.	9. Evaluation commonly is interwoven with the presentation. Clear evaluation plans help ensure measurability of goals and increase the likelihood that the nurse will recognize spontaneous opportunities for evaluation and respond appropriately to them.
10. Communicate the teaching strategy to other critical care professionals involved in the patient's care.	10. Communication enhances consistency of information provided by caregivers, permits appropriate reinforcement, and minimizes unnecessary repetition.
11. Identify and document long-range learning needs. When the patient is transferred from the critical care unit, communicate learning needs to colleagues on the receiving unit and arrange for continuation of the teaching plan.	11. The patient's condition, extensiveness of learning needs, and the busy CCU atmosphere make it difficult for the patient to complete necessary learning before being transferred. Documentation and communication of long-range learning needs allow personalization of ongoing educational efforts.

(continued)

Interventions	Rationales
12. Additional individualized interventions: ________	12. Rationales: ________

Target outcome criteria
According to individual readiness, the patient will identify priority learning needs.

Nursing diagnosis: *Potential knowledge deficit related to inadequate or ineffective implementation of teaching plan*

NURSING PRIORITY: Implement an individualized teaching plan that maximizes learning, retention, and compliance.

Interventions	Rationales
1. Incorporate teaching into other nursing activities. Be alert for serendipitous teaching opportunities; for example, use symptomatic episodes (such as an insulin reaction in a new diabetic) to help the patient and family learn to identify symptoms.	1. The hectic pace of most critical care units allows little time for extended teaching sessions. Incorporating teaching into other activities increases the likelihood of accomplishing it and contributes to an atmosphere of naturalness and informality. Activity-related teaching also reinforces learning (for example, teaching stoma care whenever the stoma is visible). The immediacy of a symptomatic episode makes it a powerful teaching tool for establishing the importance of the patient's and family's active involvement in the learning process.
2. Present yourself as enthusiastic, knowledgeable, and approachable.	2. Enthusiasm is contagious. Presenting yourself as knowledgeable increases credibility, and maintaining approachability allows the patient to feel comfortable capitalizing on your expertise.
3. Present manageable amounts of information at any one time.	3. Too much information at one time causes confusion. The patient may lose sight of key points.
4. Provide simple explanations, using easy-to-understand terminology.	4. Medical and nursing jargon distances the patient and family members. Intricate explanations may confuse or overwhelm them.
5. Use review and repetition judiciously, considering individual factors.	5. Physiologic changes, pain medications, anxiety, the CCU environment, and the patient's age may contribute to a short attention span and poor retention. (Elderly persons commonly have difficulty remembering details.)
6. Before planned teaching, assess for physiologic needs (such as thirst or urge to void) and intense emotions. Meet any physiologic needs first, and encourage the patient to express any strong emotions.	6. Unmet physiologic needs and strong emotions interfere with the ability to concentrate on learning.
7. Provide opportunities for immediate application of learning. For example, when teaching pulse-taking, show the patient, then have him count your radial pulse while you take your carotid pulse for comparison.	7. Immediate application improves retention.
8. Ask for feedback: Were the words understandable? Was the presentation too fast, too slow, too much, or too little? Adjust terminology, pace, and amount of information accordingly.	8. The patient may be reluctant to reveal lack of understanding. Soliciting feedback demonstrates respect for the learner and permits adjustments before the patient becomes lost, overwhelmed, or bored.

Interventions	Rationales
9. Be alert for signs of pain, fatigue, confusion, or boredom, such as fidgeting, yawning, lack of eye contact, grimacing, or agitation.	9. These nonverbal signs may provide clues to the need for modification or conclusion of the current teaching session.
10. Promote a positive outlook; solicit feelings and convey confidence in the patient's ability to learn.	10. The patient may initially feel overwhelmed and insecure about his ability to learn because of the magnitude, urgency, or unfamiliarity of necessary adaptations to illness.
11. Encourage active participation. Use interactive teaching methods.	11. Adults learn best when actively involved. Active participation also facilitates changes needed to allow recovery from or adaptation to the patient's disorder.
12. Document teaching sessions. Communicate progress to appropriate caregivers.	12. Documentation provides a teaching record for legal purposes and enhances continuity of teaching among caregivers.
13. Additional individualized interventions: ________	13. Rationales: ________

Target outcome criteria
According to individual readiness, the patient will:
- indicate interest in learning during care activities
- provide relevant feedback to teachers.

Nursing diagnosis: *Potential knowledge deficit related to lack of modification of teaching as needed*

NURSING PRIORITIES: (a) Evaluate learning and (b) modify teaching when appropriate.

Interventions	Rationales
1. During and after teaching, determine what learning has occurred. For example, observe the patient, ask questions, or have the patient demonstrate a new skill.	1. Determining learning accomplishment permits resolution of some learning needs and provides guidance for meeting others.
2. With the patient, compare learning against previously identified goals.	2. Comparison indicates whether goals have been achieved or whether their appropriateness should be reevaluated.
3. Modify the teaching plan as indicated by unmet goals or new learning needs.	3. Frequent evaluation and modification of the teaching plan ensures that the teaching is tailored to individual learning capabilities and ongoing learning needs.
4. Refer the patient and family to health care agencies and community agencies, as appropriate, before discharge.	4. Needs not met by the time of discharge require further follow-up.
5. If the patient is noncompliant, evaluate why. Refer to the noncompliance problem in the "Congestive Heart Failure" care plan in *Medical-Surgical Care Plans* for further information.	5. The patient has the right to control his own life, including the right to reject treatment or teaching. In many cases, the patient has valid reasons for noncompliance; for example, the need to focus energy on meeting basic needs for food, clothing, and shelter may rule out time-consuming self-care practices. The noncompliance problem details the assessment of intractable behavior and appropriate interventions.

(continued)

Interventions

6. Additional individualized interventions: ________

Rationales

6. Rationales: ________

Target outcome criteria

According to individual readiness, the patient will:
- demonstrate learning
- display minimal anxiety about self-care
- express satisfaction with learning needs met
- display realistic appraisal of continuing learning needs
- identify appropriate learning resources.

Transfer planning

NURSING TRANSFER CRITERIA

Upon transfer, documentation shows evidence of:
- identification of learning needs
- teaching accomplished during unit stay
- continuing learning needs communicated to receiving staff.

PATIENT-FAMILY TEACHING CHECKLIST

Document evidence that patient and family demonstrate understanding of:

__ key pathophysiologic aspects of the disorder
__ signs and symptoms requiring medical attention
__ dietary modifications, if appropriate
__ medications
__ other therapies
__ community resources for adjustment to life-style changes.

DOCUMENTATION CHECKLIST

Using outcome criteria as a guide, document:

__ assessment of readiness for learning
__ identification of factors that may inhibit learning
__ identification of learning goals
__ response of patient and family to teaching plan
__ problems encountered in teaching
__ evaluation of learning.

ASSOCIATED CARE PLANS

Acute Pain
Ineffective Coping
(Also see the care plan for the specific disorder.)

REFERENCES

Alfaro, R. *Application of Nursing Process.* Philadelphia: J.B. Lippincott Co., 1986.

Carpenito, L. *Nursing Diagnosis: Application to Clinical Practice.* Philadelphia: J.B. Lippincott Co., 1983.

Gordon, M. *Nursing Diagnosis: Process and Application,* 2nd ed. New York: McGraw-Hill Book Co., 1987.

Hochbaum, G. "Patient Counselling vs. Patient Teaching," *Topics in Education for Self-Care* 2(2), July 1980.

Scalzi, C., and Burke, L. "Education of the Patient and Family," in *Cardiac Nursing.* Edited by Underhill, S., et al. Philadelphia: J.B. Lippincott Co., 1982.

Watkins, L., and Odegaard, V. "Preparation for Cardiac Catheterization: Tailoring the Content of Instruction to Coping Style," *Heart & Lung* 15(4):382-89, 1986.

Nutritional Deficit

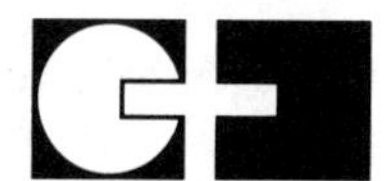

Introduction

DEFINITION AND TIME FOCUS

A nutritional deficit exists when a patient does not ingest or absorb the nutrients necessary to meet metabolic needs. Adequate nutrition is vitally important in recovering from critical illness. Besides glucose needs for cellular metabolism and energy production, many other nutritional needs exist. For example, calories, protein, and potassium are necessary to rebuild injured tissue; proteins, fatty acids, and phosphate are necessary to fight infection; and trace elements are necessary for optimal functioning of enzyme systems. This care plan focuses on the critically ill patient whose survival and recovery may be threatened by inadequate nutrition.

ETIOLOGY AND PRECIPITATING FACTORS

- contraindications to eating, as with peptic ulcer or pancreatitis
- decreased appetite
- inability to chew, as with jaw wiring or poor dentition
- impaired swallowing, as with cerebrovascular accident (CVA) or coma
- preexisting malnutrition, as with cancer or anorexia nervosa
- decreased GI motility, as with paralytic ileus
- failure to absorb nutrients, as with malabsorption syndrome or ulcerative colitis
- hypermetabolic state, as with burns or trauma

Focused assessment guidelines

NURSING HISTORY (Functional health pattern findings)

Health perception–health management pattern

- may have history of chronic GI disorder
- may have preexisting debility
- may be acutely ill with increased nutritional needs

Nutritional-metabolic pattern

- may complain of anorexia, indigestion, nausea, or vomiting
- may report difficulty or pain on swallowing
- may refuse to eat

Activity-exercise pattern

- may report weakness or lack of energy

Cognitive-perceptual pattern

- may complain of abdominal pain

Coping-stress tolerance pattern

- may complain of or display depression

PHYSICAL FINDINGS

General appearance

- emaciation (if preexisting malnutrition exists)
- weakness

Gastrointestinal

- weak mastication or swallowing muscles
- inflamed oral cavity or tongue
- vomiting
- absent bowel sounds
- diarrhea

Neurologic

- lethargy
- decreased level of consciousness
- paresthesias
- confusion
- disorientation

Integumentary

- subcutaneous fat loss
- dry, scaly skin
- poor skin turgor
- sparse, lackluster, or easily plucked hair
- dry, cracked lips
- thin, brittle nails

Musculoskeletal

- weakness
- body weight at least 20% below ideal weight for height and frame
- poor muscle tone
- muscle wasting

DIAGNOSTIC STUDIES

Note: The body has two types of protein stores—muscle protein and visceral protein (crucial protein stores in plasma proteins, hemoglobin, clotting factors, hormones, antibodies, and enzymes). Muscle protein is assessed via such anthropometric measures as height-weight index, creatinine-height index, mid-upper arm circumference (MAC) and midarm muscle circumference (MAMC). Visceral protein is assessed through such laboratory measures as total lymphocyte count and serum albumin and transferrin levels, and total iron-binding capacity.

- Serum electrolyte levels are obtained as baseline values and to guide replacement therapy; in patients with malnutrition, they typically reveal hyponatremia, hypokalemia, hypomagnesemia, and hypophosphatemia.
- A 24-hour urinary urea nitrogen (UUN) excretion test may reveal increased nitrogen losses, indicating excessive protein catabolism.

• Nitrogen balance measurements are obtained by comparing UUN excretion with nitrogen intake (calculated from protein intake). In malnutrition, negative nitrogen balance reveals catabolic state. A positive nitrogen balance of 2 to 3 g is ideal; in severe illness, zero nitrogen balance may be the realistic maximum attainable.
• Serum transferrin test measures level of a protein synthesized in the liver; decreases correlate with malnutrition severity.
• Total iron-binding capacity test measures the ability of iron to bind with and transport transferrin in the blood.
• Serum albumin test is not a reliable early indicator; late decreases correlate with malnutrition severity.
• Total lymphocyte count may reveal decreased levels, indicating inadequate antibody production and impaired immunocompetence.
• Creatinine-height index, which shows the relationship between creatinine level and patient's height, correlates with extent of protein depletion; increased creatinine excretion indicates skeletal muscle breakdown.
• Basal energy expenditure, which estimates the calories needed daily to maintain weight at rest, is determined by the Harris-Benedict equation. This equation uses height, weight, age, sex, and activity level and general injury type to calculate caloric intake necessary to promote anabolism.
• Height-weight ratio, if less than predicted values, may indicate the degree of protein-calorie malnutrition. Weight data may be difficult to evaluate because of unstable volume status in the critically ill patient.
• Triceps skinfold measurements may show decreased values, indicating depletion of body fat reserves; these are difficult to evaluate if the patient has edema or cannot sit.
• MAC and MAMC, if less than predicted values, may correlate with degree of depleted body fat reserves and skeletal muscle mass; these are difficult to evaluate if the patient has edema or cannot sit.
• Antigen skin testing may yield a decreased or absent reaction that indicates impaired cell-mediated immunity.

POTENTIAL COMPLICATIONS
• reduced immunocompetence
• electrolyte imbalances
• poor wound healing

Nursing diagnosis: *Nutritional deficit related to difficulty chewing or swallowing, sore throat after endotracheal extubation, or dry mouth*

NURSING PRIORITY: Compensate for eating difficulties.

Interventions	Rationales
1. Assess and document causes. Initiate referrals as appropriate, for example, to dentist or speech pathologist.	1. Some eating difficulties call for diagnosis or interventions beyond the scope of nursing. Early referrals help resolve the problem. For example, a dentist may be able to diagnose jaw pain or a speech pathologist may be able to teach swallowing techniques.
2. Assess level of consciousness and ability to chew and swallow, and check for gag reflex.	2. Alertness, ability to chew and swallow, and a gag reflex determine if the patient can safely ingest nutrients orally.
3. In collaboration with the dietitian and as ordered, provide a diet appropriate to the patient's abilities, for example, liquids, soft foods, or food requiring little cutting.	3. Provision of an appropriate diet minimizes patient frustration when eating.
4. If the patient has a sore mouth or throat, obtain an order for viscous lidocaine. If the patient has been extubated recently, explain that the sore throat usually resolves spontaneously within a few days.	4. Use of viscous lidocaine, a topical anesthetic, reduces discomfort. Knowing that the sore throat, common after extubation, will probably disappear after extubation may increase the patient's tolerance to the discomfort.
5. Place the patient sitting upright for meals, with his head flexed forward about 45 degrees, unless contraindicated.	5. This position maintains esophageal patency, facilitates swallowing, and minimizes the aspiration risk.
6. Have suction equipment available nearby but out of the patient's sight. Suction food, fluids, and accumulated saliva, as needed.	6. If the patient has sudden difficulty swallowing, prompt suctioning prevents aspiration. Keeping the equipment out of sight creates a more pleasant eating environment.

Interventions	Rationales
7. Provide assistance, as needed. If the patient had a stroke, place food on the unaffected side of the mouth.	7. Providing assistance increases food intake. Placing the food on the unaffected side facilitates use of the tongue to move food toward the back of the mouth.
8. Document feeding technique and food intake.	8. Documenting the technique provides for continuity of care; records are necessary to monitor the adequacy of food intake.
9. Additional individualized interventions: ____________ ____________	9. Rationales: ____________ ____________

Target outcome criteria
According to individual readiness, the patient will:
- eat the prescribed diet
- swallow without choking.

Nursing diagnosis: *Nutritional deficit related to anorexia*

NURSING PRIORITY: Promote appetite.

Interventions	Rationales
1. Assess possible causes of anorexia, such as nausea and vomiting, unpleasant sights and odors, depression, and medications.	1. Accurate identification of anorexia's cause facilitates selection of appropriate interventions.
2. Provide a pleasant eating environment. For example, place an emesis basin nearby but out of direct sight (if someone will be staying at the bedside); remove tissues containing sputum.	2. Removal of noxious sights and smells decreases anorexia, nausea, and vomiting.
3. Before meals, provide rest; administer analgesics or antiemetics, as needed and ordered; avoid painful procedures; and provide oral hygiene.	3. Adequate rest conserves the energy necessary to eat. Analgesics, antiemetics, and avoidance of painful procedures remove the distracting influences of pain, nausea, and emotional stress. Oral hygiene removes unpleasant tastes.
4. Emphasize the importance of eating. Use positive terms when presenting food; for example, "Here's a milkshake to help you regain your strength," rather than "Do you think you'll be able to keep this down?"	4. Emphasizing the importance of eating encourages the patient to eat despite anorexia. Positive terms capitalize on the power of suggestion to influence the subconscious mind.
5. Provide social interaction during meals, preferably with family and friends.	5. Social interaction increases food intake by providing a pleasant distraction from anorexia. Involving family and friends strengthens interpersonal bonds and provides a concrete way for them to contribute to the patient's recovery.
6. Offer small, frequent feedings of highly nutritious foods, including the patient's preferences whenever possible.	6. Small meals promote prompt gastric emptying, lessening anorexia and nausea. When food intake is low, every mouthful must count toward meeting nutrient needs.
7. Limit fluid intake at mealtimes.	7. Large amounts of fluid distend the stomach, causing early satiety and promoting nausea.
8. If the patient begins to feel nausea, encourage slow deep breathing. If vomiting occurs, document the amount and type of emesis. Provide oral hygiene afterward.	8. Deep breathing helps to diminish the vomiting reflex. Documentation of emesis is necessary to maintain accurate intake and output records and to evaluate the adequacy of oral nutrition.

(continued)

Interventions	Rationales
9. Praise the patient for signs of increased appetite.	9. Praise acknowledges the patient's efforts to overcome anorexia and reinforces desired behavior.
10. Additional individualized interventions: ____________	10. Rationales: ____________

Target outcome criteria
According to individual readiness, the patient will eat and retain at least three quarters of prescribed diet.

Collaborative problem: *Nutritional deficit related to inability to digest nutrients or hypermetabolic state*

NURSING PRIORITY: Provide nutrients in a form that can be assimilated.

Interventions	Rationales
1. Stay alert for patients with increased nutrient needs, such as those with trauma, burns, infection, surgical wounds, and fever. Also observe all patients for indicators of possible inability to absorb nutrients, such as diarrhea.	1. In the hectic environment of the critical care unit, the patient's nutrient needs may be easily overlooked because of more immediate needs. Early recognition of patients with decreased absorptive ability or increased needs helps provide adequate nutrition before debilitation occurs.
2. Collaborate with the dietitian, nutritional support team, and doctor to obtain a comprehensive nutritional assessment.	2. A comprehensive assessment includes anthropometric and laboratory measurements performed by colleagues with special nutritional expertise. These measurements document the type and degree of nutritional deficit and provide guidelines for selecting appropriate nutritional interventions.
3. Assess and document bowel sounds and abdominal distention every 4 hours.	3. Bowel sounds indicate whether the patient can tolerate enteral feedings or whether parenteral feedings are necessary. Abdominal distention suggests paralytic ileus.
4. Collaborate with nutritional experts to establish nutrient requirements, depending on whether the following exist:	4. Nutrient requirements vary depending on whether the patient is merely nutritionally depleted or is experiencing a hypermetabolic state.
• starvation	• Early starvation is characterized by various compensatory mechanisms, including glycogenolysis, lipolysis, proteolysis, and gluconeogenesis. Rapid catabolism produces rapid weight loss, osmotic diuresis, and urinary nitrogen loss. After approximately 10 days, the metabolic rate slows and weight loss continues at a slower rate while the body uses fat as its primary energy source. After several months, exhaustion of fat stores causes the body to use visceral protein for energy.
• hypermetabolism.	• The release of catecholamines, glucocorticoids, and mineralocorticoids in response to stress cause the traumatized or infected patient to develop greater glucose mobilization than the starved patient. Rapid weight loss and osmotic diuresis are delayed for approximately 24 to 48 hours after trauma.

(continued)

NURSING CONSIDERATIONS IN TPN

■ **Definition:** Total parenteral nutrition (TPN) is the delivery of complete nutrition via I.V. infusion of glucose, amino acids, fats, vitamins, and trace elements in sufficient quantities to replenish body stores and prevent catabolism.

■ **Usual nutrient requirements for critically ill patients**
- calories—3,000 to 4,000 cal/day
- protein—0.8 to 2 gm/kg/day
- fat—30% of nonprotein calories
- trace elements—variable, supplied by trace element formula added to solution
- vitamins—variable, supplied by 10 ml/day of multivitamin preparation added to solution.

■ **Catheter insertion**: After using a local anesthetic, the doctor inserts the catheter into the subclavian or internal jugular vein and positions the tip in the superior vena cava. He then sutures the catheter in place and applies an occlusive dressing. Nursing responsibilities include the following:
- Position the patient in Trendelenburg's position, with his head turned away from the insertion site.
- Monitor the patient for shock or respiratory distress, which may result from pneumothorax, air embolism, or other potential complications of central line insertion.
- Obtain a chest X-ray immediately to verify placement before starting TPN infusion.

■ **Catheter care**: Follow unit protocol for dressing changes, tubing changes, and filter use. When changing the dressing, observe the site for signs of infection and suture integrity. Monitor the patient for leakage around the catheter, swelling around the catheter site, increased collateral vein visibility, chest pain, and inability to withdraw blood from the catheter. These signs may indicate catheter displacement or clotting.

■ **Routine monitoring:** Measure urine glucose and ketone levels every 6 hours. Maintain urine glucose level at 1+ to 4+.
- Monitor blood glucose level daily. Maintain at 100 to 200 mg/dl. Values over 200 mg/dl indicate the need for insulin administration or presence of a new stressor, such as sepsis.
- Monitor weight daily. Generally, maintain weight gain at <0.5 lb/day; values exceeding that may indicate fluid retention.
- Monitor intake and output; maintain approximate balance.
- Monitor serum electrolyte levels, visceral protein measurements, and other laboratory tests as ordered (typically, daily until patient's stable and then 2 to 3 times a week).

■ **Solution delivery**: Nursing goals include preventing rebound hypoglycemia, minimizing fibrin deposition within the catheter, and detecting allergic responses to supplemental fat emulsions.
- Deliver the solution at a constant rate, using an infusion pump.
- Infuse TPN only; do not use the line for administering medications or obtaining blood samples.
- Change the solution every 24 hours; do not hang cloudy or precipitated solution.
- If solution flow stops and cannot be restarted promptly, hang 10% dextrose in water at another site and obtain medical assistance. During cardiopulmonary resuscitation, administer 50% dextrose solution I.V., as ordered. Once the flow is reestablished, do not increase the infusion rate in order to catch up with the schedule.
- If administering a 3-in-1 solution of glucose, protein, and fat, replace the solution if fat separation occurs. If a separate fat solution is administered, infuse at a rate of 1 ml/minute for the first 15 minutes and observe for dyspnea, chest or infusion site pain, and other evidence of allergic reaction.
- Administer insulin separately, as ordered, for a diabetic patient or for a patient suffering increased physiologic stress, for example, from surgery.

■ **Complications:** Observe constantly for the following complications and, as needed, obtain medical reevaluation:
- hypoglycemia—monitor for weakness, agitation, tremors, personality changes, blood glucose level <60 mg/dl, urine negative for glucose and ketones
- hyperglycemia—monitor for headache, confusion, lethargy, thirst, acetone breath, diuresis, blood glucose level >200 mg/dl, urine positive for glucose and ketones
- hyperosmolar overload—monitor for lethargy, headache, seizures, thirst, blood glucose level >600 mg/dl, urine positive for glucose but negative for ketones
- fluid volume excess—monitor for crackles, neck vein distention, hypertension, edema
- electrolyte imbalances—see Appendix C, "Fluid and Electrolyte Imbalances," for signs of hyponatremia, hypokalemia, hypocalcemia, and hypomagnesemia; also observe for weakness, encephalopathy, and poor infection resistance, which may indicate hypophosphatemia
- protein overload—monitor for elevated blood urea nitrogen and creatinine levels
- infection—monitor for temperature >101° F, tachypnea, tachycardia, chills, diaphoresis, blood glucose level >200 mg/dl, glycosuria, white blood cell count >10,000/mm³.

■ **Discontinuation of TPN**: When oral fat intake reaches 10 g/day, fat emulsions may be discontinued. When oral calorie intake reaches 1,000 calories/day, TPN may be discontinued. Before discontinuing, taper the infusion rate to 50 ml/hour for 4 hours to allow the body to adjust and appetite to return.

Interventions	Rationales
5. Provide the appropriate nutritional replacement, as ordered. Options include the following:	5. Nutritional replacement methods vary depending on the patient's needs.
• enteral feeding (via nasogastric, gastrostomy, or jejunostomy tubes), such as:	• Enteral feeding is preferred for the patient with a functioning GI tract.
□ meal replacements	□ Meal replacements are nutritionally complete but require digestive and absorptive abilities.
□ nutrient supplements	□ Supplements, although nutritionally incomplete, can replace one or more specific nutrients.
□ defined-formula diets;	□ Defined-formula diets are nutritionally complete and require little digestion.
• parenteral nutrition, which may consist of one or both of the following:	• Parenteral nutrition is appropriate for patients who cannot meet nutritional needs through GI absorption.
□ peripheral venous nutrition	□ Peripheral venous nutrition may be prescribed if calorie needs are relatively low and if relatively short-term GI dysfunction is anticipated.
□ central venous nutrition, also known as total parenteral nutrition (TPN).	□ TPN is appropriate for patients with relatively high calorie needs because TPN solutions have greater calorie and protein content than peripheral venous solutions.
6. If the patient is receiving tube feedings:	6. Nursing measures for tube feedings are designed to facilitate absorption and prevent complications.
• Check tube placement before each feeding.	• Checking tube placement confirms that the tube is in the stomach or jejunum, as appropriate. With a nasogastric tube, checking proves essential to ensure that it has not migrated upward into the trachea.
• Keep the head of the bed elevated during and for 1 hour after feedings.	• Elevation prevents reflux of solution into the esophagus.
• Begin with small amounts of dilute solution. Increase the amount and concentration as tolerated, within prescribed parameters.	• Large amounts of concentrated solution may provoke osmotic diarrhea. Gradual increases allow time for the GI system to adapt to the increased volume and solute load.
• Use a continuous infusion pump, as ordered.	• Delivery with a continuous infusion pump is less likely to provoke diarrhea.
7. If the patient is receiving TPN, ensure delivery of the prescribed solutions and monitor for complications. Refer to *Nursing Considerations in TPN*, page 57, for details.	7. TPN is a complex therapy with numerous nursing considerations.
8. Additional individualized interventions: ____________	8. Rationales: ____________

Target outcome criteria

Within 7 days of admission, the patient will:
- tolerate enteral or parenteral feedings without adverse effects
- gain up to 1 kg/week.

Transfer planning

NURSING TRANSFER CRITERIA

Upon transfer, documentation shows evidence of:
- assessment of nutritional status
- implementation of appropriate nutritional support.

PATIENT-FAMILY TEACHING CHECKLIST

Document evidence that patient and family demonstrate understanding of:

___ importance of nutrition to recovery
___ rationale for selection of specific nutritional support method.

DOCUMENTATION CHECKLIST

Using outcome criteria as a guide, document:
__ clinical status on admission
__ significant changes in status
__ pertinent diagnostic test findings
__ specific nutritional support method
__ tolerance of method
__ complications, if any
__ daily nutritional intake
__ medications administered, if any
__ attitude toward eating
__ patient-family teaching
__ transfer planning.

ASSOCIATED CARE PLANS

See the care plan for the specific disorder.

REFERENCES

Butterworth, C., and Weinsier, R. "Malnutrition in Hospitalized Patients: Assessment and Treatment," in *Modern Nutrition in Health and Disease.* Edited by Goodhart, R., and Shils, M. Philadelphia: Lea & Febiger, 1980.

Carpenito, L. *Nursing Diagnosis: Application to Clinical Practice*. Philadelphia: J.B. Lippincott Co., 1983.

Elwyn, D. "Nutritional Requirements of Adult Surgical Patients," *Critical Care Medicine* 8:10-36, 1980.

Holloway, N., and Forlaw, L. "Nourishment of the Critically Ill," in *Nursing the Critically Ill Adult,* 3rd ed. Edited by Holloway, N. Menlo Park, Calif.: Addison-Wesley Publishing Co., 1988.

Keithley, J. "Infection and the Malnourished Patient," *Heart & Lung* 12:23-27, January 1983.

Keithley, J. "Nutritional Assessment of the Patient Undergoing Surgery," *Heart & Lung* 14:449-455, 1985.

Lederer, J., et al. *Care Planning Pocket Guide: A Nursing Diagnosis Approach.* Menlo Park, Calif.: Addison-Wesley Publishing Co., 1986.

Moran, M., and Powell, C. "Total Parenteral Nutrition," in *Medical-Surgical Care Plans.* Edited by Holloway, N. Springhouse, Pa.: Springhouse Corp., 1988.

Stotts, N., and Friesen, J. "Understanding Starvation in the Critically Ill Patient," *Heart & Lung* 11:469-78, 1982.

Taylor, C., and Cress, S. *Nursing Diagnosis Cards.* Springhouse, Pa.: Springhouse Corp., 1987.

Sensory-Perceptual Alteration

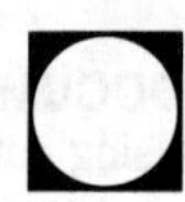

Introduction

DEFINITION AND TIME FOCUS

A sensory-perceptual alteration is a change in the patient's experience of his surroundings. Such alterations may affect a patient's overall well-being in numerous ways. The critical care unit environment, the physiologic manifestations of critical illness, and the psychological stress caused by the hospitalization may have a severe cumulative effect unless astute anticipatory intervention is initiated.

Most critical care nurses are familiar with the phenomenon of ICU (intensive care unit) psychosis. Such a distressing response may be averted or minimized by careful assessment and attention to modifiable aspects of the patient's environment. Family members may be a particularly helpful resource for nursing care planning for this problem because they can provide guidance about the patient's usual home environment and sensory-perceptual abilities. Intervention for this problem, perhaps more than for any other nursing diagnosis, must be individually tailored to the patient's subjective view of his situation.

ETIOLOGY AND PRECIPITATING FACTORS*

- altered environment (excessive or insufficient stimuli)
- altered sensory reception, transmission, or integration
- chemical alterations (endogenous or exogenous)
- psychological stress

Focused assessment guidelines

NURSING HISTORY (Functional health pattern findings)

The patient with a sensory-perceptual alteration may be unable to provide meaningful subjective data for assessment purposes. The patient's family may be especially helpful in providing information about baseline mental status and normal activities and interests. Although findings may vary widely among individuals, the following are common findings associated with sensory-perceptual alteration.

Health perception–health management pattern

- may express unrealistic ideas regarding condition

Nutritional-metabolic pattern

- may display reduced appetite or apathy about food

Activity-exercise pattern

- may complain of insomnia and/or fatigue
- may engage in wandering behavior
- may become hyperactive

Cognitive-perceptual pattern

- commonly demonstrates impaired judgment
- may demonstrate loss of time sense
- may demonstrate memory impairment
- is likely to exhibit reduced attention span
- may misidentify familiar persons
- may display increased need for pain medications

Self-perception–self-concept pattern

- may assume all external stimuli have reference to self (ideas of reference)
- commonly verbalizes paranoid ideas
- may express suicidal thoughts

Coping-stress tolerance pattern

- may withdraw from others in response to perceived threat
- may become increasingly demanding or make repeated requests for minor needs
- may exhibit obsessive or compulsive behavior, such as constant rearrangement of familiar items on bedside table
- may be unable to make decisions
- may exhibit aggressive behavior or make verbal or sexual overtures
- may respond to minor frustration or annoyance by crying or becoming enraged

PHYSICAL FINDINGS

Physical manifestations of sensory-perceptual alteration may vary widely, depending on the patient's underlying condition and other factors. The findings listed below, however, may indicate such an alteration is present, and the astute nurse will be alert to such cues.

General appearance

- nervous mannerisms
- anxious facial expression
- flat affect

Neurologic

- restlessness
- irritability
- combativeness
- confusion
- nystagmus
- delusions or hallucinations
- psychosis
- depression

Cardiopulmonary

- cardiac dysrhythmias (associated with sleep deprivation)

*From McLane, M. *Classification of Nursing Diagnosis: Proceedings of the Seventh NANDA Conference.* St. Louis: C.V. Mosby Co., 1987, p. 502.

Respiratory
- hyperventilation or other physiologic manifestations of tension or anxiety
- reduced ventilatory response to hypoxia and hypercapnia (associated with sleep deprivation)

Musculoskeletal
- increased muscle tension
- hand tremors

DIAGNOSTIC STUDIES
No laboratory tests or diagnostic procedures exist specifically for patients with sensory-perceptual alteration; however, any patient with altered mental status for any reason should be evaluated for possible toxic, endocrine, or metabolic causes for his symptoms.

POTENTIAL COMPLICATIONS
- acute brain syndrome
- physical injury from confusion
- crisis state

Nursing diagnosis: *Sensory-perceptual alteration related to excessive and/or insufficient environmental stimuli**

NURSING PRIORITIES: (a) Promote normal processing and integration of environmental cues, and (b) control stimuli for maximum therapeutic effect.

Interventions	Rationales
1. Assess the unit environment. Evaluate the type, quantity, duration, frequency, and clarity of auditory, visual, olfactory, tactile, and gustatory stimuli in the unit environment. Consider having the nursing staff periodically role-play as patients, as unit census permits.	1. The patient in the critical care unit is subjected to a dramatic reduction in some types of stimuli (visual, gustatory, tactile) and an increase in other types (auditory). Such changes, particularly when the patient's ability to perceive, integrate, and cope with new information is impaired by physiologic stress, may result in significant mental status alterations. Staff awareness of the environment to which most patients are constantly exposed is essential for effective intervention on the patient's behalf. Nurses may become so habituated to the work environment that their sensitivity to its effects on patients is reduced. Role-playing as a patient may promote increased awareness and provide information to guide interventions.
2. Assess the patient's normal prehospitalization routines, including the general home environment, activity, diet, and sleep patterns. Ask the family to provide information regarding specific personal habits or preferences, such as reading before bedtime or leaving the television or radio on during waking hours. Ask the patient or family to describe a typical 24-hour period. As feasible, modify care routines and the unit environment to resemble the patient's home surroundings.	2. Careful assessment of the patient's usual prehospitalization surroundings is essential to making appropriate adjustments. A description of the customary 24-hour routine provides valuable information about the interrelationship and significance of various aspects of the patient's life. Modifications of routines and surroundings may promote a sense of security.
3. Orient the patient and family to the unit, explaining structure and routines. At the same time each day, review with them the day's activity plan and instruct them regarding special procedures or changes that are anticipated. As much as possible, prepare the patient and family in advance for change of any kind. Attempt to provide continuity in staffing.	3. Structure and routine provide the patient with a foundation to aid in interpreting and processing unfamiliar environmental cues. Reviewing plans at the same time each day reinforces the routine and increases security. Advance preparation allows the patient and family to integrate and cope with change more effectively. Continuity of staffing adds to the patient's repertoire of familiar information.

*The large number of interventions for sensory-perceptual alteration have been grouped into problems according to etiology.

(continued)

Interventions	Rationales
4. Provide cues to orientation and reinforce them frequently while providing care. Ensure, for example, that a large clock and calendar are placed within the patient's visual field; wear easily read name tags and introduce yourself to the patient at least once a shift until familiarity is established. For patients with visual deficits, always introduce yourself when approaching the bedside, before touching the patient. For patients without visual impairments, encourage the family to bring in photographs or other small items from home to place on the wall or at the bedside.	4. Reality testing requires input of familiar, predictable, and meaningful external informational cues. Without such orientation guides, internal and external events may become confused. Studies have shown that even normal, healthy individuals experience sensory-perceptual alterations when subjected to bed rest and its attendant sensory-perceptual deprivation. Even a few familiar items from home, particularly photographs of loved ones, may help the patient maintain orientation and reduce the alienation patients experience in the strange environment of the critical care unit.
5. Control environmental stimuli, as possible, to provide an environment that is secure and meaningful for the patient. Pay particular attention to the type and level of unit noise, ensuring that extraneous conversation is kept to a minimum. Encourage questions and provide interpretation of unfamiliar sensory stimuli as part of the patient's orientation to the unit, for example, "That beeping sound is an alarm on a patient's I.V. monitor," or "The hissing you hear is a machine that helps another patient to breathe."	5. Studies have shown that ambient noise in critical care units is very distressing to a patient, increasing muscle tension and diastolic pressure and contributing to sleep disturbances. Nurse, staff, and visitor conversations may be even more disruptive to normal rest and sleep than the steady noise from the many pieces of equipment. Without normal sensory stimulation, the critical care patient commonly interprets all overheard conversations as pertaining to him. For example, the patient who overhears a staff conversation about a surgical procedure may assume he is to undergo such a procedure. Interpreting unfamiliar stimuli and answering all questions increases security and promotes adaptation to the unit environment.
6. As the patient's condition permits, encourage family participation in care. Explain the potential benefits of family-patient contact even when patient is unresponsive. Speak to the patient when providing care, using touch generously unless patient appears uncomfortable with physical contact.	6. Family contact decreases the strangeness of the environment and promotes orientation. Even patients who appear unconscious may continue to process environmental input, particularly sounds. Familiar verbal and tactile stimuli reduce sensory deprivation and provide reassurance. Touching the patient is one way of acknowledging the human dimension of care, which the patient may otherwise perceive as secondary in the high-technology critical care setting.
7. Schedule care to provide uninterrupted sleep cycles of 2 hours or more by:	7. The function of sleep is unknown, but it may help maintain central nervous system control of various homeostatic mechanisms. Some theories postulate that sleep is essential for normal processing and integration of information. Studies of critical care unit patients have shown a 33% decrease in the mental status of sleep-deprived patients. The following procedures help minimize these effects.
• grouping necessary procedures	• Grouping procedures minimizes interruption of normal sleep cycles, which usually last 90 to 120 minutes.
• using continuous monitoring devices to check routine vital signs and other parameters	• Monitoring devices do not require awakening the patient.
• scheduling planned sleep times, as possible, to coincide with usual home pattern	• Once the patient's usual rhythm is disrupted, it is more difficult to reestablish an effective sleep pattern.
• minimizing noise (especially sudden loud sounds), setting alarms as low as safety allows, and turning off equipment when not in use	• Even sounds that do not cause the patient to awaken completely may disrupt the normal sleep cycle. Abrupt loud sounds are more likely to cause awakening, though even continuous, low-level noise may alter the normal pattern.
• evaluating for possible effects of medications on the sleep pattern and discussing their probable benefits and risks with the doctor, as appropriate	• Many medications, including morphine, phenobarbital, and diazepam, may decrease rapid eye movement (REM) sleep. REM sleep is considered essential to normal psychological functioning. The greatest amount of REM sleep occurs toward the end of a sleep period.

Interventions	Rationales
• providing eyeshades, earplugs, extra blankets or pillows, and other comfort measures	• Most people find it difficult to sleep in lighted areas. Reducing stimulation and providing comfort measures help achieve sleep.
• teaching relaxation techniques, such as imagery, progressive muscle relaxation, massage, and deep breathing.	• Relaxation aids in falling asleep.
8. Assess the patient's mental status daily, noting particularly any alteration in orientation or memory. Be especially observant for indications of sensory-perceptual alteration in elderly patients and in children.	8. Patients who develop ICU psychosis have a higher mortality than those who do not. Early detection of possible signs and symptoms allows for preventive intervention. Older and younger patients are most susceptible to the effects of significant sensory-perceptual changes.
9. When leaving the bedside, always explain to the patient where you are going and approximately when you will return.	9. Knowing what to expect from the nurse decreases free-floating anxiety and provides a time reference for the patient.
10. Additional individualized interventions: ______	10. Rationales: ______

Target outcome criteria

Within 24 hours, the patient will:
- verbalize understanding of unit routines
- know the names of two nurses
- experience at least one uninterrupted sleep cycle of 2 hours or more.

Nursing diagnosis: *Sensory-perceptual alteration related to altered sensory reception, transmission, and/or integration*

NURSING PRIORITY: Minimize or compensate for sensory-perceptual deficits.

Interventions	Rationales
1. Assess for conditions in which sensory reception, transmission, or integration is likely to be impaired, such as old age, neurologic abnormalities, use of neuromuscular blocking agents, visual or hearing problems, immobilization, endotracheal intubation, tracheostomy and mechanical ventilation, altered level of consciousness, depression, or anxiety. If such conditions are present, identify the type and level of dysfunction, if possible, and note in the care plan or post a notice near the patient's bed, for example, "Deafness in right ear, full hearing in left" or "Speak slowly."	1. Evaluation for risk factors permits early intervention to avert severe sensory deprivation and its distressing sequelae.
2. Consult the medical history for additional pertinent data regarding specific deficits, such as anatomic site and physiologic effects of cerebrovascular accident. Tailor care accordingly.	2. Attempting to implement interventions that are inappropriate to the patient's functional level may increase frustration and reduce the patient's motivation to communicate.
3. Ensure that a patient's glasses or hearing aid is accessible. Consider using mirrors to expand visual access if immobilization devices restrict movement.	3. Accurate visual and auditory perceptions are the patient's primary connections to the external world and enhance reality orientation.

(continued)

Interventions

4. For any patient with altered mentation or consciousness, provide reality orientation at regular, planned intervals, at least every 8 hours. Include the time, day, date and year, location, and a brief explanation of the patient's immediate circumstances. Continue to provide such information on a regular basis, even if the patient is unresponsive, until the patient can repeat it back on request.

Rationales

4. Reality orientation provides an essential anchor to reality and a sense of security for patients recovering from altered consciousness, who commonly are uncertain even whether they are dead or alive. Numerous case studies reveal that even unresponsive patients are receptive to auditory stimuli and frequently remember conversations even after a prolonged coma.

5. Additional individualized interventions: ____________

5. Rationales: ____________

> **Target outcome criteria**
> Within 8 hours of admission and then daily, the patient will repeat baseline reality orientation information when asked.

Nursing diagnosis: *Sensory-perceptual alteration related to endogenous or exogenous chemical alterations*

NURSING PRIORITY: Identify and treat possible causes of biochemical alteration.

Interventions

1. Assess for conditions that may contribute to chemically induced sensory-perceptual alterations, such as the therapeutic medication regimen, drug intoxication, diabetes, or other metabolic disorders, or electrolyte and acid-base imbalances. Collaborate with the doctor to treat the underlying cause(s).

Rationales

1. Appropriate intervention to decrease the effects of sensory-perceptual changes depends upon accurate identification of their cause(s).

Interventions

2. Provide appropriate, accurate explanations to the patient and family about the effects of psychotropic medications or other chemical causes of sensory-perceptual alteration.

Rationales

2. The patient and family may be alarmed or ashamed about chemically induced behavior. Providing explanations and displaying an attitude of acceptance promotes trust and open communication.

3. Additional individualized interventions: ____________

3. Rationales: ____________

> **Target outcome criteria**
> Throughout the critical care unit stay, the patient will:
> • display a clear sensorium
> • make verbal statements congruent with reality.

Nursing diagnosis: *Sensory-perceptual alteration related to psychological stress*

NURSING PRIORITY: Promote effective coping.

Interventions	Rationales
1. Be aware of the patient's needs for personal space. Ask permission and provide explanations before performing procedures. Provide effective screening to protect the patient's privacy.	1. Everyone is protective of his unconsciously defined personal boundaries, which help an individual maintain ego integration. In the critical care setting, these boundaries are constantly assaulted by invasive tubing, procedures, and noise the patient cannot control. Even small measures to acknowledge these boundaries may reduce stress from loss of control.
2. See the "Ineffective Coping" care plan, page 26.	2. The "Ineffective Coping" care plan contains detailed interventions applicable to the care of the patient experiencing psychological stress.
3. Additional individualized interventions: ________	3. Rationales: ________

Target outcome criteria
Throughout the critical care unit stay, the patient will:
• express feelings regarding stressors
• display relaxed posture and facial expression.

Transfer planning

NURSING TRANSFER CRITERIA

Upon transfer, documentation shows evidence of:
• identification of specific sensory-perceptual alterations, if present
• successful resolution or ongoing treatment of the problems.

PATIENT-FAMILY TEACHING CHECKLIST

Document evidence that patient and family demonstrate understanding of:
___ signs and symptoms of sensory-perceptual alteration
___ causes of sensory-perceptual alterations
___ reality orientation measures
stress-reduction measures
___ measures to promote sleep.

DOCUMENTATION CHECKLIST

Using outcome criteria as a guide, document:
___ clinical status on admission
___ significant changes in status
___ pertinent diagnostic test findings
___ reality orientation measures
___ sleep status
___ family participation in care
___ patient-family teaching
___ transfer planning.

ASSOCIATED CARE PLANS

Acute Pain
Impaired Physical Mobility
Ineffective Coping
Knowledge Deficit

REFERENCES

Brewer, M.J. "To Sleep or Not To Sleep: The Consequences of Sleep Deprivation," *Critical Care Nurse* 5(6):35-41, 1985.
Burgener, S. "Circadian Rhythms: Implications for Evaluation of the Critically Ill Patient," *Critical Care Nurse* 5(5):43-48, 1985.
Hudak, C., et al. *Critical Care Nursing: A Holistic Approach,* 4th ed. Philadelphia: J.B. Lippincott Co., 1986.
Kartmann, J. "Sleep and the Elderly Critical Care Patient," *Critical Care Nurse* 5(6):52-57, 1985.
Kenner, C., Guzzetta, C., and Dossey, B. *Critical Care Nursing: Body-Mind-Spirit,* 2nd ed. Boston: Little, Brown & Co., 1985.
Snyder-Halpern, R. "The Effect of Critical Care Unit Noise on Patient Sleep Cycles." *Critical Care Quarterly* 7(1):41-51, March 1985.

Craniotomy

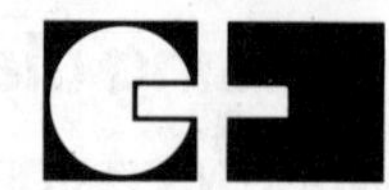

DRG information

DRG 001 Craniotomy. Age over 17, Except for Trauma.
Mean LOS = 14.2 days
Principal procedures include:
- biopsy of brain or cerebral meninges
- excision of brain or skull lesion
- clipping or repair of cerebral aneurysm
- insertion of ventricular shunt
- repair of arteriovenous fistula
- incision of brain or cerebral meninges
- incision or excision of intracranial vessels.

DRG 002 Craniotomy for Trauma. Age over 17.
Mean LOS = 12.6 days
Principal diagnoses include:
- concussion
- skull fracture
- hemorrhage (subarachnoid, subdural, or extradural) following injury
- cerebral laceration or contusion
- fracture of vertebral column with spinal cord injury.

Additional DRG information: These diagnoses must be treated surgically; see DRG 001 for examples of procedures.

DRG 003 Craniotomy. Age 0 to 17.
Mean LOS = 12.7 days
Principal procedures for DRG 003: see principal procedures listed under DRG 001.

Introduction

DEFINITION AND TIME FOCUS

Craniotomy, the most common neurosurgical procedure, is the surgical opening of the skull to provide access to the brain. It is performed to treat intracranial disease; for example, to remove tissue for biopsy or to remove a mass lesion (a substance occupying the cranial cavity and compromising either the space or the integrity of the brain). The surgery involves making a series of small holes, called burr holes, in the cranium with a special drill, then cutting between the holes to allow removal of a flap of bone and scalp. At the end of the surgery, the flap is replaced and the muscle and scalp are realigned and sutured.

Although the surgical approach depends on the location of the lesion, surgery is performed in two general areas. In the supratentorial craniotomy, the cranium is incised above the tentorium (the fold of dura mater that separates the cerebral cortex from the cerebellum and brain stem). This approach is used for lesions in the frontal, parietal, temporal, and occipital lobes of the cerebral hemispheres. The infratentorial approach, in which the cranium is incised below the tentorium, is used for lesions in the brain stem (midbrain, pons, and medulla) and cerebellum.

A craniotomy may be an emergency procedure for removal of a rapidly expanding lesion, such as an epidural hematoma or intracranial abscess, or an elective procedure in situations where the growth rate of the space-occupying lesion has been slow, such as with benign tumors. This clinical plan focuses on the immediate preoperative and postoperative care of a patient undergoing an elective craniotomy.

ETIOLOGY AND PRECIPITATING FACTORS

- presence of tumors, abscesses, aneurysms, chronic hematomas, cysts, or arteriovenous malformations
- any condition requiring repair of a cerebral injury

Focused assessment guidelines

NURSING HISTORY (Functional health pattern findings)

Health perception–health management pattern

- may have history of headache that is worse on arising in the morning and is aggravated by movement or straining at stool
- may have experienced personality changes
- may have experienced mental changes or mood swings
- may be at increased risk because of age (adults are at increased risk)
- may be at increased risk because of family or personal history of diabetes mellitus, intolerance to previous operative procedures, history of adrenocortical steroids, or signs and symptoms of endocrine dysfunction

Nutritional-metabolic pattern

- may report vomiting

Activity-exercise pattern

- may have been hospitalized and on bed rest
- may have been restricted in physical activity as a result of motor or sensory deficits

Cognitive-perceptual pattern

- may have experienced changes in vision, hearing, touch, taste, or smell depending on location and duration of lesion
- may experience language and memory problems with chronic lesion

Self-perception–self-concept pattern

- if undergoing radiation or chemotherapy for chronic lesion, may have negative self-image because of body disfigurement
- may express anger, embarrassment, or denial

Role-relationship pattern
• depending on duration of lesion, may have alteration in role of spouse and breadwinner

Sexuality-reproductive pattern
• depending on location of lesion, may have impaired sexual functioning

Coping–stress tolerance pattern
• may exhibit ineffective coping patterns
• may have anticipatory grieving for loss

Value-belief pattern
• may have delayed seeking medical attention because of fear of the unknown, surgery, and possibility of death
• may feel frustrated with health care system if diagnosis was delayed because of vague symptoms

PHYSICAL FINDINGS
Note: Signs and symptoms depend on the lesion's site. The following are general findings that would indicate cerebral dysfunction.

Neurologic
• decreased level of consciousness
• mental changes, such as impaired memory, lack of initiative, or mood changes
• visual deficits, such as decreased visual acuity, blurred vision, diplopia, or changes in extraocular eye movements
• sensory deficits
• motor deficits
• seizures
• papilledema
• cranial nerve dysfunction

Gastrointestinal
• vomiting

DIAGNOSTIC STUDIES
• complete blood count—decreased hemoglobin may indicate anemia or blood dyscrasia as well as the need for blood transfusion before surgery to ensure adequate transport for oxygen in the blood. Increased white blood cell (WBC) count may signify the beginning of infection or an abscess, which is a contraindication for surgery (unless the abscess is in the brain).
• blood urea nitrogen, serum creatinine—used to monitor renal function; increased values may indicate an impaired ability to cope with the sodium and water retention that result from the body's stress reaction to surgery.
• electrolyte analyses—used to monitor fluid status and detect hypokalemia and hyperkalemia. Patients may develop diabetes insipidus or syndrome of inappropriate secretion of antidiuretic hormone.
• fasting blood glucose levels—used to detect diabetes mellitus, which would require control before and after surgery
• typing and cross matching blood—makes blood more readily available if the patient requires blood replacement from surgical loss
• computed tomography (CT) scan—used to diagnose cerebral lesions, such as hematomas, tumors, cysts, hydrocephalus, cerebral atrophy, cerebral infarction, and cerebral edema. Serial scanning may be done before and after surgery
• cerebral angiography—used to diagnose cerebrovascular aneurysms, cerebral thrombosis, hematomas, tumors with increased vascularization, vascular plaques or spasm, arteriovenous malformations, cerebral fistulas, or cerebral edema
• radionuclide imaging studies (brain scan)—used to diagnose intracranial masses such as malignant or benign tumors, abscess, cerebral infarctions, intracranial hemorrhage, arteriovenous malformations, or aneurysms. They have been largely replaced by CT scans.
• magnetic resonance imaging—used to assess brain edema, hemorrhage, infarction, blood vessels, and tumors and to measure fluid flow
• chest X-ray—can rule out congestion, pneumonia, atelectasis, or other pulmonary pathology that would compromise respirations
• EKG—can detect cardiac abnormalities, such as dysrhythmias, that would be aggravated by the stress of a long surgical procedure and drug therapy

POTENTIAL COMPLICATIONS
• increased intracranial pressure
• shock (hemorrhagic, hypovolemic, or from intracranial bleeding)
• atelectasis
• pneumonia
• seizures
• diabetes insipidus
• meningitis
• wound infection
• neurologic deficits
• loss of corneal, pharyngeal, or palatal reflexes
• cardiac dysrhythmias
• thrombophlebitis
• hyperthermia
• postoperative hydrocephalus
• GI ulceration and bleeding

Nursing diagnosis: *Preoperative knowledge deficit related to impending craniotomy*

NURSING PRIORITY: Prepare the patient and family for the craniotomy.

Interventions	Rationales
1. Implement the measures in the "Knowledge Deficit" care plan, page 45, as appropriate.	1. The "Knowledge Deficit" care plan contains detailed, general information about teaching. This plan covers only specific information about craniotomy.
2. Assess what the patient and family already know about the impending craniotomy and what they want to know. Consider the patient's educational level, level of consciousness, mental changes, and memory loss. As appropriate, ask the patient or family what has been learned from the doctor, other family members, or anyone else who has had a craniotomy.	2. Level of consciousness, mental changes, or memory loss affect the patient's knowledge base. Although the doctor should have informed the patient and family about the procedure and potential complications, anxiety, memory loss, or limited comprehension may interfere with understanding and retention. Also, the patient and family may have limited or confusing information from various sources. Assessing the knowledge base allows the nurse to reinforce appropriate information, correct misconceptions, and fill in gaps in knowledge.
3. Describe the preoperative procedure, including: neurologic assessment, weight measurement, nothing by mouth after midnight, hair washing, and the possibility that long hair will be braided.	3. Knowing what to expect usually decreases anxiety.
4. Explain that the hair is cut and the scalp shaved in the operating room. Explain the rationale and allow time for the patient to express his feelings. If the operating room personnel are willing to save the patient's hair, ask the patient if this is desired. Explain to the patient that he may request that all hair be shaved, to promote uniform regrowth. If possible, have the family present during this explanation.	4. Hair is an important component of body image and self-concept. Having the hair cut may be extremely distressing to the patient. Knowing why it must be removed and that it may be saved may alleviate some of the distress and sense of loss. Allowing time for the patient to express his feelings conveys your sensitivity and validates the patient's feelings. Having the family present may provide the emotional support necessary to cope with this situation and prepare them for the way the patient will appear after surgery.
5. Discuss the critical care unit environment and the effects of the craniotomy during the immediate postoperative period. Mention that headaches and altered consciousness may occur.	5. Knowing in advance about the critical care unit environment may increase the patient's sense of security when he awakens after surgery. Knowing that headaches and altered consciousness are common after the operation may help decrease the patient's and family's anxiety.
6. Encourage the patient and family to express fears and concerns about the impending surgery.	6. Fear of death, anxiety over other possible outcomes, and anticipatory grieving for the possible loss of body function interfere with the learning process. Providing an environment where the patient is comfortable discussing these feelings may help facilitate the learning process and reduce preoperative and postoperative anxiety.
7. Additional individualized interventions: ______	7. Rationales: ______

Target outcome criteria

Before surgery, the patient and family will:

- verbalize understanding of the upcoming surgery and its potential effects and complications
- describe their anxieties and how they are coping with them.

Collaborative problem: *Potential cerebral ischemia related to increased intracranial pressure*

NURSING PRIORITIES: (a) Decrease intracranial pressure and (b) minimize fluctuations in cerebral perfusion pressure.

Interventions	Rationales
1. Implement the measures in the "Increased Intracranial Pressure" care plan's problem on potential cerebral ischemia, page 84.	1. Numerous problems may raise intracranial pressure to dangerous levels after a craniotomy, including surgical trauma, cerebral edema, blood pressure fluctuations, and nursing activities. The care plan for "Increased Intracranial Pressure" covers this problem in detail.
2. Additional individualized interventions: ____________	2. Rationales: ____________

Nursing diagnosis: *Potential for infection related to surgery, invasive techniques, continuous intracranial monitoring, ventricular drains, or cerebrospinal fluid leakage*

NURSING PRIORITY: Prevent or promptly detect signs of infection.

Interventions	Rationales
1. Implement the measures in the "Increased Intracranial Pressure" care plan's problem on potential for infection, page 87.	1. The "Increased Intracranial Pressure" care plan provides general measures for prevention, assessment, and treatment of infection. This plan discusses additional care specific to the craniotomy patient.
2. Administer antibiotics as ordered, usually immediately before surgery begins.	2. Wound infection occurs in 0.7% to 5.7% of neurosurgical patients. Prophylactic antibiotic administration helps prevent infection by establishing the optimal tissue concentration of antibiotic before possible contamination. Antibiotic administration also may be repeated during a lengthy procedure. Antibiotics may be discontinued at the completion of surgery.
3. Assess for respiratory infection: • auscultate lungs every 2 hours and as necessary for adventitious sounds • assess sputum for color, consistency, amount, and odor; culture if necessary • observe for temperature elevation and WBC elevation.	3. The overall pulmonary infection rate in the neurosurgery patient is 13% to 16%. Impaired mobility, characteristic of the surgical and postoperative period, compromises the respiratory system by increasing stasis of secretions, promoting atelectasis, and producing generalized hypoxia. To decrease intracranial pressure (ICP), the patient's fluid balance is maintained slightly dehydrated. Dehydration increases the tenacious nature of the sputum, increasing the risk of consolidation and pneumonia. Adventitious lung sounds, purulent or foul-smelling sputum, fever, and WBC elevation strongly suggest the development of pulmonary infection.
4. Observe the surgical wound daily for signs and symptoms of infection, such as redness, edema, suture stretch, pigskin appearance of the epidermis, tenderness, or drainage. Also observe for systemic manifestations, including fever, malaise, leukocytosis, or tachycardia.	4. Scalp margin necrosis, wound dehiscence, cerebrospinal fluid (CSF) leakage, presence of a drain and monitoring device, possible scratching and manipulation by the patient, and environmental factors increase the risk of wound infection in the postcraniotomy patient. A stitch abscess may appear before a major wound infection. A true wound infection rarely occurs before the second postoperative day and usually occurs within the first 2 weeks.

(continued)

Interventions

5. Assess constantly for signs and symptoms of meningitis, such as temperature elevation, lethargy, severe headache, nausea and vomiting, nuchal rigidity, positive Kernig's sign, photophobia, irritability, decreased level of consciousness, or generalized seizures. Assist with CT scan and lumbar puncture if necessary.

Rationales

5. Patients at risk for developing this acute inflammation of the meninges of the brain or spinal cord include those with cranial or spinal wound infections, CSF fistulae following operative procedures on the dura mater, and subarachnoid bolts or ventricular drains. All of these risk factors for meningeal contamination may apply to the postcraniotomy patient. Abnormal lumbar puncture (LP) findings typically confirm the diagnosis. These findings include a positive culture, an elevated opening pressure of 200 to 700 mmH_2O, WBC count increased from 10 to 1,000 cells/mm^3, an increased protein count, decreased glucose and chloride levels, and, in purulent bacterial meningitis, a tan or milky appearance of the fluid. A CT scan may be done before the LP to determine the risk of brain herniation from the sudden removal of CSF from the spinal canal.

6. Additional individualized interventions: ______________________

6. Rationales: ______________________

Target outcome criteria

By 72 hours after surgery, the patient will:
- have a normal temperature and WBC count
- display negative cultures
- manifest no signs or symptoms of infection.

By the time of transfer, the patient will have no signs or symptoms of wound infection.

Nursing diagnosis: *Potential for impaired gas exchange related to decreased level of consciousness, neurologic deficits, effects of anesthesia, immobility, altered respiratory patterns, and tenacious secretions associated with fluid loss and decreased fluid intake*

NURSING PRIORITY: Maintain effective gas exchange.

Interventions

1. Implement the measures discussed in the "Increased Intracranial Pressure" care plan in the "Potential for respiratory failure" collaborative problem, page 89.

Rationales

1. The neurosurgical patient requires meticulous respiratory assessment, support of oxygenation and ventilation, and pulmonary hygiene. The measures used to provide airway and ventilation care are those discussed in the "Increased Intracranial Pressure" care plan.

2. Additional individualized interventions: ______________________

2. Rationales: ______________________

Nursing diagnosis: *Potential for injury related to decreased level of consciousness, effect of anesthetics, seizure activity, and/or drug therapy*

NURSING PRIORITY: Prevent injury.

Interventions	**Rationales**
1. Implement the measures discussed in the "Increased Intracranial Pressure" care plan in the "Potential for injury" nursing diagnosis, page 92.	1. Although the factors creating the potential for injury for the neurosurgical patient differ somewhat from those for the patient with increased intracranial pressure, the measures used to protect them are the same.
2. Additional individualized interventions: ______	2. Rationales: ______

Collaborative problem: *Potential for fluid volume excess related to physiologic stress response to surgery, steroid therapy, or syndrome of inappropriate secretion of antidiuretic hormone*

NURSING PRIORITY: Maintain the patient in a slightly dehydrated state.

Interventions	**Rationales**
1. Implement the measures discussed in the "Increased Intracranial Pressure" care plan in the "Potential for fluid volume excess" nursing diagnosis, page 91.	1. That care plan discusses potential for fluid volume excess in detail.
2. Additional individualized interventions: ______	2. Rationales: ______

Collaborative problem: *Potential for fluid volume deficit related to diuretic therapy, fluid restriction, diabetes insipidus, hyperthermia, or GI suction*

NURSING PRIORITY: Maintain fluid volume within prescribed limits.

Interventions	**Rationales**
1. Implement the measures discussed in the "Increased Intracranial Pressure" care plan in the "Potential for fluid volume deficit nursing diagnosis," page 90.	1. Diabetes insipidus most commonly occurs in postneurosurgery patients. The "Increased Intracranial Pressure" care plan discusses this problem in detail.
2. Additional individualized interventions: ______	2. Rationales: ______

Nursing diagnosis: *Disturbed self-concept: body image related to hair loss, possible disruption in sensory or motor function, or possible alteration in personality and thought processes*

NURSING PRIORITIES: (a) Promote a healthy body image and (b) minimize damage to self-concept.

Interventions	Rationales
1. Encourage the patient to express his feelings, beliefs, and concerns about changes resulting from the diagnosis and craniotomy. Offer emotional support, as appropriate, based on knowledge of diagnosis and success of surgery.	1. The patient may have fears or misconceptions that can be clarified. Some residual effects of surgery are temporary. Recovery may be slow (months or years).
2. Implement measures to minimize the patient's reaction to loss of hair and to the misshapen skull, if a bone flap was removed.	2. Specific interventions to minimize the body image changes may make the patient feel less self-conscious.
• Provide surgical cap or scarf to wear; encourage usual grooming, makeup habits, and using a wig; reinforce that hair will grow back.	• These measures to improve appearance and awareness of the temporary nature of alterations in body image may encourage greater acceptance of the changes.
• Use therapeutic touch and frequent visits.	• Therapeutic touch and frequent visits convey acceptance of the patient as a worthwhile person, which may facilitate the patient's self-acceptance.
3. Provide appropriate stimuli: • Place the patient in a room with a window, if possible. • Provide a clock and calendar. • Provide objects of interest to the patient, such as photographs of loved ones. • Play the radio, tapes, or TV, if desired. • Talk with the patient. • Encourage the family to interact with the patient.	3. The measures listed provide stimulation and reality orientation. Talking with the patient and encouraging family interaction are particularly important because they reinforce a sense of human connection in what may otherwise seem to be a surreal world in the critical care unit.
4. Implement the measures in the "Impaired Physical Mobility" care plan, page 33, as appropriate. Encourage participation in self-care, occupational therapy, daily living activities, and ambulation, as permitted.	4. The measures in this care plan prevent deformities and other complications associated with the enforced immobility associated with major surgery. Maintaining motor function, muscle strength, and joint mobility are particularly important in preserving the patient's ability to benefit from later rehabilitation programs. Participation in the listed activities foster the patient's belief that independence can be reestablished.
5. Additional individualized interventions: ____________	5. Rationales: ____________

Target outcome criteria

Within 5 to 7 days after surgery, the patient will:

- verbalize feelings of self-worth
- participate in self-care
- demonstrate an interest in personal appearance
- demonstrate an interest in occupational therapy, activities of daily living, and a potential rehabilitation program.

Nursing diagnosis: *Postoperative knowledge deficit related to follow-up care*

NURSING PRIORITY: Provide early teaching regarding rehabilitation and follow-up care.

Interventions	Rationales
1. Implement measures in the "Knowledge Deficit" care plan, page 45, as appropriate. Defer formal teaching until after transfer from the unit.	1. During the stay in the critical care unit, the craniotomy patient usually is too ill for a structured teaching program, and the patient's and family's attention is directed toward more immediate needs. Formal teaching is best accomplished after the patient's condition has stabilized and he is transferred to a more conducive teaching environment.
2. Provide informal teaching, as appropriate. Encourage questions, provide brief explanations about the current situation, and clarify misconceptions.	2. Capitalizing on informal opportunities conveys a willingness to meet the patient's and family's immediate learning needs.
3. Identify and document long-range teaching needs as the patient or family raises or displays them. Upon the patient's transfer to the medical-surgical unit, communicate these needs to the receiving staff.	3. Planning for discharge teaching is most effective when an awareness of its importance pervades all phases of care. Documentation and colleague-to-colleague communication enhance continuity of care.
4. Provide information to the patient and family about community agencies and support groups, such as head injury support groups, vocational rehabilitation, and the American Cancer Society.	4. These organizations provide many forms of support for patients and families. In many cases, their credibility allows them to provide invaluable practical information on long-range education and rehabilitation. Knowing that others have coped with similar experiences may provide a sense of rapport and trust that facilitates the learning necessary to adjust successfully to cranial surgery and possible residual deficits.
5. Additional individualized interventions: ____________	5. Rationales: ____________

Target outcome criteria

By the time of transfer, the patient and family will:
- verbalize questions
- express satisfaction with the staff's willingness to answer questions
- begin identifying long-range learning needs.

Transfer planning

NURSING TRANSFER CRITERIA

Upon transfer, documentation shows evidence of:
- stable vital signs
- stable neurologic function
- intracranial pressure within normal limits
- healing incision
- headache controlled by oral analgesics
- absence of pulmonary, cardiovascular, or GI complications
- normal fluid and electrolyte balance
- absence of infection
- absence of fever.

PATIENT-FAMILY TEACHING CHECKLIST

Document evidence that patient and family demonstrate understanding of:

___ diagnosis and extent of surgery
___ extent of neurologic deficits, if present
___ extent and demands of the rehabilitation process
___ need for continued family support.

DOCUMENTATION CHECKLIST

Using outcome criteria as a guide, document:

___ clinical status on admission
___ significant changes in status
___ pertinent laboratory and diagnostic test findings
___ fluid intake and output
___ neurologic status
___ neurologic deficits, if present
___ GI bleeding, if any
___ wound condition
___ seizure activity, if any
___ rehabilitation program needs.

ASSOCIATED CARE PLANS

Acute Pain
Impaired Physical Mobility
Ineffective Coping
Knowledge Deficit
Nutritional Deficit
Sensory-Perceptual Alteration

REFERENCES

Gordon, M. *Nursing Diagnosis, Process and Application,* 2nd ed. New York: McGraw-Hill Book Co., 1987.

Hickey, J.V. *The Clinical Practice of Neurological and Neurosurgical Nursing,* 2nd ed. Philadelphia: J.B. Lippincott Co., 1987.

Kee, J.L. *Laboratory and Diagnostic Tests with Nursing Implications,* 2nd ed. East Norwalk, Conn.: Appleton & Lange, 1987.

Lewis, S.M., and Collier, I.C. *Medical-Surgical Nursing Assessment and Management of Clinical Problems,* 2nd ed. New York: McGraw-Hill Book Co., 1987.

Ulrich, S.P., et al. *Nursing Care Planning Guides, A Nursing Diagnosis Approach.* Philadelphia: W.B. Saunders Co., 1986.

Wotzka-Lagaard, M. "Craniotomies: Procedures, Problems, and Interventions," in *Acute Neuroscience Nursing Concepts and Care.* Edited by Lundgren, J. Boston: Jones and Bartlett Publishers, Inc., 1986.

Guillain-Barré Syndrome

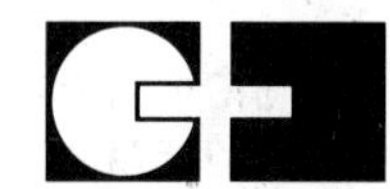

DRG information

DRG 018 Cranial and Peripheral Nerve Disorders.
With Complication or Comorbidity (CC).
Mean LOS = 6.3 days
Principal diagnoses include:
- disorders of cranial or peripheral nerves
- mononeuritis of upper or lower limb
- neuritis or radiculitis of brachial or unspecified nerve
- various types of neuropathy (including Guillain-Barré syndrome)
- various types of polyneuropathy.

DRG 019 Cranial and Peripheral Nerve Disorders.
Without CC.
Mean LOS = 4.5 days
Principal diagnoses include select principal diagnoses listed under DRG 018.

Introduction

DEFINITION AND TIME FOCUS

Guillain-Barré syndrome, also known as acute idiopathic polyneuritis and Landry–Guillain-Barré–Strohl syndrome, is a demyelinating disorder affecting the peripheral nervous system. Guillain-Barré syndrome, first described in 1859, is diagnosed typically when the patient complains of sudden weakness or paralysis of the legs that progresses upward symmetrically. Its cause is unknown; however, the disorder may result from an autoimmune response in which sensitized lymphocytes infiltrate the peripheral nervous system and produce demyelination, edema, and inflammation. The destruction of the myelin sheath, which increases impulse transmission by allowing impulses to jump from node to node along the axon, results in slowed conduction or, if significant edema is present, complete blockage of impulse transmission.

Commonly, the disorder causes progressive loss of function over 2 to 3 weeks, at which time the patient may require ventilatory support because of respiratory paralysis. However, the symptoms are potentially reversible because the myelin sheath can regenerate; full recovery without residual deficits eventually occurs in about 75% of cases. Complete recovery is a slow process and commonly takes 18 to 24 months from the onset of symptoms. This care plan focuses on the patient who is admitted to the critical care unit with a diagnosis of Guillain-Barré syndrome.

ETIOLOGY AND PRECIPITATING FACTORS

- idiopathic origins
- possible link to autoimmune factors
- immunizations (vaccinations for smallpox, tetanus, influenza, and measles have been implicated in the syndrome)
- possible climate factors (higher incidence in autumn in some areas)
- viral illnesses
- immunosuppression (Hodgkin's disease and other lymphomas may increase risk)

Focused assessment guidelines

NURSING HISTORY (Functional health pattern findings)

Health perception–health management pattern

- typically, complains of sudden, symmetric weakness of legs, increasing and ascending over several days
- usually, has experienced self-limiting, mild respiratory or GI illness 2 to 3 weeks before onset of symptoms
- may note frequent paresthesias before onset of weakness, such as a "stocking-and-glove" numbness and tingling
- may have difficulty speaking

Nutritional-metabolic pattern

- may complain of dysphagia

Elimination pattern

- usually, retains sphincter control; may become incontinent if autonomic nervous system involvement develops

Activity-exercise pattern

- commonly, notes leg weakness or paralysis that progresses upward to trunk, arms, and head
- uncommonly, reports that arms were affected first
- may present complaining of injuries from falling
- may complain of shortness of breath
- uncommonly, complains of easy fatigability

Cognitive-perceptual pattern

- may note pain in arms and legs
- may describe altered position sense

Coping–stress tolerance pattern

- likely to express extreme anxiety over progression of symptoms

Self-perception–self-concept pattern

- likely to complain of feelings of helplessness

PHYSICAL FINDINGS

Cardiovascular

- hypotension or hypertension (if autonomic nervous system involved)
- tachydysrhythmias or bradydysrhythmias (if autonomic nervous system involved)

Pulmonary

- diminished breath sounds
- difficulty clearing secretions
- shallow respirations
- use of accessory muscles

Neurologic

- diminished or absent deep tendon reflexes
- symmetrical paralysis or paresis
- loss of position and vibration sense
- dysphagia
- facial paralysis

Musculoskeletal

- ascending weakness or flaccid paralysis of arms and legs
- tenderness to deep palpation of leg or arm muscles

DIAGNOSTIC STUDIES

Diagnosis of Guillain-Barré syndrome is based primarily on clinical findings and progression of symptoms; no specific diagnostic tests exist.

- routine blood studies—may reveal no significant abnormalities
- lumbar puncture—reveals classic findings of albuminocytologic dissociation (elevated protein level of >45 mg/100 ml and normal white blood cell count of 5 to 10/mm^3). Serial punctures are commonly performed to monitor disease course; cerebrospinal fluid protein level may not reveal elevation until 1 to 2 weeks after onset of symptoms
- electromyography studies—reveal denervated areas; recordings show repetitive firing of single units rather than normal sectional activity (may not appear until 2 weeks after onset of symptoms)
- nerve conduction velocity tests—reveal marked reduction in conduction speed
- pulmonary function studies—provide baseline data for evaluating degree of respiratory impairment. Usually, decreased vital capacity (<15 to 20 ml/kg) is revealed

POTENTIAL COMPLICATIONS

- respiratory failure (occurs in 25% of patients)
- thrombophlebitis
- pulmonary embolus
- ileus
- gastric dilatation
- atelectasis
- pneumonia
- skin breakdown
- urinary tract stones and infection
- GI bleeding
- septicemia
- autonomic dysfunction and dysrhythmias
- muscle atrophy
- ineffective coping

Collaborative problem: *Potential respiratory failure related to weakness or paralysis of respiratory muscles*

NURSING PRIORITY: Maintain adequate ventilatory status.

Interventions	Rationales
1. Assess airway patency, breath sounds, respiratory rate and effort, ability to count slowly from 1 to 10, skin color, chest excursion, and vital capacity (VC) at least every 2 hours. Immediately report dyspnea, increasing restlessness, increasing use of diaphragmatic and accessory muscles, cyanosis, decreased breath sounds, shallow or irregular respirations, and VC of <15 to 20 ml/kg or reduced respiratory effort.	1. Respiratory failure can occur subtly but rapidly in Guillain-Barré patients, and about 25% develop significant pulmonary problems. As muscular paralysis ascends, the phrenic nerve may become involved, affecting diaphragmatic excursion and impairing the patient's ability to maintain an adequate tidal volume and clear secretions from the airway.
2. Encourage hourly coughing and deep breathing, and assist with pulmonary hygiene measures (postural drainage, percussion, and incentive spirometry). Monitor carefully for development of fever, crackles, or areas of consolidation.	2. Reduced ventilatory capacity and resultant stasis of secretions may lead to atelectasis or pneumonia. Pulmonary hygiene measures help promote airway clearance. Coughing may lead to microatelectasis from the associated increase in intrathoracic pressure, if not followed by deep breathing to reexpand collapsed alveoli.

Interventions

3. Obtain and monitor arterial blood gas (ABG) values, as ordered. Report changes or abnormal findings promptly. Consider using a pulse oximeter to monitor oxygen saturation.

Rationales

3. Ventilatory support is indicated if the patient's PCO_2 increases 10 to 15 mmHg or if the PO_2 decreases 10 to 15 mm Hg compared to normal ranges. ABG values are a helpful adjunct to clinical observation of repsiratory status. Pulse oximetry provides ongoing monitoring without invasive procedures.

4. Prepare to assist with endotracheal intubation or tracheotomy if vital capacity falls below 800 ml or if the patient cannot clear secretions.

4. In many cases, positive-pressure mechanical ventilation is necessary during the acute phase.

5. Suction as necessary, providing supplemental oxygen.

5. Careful suctioning, as indicated, helps avert mucus plugs or pulmonary infection from secretion stasis. Also, suctioning may be required because of facial or glossopharyngeal nerve involvement, which may cause drooling and impaired swallowing.

6. Every 2 to 4 hours, monitor vital signs and neurologic status, including level of consciousness, muscle strength, and ability to gag, cough, and swallow. Also monitor hemodynamic parameters and EKG findings according to Appendix A, "Monitoring Standards," or unit protocol. Assess for and immediately report the onset of sweating, flushing, altered vital signs, or dysrhythmias. If life-threatening dysrhythmias are present, institute appropriate pharmacologic treatment according to unit protocol.

6. Bradycardia, tachycardia, or blood pressure alterations may indicate hypoxemia or autonomic nervous system involvement. Reduced cranial reflex responses, lethargy, or drowsiness may indicate increased CO_2 retention from respiratory insufficiency. Sweating, flushing, or dysrhythmias may indicate autonomic nervous system involvement. Vagus nerve involvement may be responsible for life-threatening dysrhythmias.

7. When muscles of upper arms, shoulders, or swallowing show reduced function, be particularly vigilant for indications of respiratory changes.

7. These muscle groups are commonly affected just before breathing muscles; dysfunction may herald impending respiratory problems.

8. If mechanical ventilation is required, maintain ventilator settings and monitor ABG levels. Teach patient and family about ventilator use and alarm systems. Reassure patient and family that mechanical ventilation is usually temporary and that as the patient's condition improves, he will be able to resume breathing for himself. See the "Mechanical Ventilation" care plan, page 108.

8. Ventilator settings should be correlated with ABG levels reflective of current status. Patient and family may be extremely anxious over the use of and need for mechanical ventilation. Careful explanations may decrease fear and minimize "fighting" the machine. The "Mechanical Ventilation" care plan provides details regarding care of the patient on a ventilator.

9. Additional individualized interventions: ____________

9. Rationales: ____________

Target outcome criteria

On admission, the patient will have a clear airway.
Within 4 hours, the patient will have:
- clear breath sounds
- regular respirations
- bilaterally equal chest excursion
- PO_2 >70 mm Hg
- PCO_2 of 35 to 45 mm Hg.

Nursing diagnosis: *Impaired physical mobility related to slowed or absent conduction of motor nerve impulses, resulting in weakness or flaccid paralysis*

NURSING PRIORITY: Prevent complications associated with immobility.

Interventions	Rationales
1. See the "Impaired Physical Mobility" care plan, page 33, for detailed interventions regarding positioning, range of motion exercises, skin care, infection prevention and treatment, elimination aids, and promotion of circulation.	1. The "Impaired Physical Mobility" care plan contains interventions for preventing complications associated with prolonged immobility. Patients with Guillain-Barré syndrome are at increased risk for the following immobility-related problems: infections, thromboembolic phenomena, joint contractures, muscle atrophy, skin breakdown, constipation or ileus, and urinary stones. Preventive and therapeutic measures for these complications are an essential part of caring for the patient with Guillain-Barré syndrome.
2. Alert patient and family to use caution in handling arms and legs; that is, they should be aware of risks of pressure, temperature, and, as function returns, overexertion and fatigue.	2. Reduced sensory capabilities associated with nerve dysfunction may cause the patient to be unaware of impending or actual injury. As function begins to return, caution must be taken in resuming activity, because overexertion may precipitate exacerbation.
3. Administer corticosteroids, if ordered. Monitor closely for signs and symptoms of gastric irritation, edema, hypokalemia, or other untoward effects. Be aware that steroid use may mask signs and symptoms of underlying infection.	3. Steroid use is controversial and of questionable value in reducing the inflammatory reaction that impairs mobility. Adverse reactions may negate potential benefits, so if such medication is ordered, careful monitoring is warranted.
4. Prepare the patient for plasmapheresis, if ordered.	4. Plasmapheresis has been shown to have possible benefit in chronic relapsing or in progressive Guillain-Barré syndrome. Although the reason is unknown, the procedure may remove antimyelin antibodies that are linked to the development of the disorder, possibly shortening the disease course. However, neither this nor any other treatment has been proven to have direct therapeutic effects, so monitoring and support remain the primary interventions.
5. Provide eye care, including use of artificial tears and eye protectors, as needed.	5. Trigeminal nerve impairment may cause the loss of corneal sensation. Facial nerve involvement commonly affects eyelid function.
6. Early in the hospitalization, provide assistance with physical activities and teach the patient to use splints and assistive devices, as needed. As soon as possible, encourage the patient to resume normal activities, beginning by assuming the upright position with use of tilt table or bed adjustment. Arrange referral to a physical therapist and supervise coordination of activity program.	6. Early activity and proper positioning prevent contractures and injuries from disuse. Gradually resuming an upright position helps regain vascular tone. Venous pooling associated with bed rest may contribute to initial orthostatic hypotension when the patient resumes the upright position. Function may return asymmetrically, predisposing the patient to falls, back problems, or other injuries. A physical therapist can provide expert guidance in planning the rehabilitation program.
7. Additional individualized interventions: ____________	7. Rationales: ____________

Target outcome criteria
On admission and continuously, the patient will:
- have intact skin
- have normal eye lubrication or protective measures instituted.

Within 3 days of admission, the patient will:
- have a bowel movement
- receive regular active or passive range of motion exercise, as condition allows.

As function returns, the patient will:
- show no exacerbation of condition
- suffer no accidental injuries.

Nursing diagnosis: *Potential nutritional deficit related to dysphagia, depression, tracheostomy, or mechanical ventilation*

NURSING PRIORITY: Provide adequate nutrition.

Interventions	Rationales
1. See the "Nutritional Deficit" care plan, page 53.	1. The "Nutritional Deficit" care plan contains interventions for assessment and support of the patient with a potential nutritional deficit.
2. If oral intake is tolerated, use techniques to help minimize choking and aspiration: • elevate patient's head and flex neck while swallowing • have suction equipment at hand and supervise patient closely during meals • provide semisolid foods; avoid liquids initially; allow patient to make choices about diet when possible.	2. Cranial nerve involvement may cause dysphagia; when patient takes food by mouth before and after acute phase of illness, care must be taken to avoid aspiration. Permitting choices, when possible, helps the patient maintain or regain a sense of self-control.
3. Administer enteral or parenteral feedings, as ordered, during acute phase of illness.	3. Adequate nutrition is essential to minimize muscle wasting, maintain the body's defenses against infection, and promote healing. During the acute phase, dysphagia may be too severe to safely permit oral intake.
4. Additional individualized interventions: ____________	4. Rationales: ____________

Target outcome criteria
By the time of transfer, the patient will:
- be receiving optimum nutritional intake, as reflected by stable weight (plus or minus 2 or 3 lb/week)
- eat without aspirating, if able to tolerate oral food intake.

Nursing diagnosis: *Powerlessness related to rapidly progressive symptoms, fear of death, altered communication, and dependency on others for basic needs*

NURSING PRIORITY: Maintain psychological equilibrium.

Interventions	Rationales
1. See the "Ineffective Coping" care plan, page 26.	1. The "Ineffective Coping" care plan provides interventions helpful in caring for the patient and family experiencing illness-related disorganization.

(continued)

Interventions

2. Provide frequent, factual explanations about condition, emphasizing the temporary, potentially reversible nature of the disorder. Prepare patient and family for potential problems of the acute phase. Point out any small improvements in the patient's condition as they occur. Encourage family members to participate in care.

Rationales

2. Depression and hopelessness are common emotional responses to the sudden losses caused by Guillain-Barré syndrome. Preparatory teaching may reduce panic as the acute phase progresses. Maintaining hope and providing encouragement throughout the extended course of the illness is an essential part of nursing care, especially because the patient usually remains alert and oriented despite functional deficits. Family participation in care provides tangible support for the patient.

3. If communication ability is impaired, arrange for use of signals (eye blinks or motion-sensor call devices) or use a writing tablet or word board. Anticipate needs; be sensitive to nonverbal cues such as facial expression.

3. The inability to communicate can be terrifying. Providing the patient with some means of signaling helps reduce anxiety.

4. Encourage the use of relaxation and stress control techniques. Emphasize that proficient use of such techniques may benefit the patient even after the disorder has resolved. Assist and teach the patient about the following, as appropriate:
• progressive relaxation
• guided imagery
• "thought-stopping" and positive affirmation
• meditation.

4. The patient who cannot do anything physically for himself may still find comfort in helping himself psychologically. Learning and practicing such techniques helps the patient maintain control and a sense of active participation in the recovery process. Relaxation techniques have been shown to be beneficial in averting many stress-related health problems.

5. Whenever possible, encourage the patient to make choices regarding care and involve the family in care planning.

5. The debilitating nature of Guillain-Barré syndrome promotes dependency and helplessness. Allowing some choices, even in small matters, increases the patient's sense of self-control and reduces powerlessness.

6. Encourage ventilation of feelings. Cultivate an attitude of acceptance. If manipulative or dysfunctional behavior occurs, try to provide the patient with increased control and choices. Encourage family members to talk to the patient, even if the patient cannot respond. Refer the patient to a mental health professional, if appropriate.

6. The losses caused by Guillain-Barré syndrome and their long-term effects on the patient's life will precipitate normal reactions of anger, depression, grieving, and even paranoia. Acceptance of feelings facilitates healthy coping behavior. Manipulative behavior is commonly an attempt to regain a sense of control. Although motor function is impaired, the patient can still hear and appreciate verbal communication. Mental health referral may be warranted for long-term supportive therapy.

7. Provide appropriate referrals to social services staff or other agencies, as needed.

7. The sudden transition from healthy, working adult to hopeless, disabled patient is frightening enough, but the patient may have additional worries about income, child care, or other arrangements. Facilitating early referrals may avert undue anxiety about such problems.

8. Provide pain relief measures, as needed, with nonnarcotic analgesics as ordered, supportive repositioning, and alternative pain control techniques. See the "Acute Pain" care plan, page 10, for details.

8. Patients with Guillain-Barré syndrome may experience varying degrees of limb pain or uncomfortable paresthesias. Unrelieved pain decreases coping ability and adds to the patient's physiologic stress. The "Acute Pain" care plan contains interventions applicable to any patient in pain.

9. Whenever possible, after the patient is physiologically stable, arrange for a transfer or attempt to create a more normal environment, for example, by permitting television, flowers, and personal items from home.

9. Normalization of the patient's environment reinforces his improving status and decreases the depersonalizing effects of the critical care setting.

10. Additional individualized interventions: ____________

____

10. Rationales: ____________

____

Target outcome criteria
Within 2 hours of admission, the patient will:
- have an effective communication method
- be pain-free.

Within 24 hours of admission, the patient will:
- participate in making choices about care
- begin expressing feelings
- display reduced anxiety and fear as evidenced by relaxed expression.

Transfer planning

NURSING TRANSFER CRITERIA

Upon transfer, documentation shows evidence of:
- spontaneous respiration
- effective airway clearance
- stable vital signs within normal limits for patient
- ABG measurements within normal limits
- effective communication ability.

PATIENT-FAMILY TEACHING CHECKLIST

Document evidence that patient and family demonstrate understanding of:
__ nature and progression of syndrome; expected prognosis
__ indications of possible exacerbation
__ relaxation and stress-reduction measures
__ activity program and use of assistive devices
__ safety precautions.

DOCUMENTATION CHECKLIST

Using outcome criteria as a guide, document:
__ clinical status on admission
__ significant changes in status
__ pertinent laboratory and diagnostic test findings
__ respiratory support measures
__ nutritional status
__ measures to prevent complications of immobility
__ communication measures
__ relaxation and stress-reduction teaching
__ activity progression
__ patient/family teaching
__ transfer planning.

ASSOCIATED CARE PLANS

Impaired Physical Mobility
Ineffective Coping
Knowledge Deficit
Mechanical Ventilation
Nutritional Deficit
Sensory-Perceptual Alteration

REFERENCES

Alspach, J.G., and Williams, S.M. *Core Curriculum for Critical Care Nursing,* 3rd ed. Philadelphia: W.B. Saunders Co., 1985.

Kenner, C.V., et al. *Critical Care Nursing: Body/Mind/Spirit,* 2nd ed. Boston: Little, Brown and Co., 1985.

Luckmann, J., and Sorensen, K.C. *Medical-Surgical Nursing: A Psychophysiologic Approach,* 3rd ed. Philadelphia: W.B. Saunders Co., 1987.

Rudy, E.B. *Advanced Neurological and Neurosurgical Nursing.* St. Louis: C.V. Mosby Co., 1984.

Thompson, J.M., et al. *Clinical Nursing.* St. Louis: C.V. Mosby Co., 1986.

Wells, S.L., and Trembley, S.F. *Critical Care Review for Nurses.* Monterey, Calif.: Wadsworth Publishing Co., 1984.

Increased Intracranial Pressure

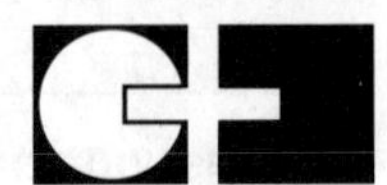

DRG information

Increased intracranial pressure (ICP) is a sign of an underlying problem and not a condition in and of itself in terms of coding guidelines. The DRG assigned for increased ICP depends entirely on the underlying cause that requires hospitalization, such as hemorrhage, hematoma, head trauma, abscess, or radiation. The LOS depends entirely on the principal diagnosis.

Introduction

DEFINITION AND TIME FOCUS

Increased ICP occurs when the components of the intracranial cavity—brain tissue, cerebral blood, and cerebrospinal fluid(CSF)—exceed the cavity's compensatory capacity. The volume of these three components usually remains relatively constant, with a normal ICP of 0 to 15 mm Hg. Autoregulatory mechanisms in the brain compensate for volume changes of the contents, so an increase in one component is counteracted by a decrease in another.

These mechanisms include displacement of CSF from the cranial cavity to the subarachnoid space surrounding the spinal cord (the primary compensatory mechanism); increased CSF reabsorption; and the reduction of cerebral blood volume by compression of the venous system, displacing venous blood from the intracranial cavity into the systemic circulation. Displacement of brain tissue without concurrent decompensation is extremely limited and occurs primarily with slowly expanding masses, such as tumors or chronic subdural hematomas.

When these autoregulatory mechanisms can no longer compensate for changes in the components of the intracranial cavity, increased ICP results. When ICP is sufficiently elevated to reduce cerebral perfusion pressure, irreversible brain damage may occur. This clinical plan focuses on the patient with acutely increased ICP.

ETIOLOGY AND PRECIPITATING FACTORS

- increase in brain volume caused by intracranial hemorrhage or hematoma, cerebral edema caused by surgical or head trauma, fast growing tumors, abscess, metabolic coma, radiation, chemotherapeutic agents, infarction, and anoxic events
- increased cerebral blood volume from loss of autoregulation; hyperthermia; vasodilation caused by hypoxemia, hypercapnia, anesthetic agents, or narcotics; venous outflow obstruction caused by compression of the internal jugular veins or intrathoracic or intraabdominal pressure; fluctuations above a mean arterial pressure (MAP) of 150 mm Hg or below 50 mm Hg
- obstruction of CSF outflow because of hematomas in the posterior fossa; brain shift and herniation; or impaired reabsorption from the subarachnoid space caused by inflammation of the meninges either by subarachnoid hemorrhage or infection, or obstruction of arachnoid villi by blood cells or bacteria

Focused assessment guidelines

NURSING HISTORY (Functional health pattern findings)

Health perception–health management pattern

- exhibits sudden onset of change in level of consciousness, ranging from flattening of affect to coma; may have loss of consciousness of less than 24 hours
- may have history of head trauma as a result of a motor vehicle accident, fall, assault, gunshot or stab wound, or recreational accidents; may be at increased risk if between ages 15 and 24 and male because of this group's higher incidence of head injury from motor vehicle accidents
- may have history of infection, particularly in the middle ear, mastoid cells, or paranasal sinuses
- may have history of receiving anesthetic agents or narcotics, radiation, or chemotherapeutic agents
- may have history of hypoxia, such as hypoventilation, apnea, chest trauma, pneumonia, or ventilation-perfusion abnormalities

Nutritional-metabolic pattern

- may report vomiting (uncommonly). If present, not preceded by nausea

Cognitive-perceptual pattern

- may report a headache (uncommon); if present, it is worse on arising in the morning. Straining or movement may increase the pain.

Self-perception–self-concept pattern

- may have feelings of anxiety or apprehension if the level of consciousness is such that the patient understands something abnormal is happening to him

PHYSICAL FINDINGS

Note: Many of the classic signs and symptoms of increased ICP now are considered indicators of brain shift and brain stem dysfunction. Clinical signs and symptoms alone are not reliable in determining if ICP is elevated, in detecting early increased ICP, or in determining the severity of increased ICP. Frequent neurologic assessment and ICP monitoring are the most reliable methods of detecting early deterioration.

Neurologic

Early stage of increased ICP:
- decreasing level of consciousness (most sensitive indicator of increased ICP), such as confusion, restlessness, or lethargy
- pupillary abnormalities, with the pupil dilating gradually and becoming slightly ovoid and sluggish, ipsilateral to the causative factor for the increased ICP
- visual deficits, such as decreased visual acuity, blurred vision, diplopia, and changes in extraocular eye movements
- motor weakness (monoparesis or hemiparesis) contralateral to the cause of the increased ICP

Later stage of increased ICP:
- coma
- pupillary abnormalities, including dilated and nonreactive (fixed) ipsilateral pupil. With herniation, pupils become bilaterally fixed and dilated.
- hemiplegia and abnormal posturing (sometimes termed decorticate or decerebrate posturing), which may be unilateral or bilateral. As death approaches, the patient becomes bilaterally flaccid.
- hyperthermia from hypothalamic injury
- loss of brain stem reflexes, including corneal, oculocephalic (doll's eyes), and oculovestibular reflexes. The oculovestibular reflex is not as readily abolished as the oculocephalic and is a more sensitive indicator of brain stem function. Gag and swallowing reflexes also are lost.
- papilledema (rarely), more common with chronically increased ICP

Cardiovascular

Later stage of increased ICP:
- Cushing's reflex (rare): rising systolic blood pressure, widening pulse pressure, and bradycardia. Pulse is full and bounding. As death approaches, pulse becomes irregular, rapid, and thready, then stops.

Pulmonary

- irregular respirations, commonly in patterns that relate to the level of brain dysfunction. Often seen in later stage of increased ICP: Cheyne-Stokes respirations, central neurogenic hyperventilation, and ataxia. May be difficult to assess with the mechanically ventilated patient.

Gastrointestinal

- vomiting (uncommon). If present, not preceded by nausea.

DIAGNOSTIC STUDIES

Note: No laboratory test for diagnosing increased ICP exists.
- arterial blood gas measurements—used to monitor patient's acid-base balance and to detect hypoxemia and hypercapnia, which increase ICP
- complete blood count (CBC)—may reveal elevated white blood cell count, which may signify beginning of infection or an abscess
- electrolyte panel—used to monitor patient's fluid status and potassium and sodium levels. Sodium is retained during stressful events whereas potassium is lost. Sodium and potassium levels also are altered in diabetes insipidus (DI) and syndrome of inappropriate antidiuretic hormone secretion (SIADH), two abnormalities that may occur with increased ICP.
- serum creatinine, blood urea nitrogen (BUN) levels—used to monitor renal function, particularly if osmotic diuretics are being administered
- glucose tolerance test—used to monitor for hyperglycemia if dexamethasone therapy is used for the increased ICP
- serum osmolality—monitors for hyperosmolality when mannitol therapy is used and aids in establishing diagnosis of DI or SIADH
- urine specific gravity—may indicate DI if low or SIADH if high
- urine glucose and acetone levels—may reveal glucose in the urine, which may be an adverse reaction to dexamethasone therapy
- computed tomography (CT) scan—can differentiate many conditions that cause increased ICP by clearly outlining ventricles and assessing size and position in relation to midline structures. CT scan is useful in diagnosing cerebral edema, hematomas caused by intracranial bleeding, abscesses, cerebral infarctions, and tumors. Serial scanning is useful in patients who deteriorate or who do not improve as rapidly as expected. It may show intracranial hematomas in patients whose initial CT scan was negative.
- skull X-rays—useful in detecting linear and depressed skull fractures and may demonstrate intracranial shifts. A high incidence of developing masses and intracranial hemorrhage occurs with linear fractures. Skull X-rays should be considered when the patient has an altered level of consciousness any time after injury, focal neurologic signs, or CSF discharge from the nose or ears.
- cerebral echoencephalography— may be used if a CT scan is not available. It is useful in detecting shifts of normally midline structures, but not reliable in generalized cerebral edema that does not produce a midline shift.
- cerebral angiography—may be done if a CT scan is not available. It will reveal space-occupying lesions, such as subdural hematoma and epidural hematoma, and cerebral edema. Because cerebral angiography is an invasive study, CT scan is preferred.
- magnetic resonance imaging (MRI)—gives clearer images of soft tissues than a CT scan and can detect brain edema, hemorrhage, infarction, and blood vessel disruptions. At this time, it has limited usefulness for increased ICP monitoring because it cannot be used by patients who are using any device that contains metal.
- ICP monitoring—may reveal values of 15 to 40 mm Hg, indicating moderately elevated ICP, or 40 mm Hg or greater, indicating severely elevated ICP.

• EKG—useful in assessing changes, such as development of tall T waves in early increased ICP that become progressively flatter or inverted with an ICP above 45 mm Hg. ST segment changes occur with transient changes in ICP and return to normal with the return of ICP to previous levels. Low levels of increased ICP produce abnormally shortened QT intervals, whereas prolonged QT intervals occur with ICP over 65 mm Hg.

POTENTIAL COMPLICATIONS

- brain herniation
- permanent neurologic deficits
- seizures
- pneumonia
- atelectasis
- GI ulceration and hemorrhage
- infection
- diabetes insipidus
- syndrome of inappropriate antidiuretic hormone secretion
- neurogenic pulmonary edema

Collaborative problem: *Potential cerebral ischemia related to fluctuations in arterial blood pressure, stressful events, nursing activities, hypoxemia, or hypercapnia*

NURSING PRIORITY: Minimize fluctuations in cerebral perfusion pressure.

Interventions	Rationales
1. Assess the patient's level of consciousness, behavior, motor and sensory function, pupillary reactions (size, position, and reactivity), and respiratory patterns every 1 to 2 hours and as necessary.	1. The factors listed in the problem may increase intracranial blood volume, CSF volume, or both and lead to cerebral ischemia. Changes in any of these parameters can alert you to a deterioration in the patient's neurologic condition. The level of consciousness is the most sensitive and reliable indicator of increasing ICP. A change in respiratory patterns is also a sensitive indicator of increased ICP as well as an early indicator of hypoxemia or hypercapnia.
2. Monitor ICP (if an ICP monitoring device is in place) and MAP continuously and compare to desirable level. Document every hour or as changes occur. Calculate cerebral perfusion pressure (CPP) as changes occur. (See Appendix A, "Monitoring Standards".)	2. ICP indicates how well the three components of the intracranial cavity are balanced. CPP is the blood pressure gradient across the brain and is calculated as the difference between the incoming MAP and the opposing mean venous blood pressure, approximately equal to the ICP (CPP = MAP − ICP). Alterations in either MAP or intracranial volume affect CPP and the integrity of brain tissue. A CPP of at least 60 mm Hg must be maintained to provide minimally adequate blood supply to the brain. A CPP of less than 30 mm Hg results in cell death and is fatal.
3. Maintain MAP at a level that will result in a CPP of 60 mm Hg or more.	3. Blood pressure must be maintained to ensure adequate CPP. Between a MAP of 60 to 160 mm Hg, the brain automatically regulates blood vessel diameter to maintain constant cerebral blood flow (CBF) and thus CPP. If the autoregulatory mechanism is lost, CBF and cerebral blood volume are passively dependent on the blood pressure and CPP, so that hypotensive episodes provoke ischemia, whereas hypertensive bursts pound fluid into the brain.
• If pharmacologic support of blood pressure is needed, administer dopamine hydrochloride (Intropin) or other vasopressors, as ordered.	• Failure to reverse systemic hypotension results in worsening cerebral ischemia and necrosis.

Interventions	Rationales
• If systemic hypertension is present, titrate fluid restriction, vasodilator administration, or other therapies according to CPP, as ordered.	• Treating hypertension may be difficult because blood pressure already may be elevated as a compensatory mechanism for ischemia. Usually, blood pressure is lowered only after ICP is controlled. CPP is considered the best guide for gauging the effects of therapies to control systemic hypertension in patients with increased ICP.
4. Monitor arterial blood gas (ABG) levels as ordered. Maintain ABG levels within prescribed parameters, typically PaO_2 >80 mm Hg and $PaCO_2$ of 25 to 30 mm Hg.	4. Hypoxemia and hypercapnia are potent vasodilators and increase CBF and ICP. Keeping the patient well-oxygenated and slightly hypocapnic helps limit CBF and therefore helps control ICP.
5. Observe ICP levels with an ICP monitoring device during activities that are known to precipitate sustained increases in ICP, such as suctioning, moving the patient, emotional upsets, noxious stimuli, arousal from sleep, coughing, sneezing, or Valsalva's maneuver.	5. Clinical symptoms of increased ICP are not always present, even when a substantial increase in pressure occurs. By maintaining an awareness of activities that precipitate spikes in ICP and monitoring ICP levels, you can terminate or modify these activities as ICP increases.
6. Instruct the alert patient to avoid the following activities: straining at stool, moving or turning in bed while holding his breath, coughing, nose blowing, and extreme hip flexion (90 degrees or more).	6. These activities increase intrathoracic and intraabdominal pressure, which is transmitted to the jugular veins, impeding cerebral venous return and increasing ICP.
7. Instruct the alert patient to avoid pushing his feet against a footboard or pushing his arms against the bed.	7. These activities produce isometric muscle contractions, which increase muscle tension without lengthening the muscle. These contractions elevate systemic blood pressure and result in increased ICP.
8. Administer pharmacologic agents, as ordered, for shivering and abnormal posturing, typically chlorpromazine hydrochloride (Thorazine) for shivering and pancuronium bromide (Pavulon) for severe abnormal posturing. Document administration and effects.	8. Shivering commonly occurs in response to hypothermia, which may be used to control ICP. Shivering is a form of isometric contraction and thus can increase ICP. Abnormal posturing also produces muscle contractions, which elevate ICP.
9. Structure the environment to reduce unpleasant stimuli: • avoid unnecessary or unintended emotionally stimulating conversation (for example, about prognosis or condition) • provide a quiet room • avoid jarring the patient's bed • provide soft stimuli, such as a soft voice, soft music, and gentle touch when necessary • space painful nursing or medical procedures • when necessary to awaken, use gentle touch and soft voice • avoid unnecessary disturbances.	9. Studies have shown that unpleasant or noxious stimuli produce increases in ICP. They also increase systemic blood pressure, which may increase ICP in the patient with poor or absent autoregulation.
10. Assess the patient's level of comfort and administer ordered medications as needed, documenting administration and effectiveness: • analgesics when permitted for headache and pain • antiemetics for nausea and vomiting • stool softeners for constipation.	10. Pain, nausea, vomiting, and constipation are noxious stimuli that increase ICP. Additionally, vomiting increases intraabdominal and intrathoracic pressure, impeding venous return from the brain.
11. Use restraints only when absolutely necessary and as ordered.	11. Restraints may stimulate the patient to struggle to be free. Both the stimulation and the resulting increased activity (producing increased heart rate and increased blood flow to the brain) elevate ICP.

(continued)

Interventions

12. Space activities when possible, especially routine care activities, such as baths, oral care, and bed changes.

Rationales

12. Research indicates that closely spaced activities have a cumulative effect, causing a greater and more prolonged elevation of increased ICP than a single activity.

13. Maintain venous drainage from the brain by proper alignment and positioning: keep the head and neck in a neutral position and the head of the bed elevated 15 to 60 degrees at all times, or as ordered.

13. Because the venous cerebral system has no valves, jugular vein compression causes increased pressure throughout the system, which impedes drainage from the brain and increases ICP. Placing the patient flat or in a Trendelenburg position prevents venous drainage as well; the Trendelenburg position actually increases blood flow to the brain. Elevating the head of the bed improves venous drainage.

14. Implement therapeutic measures, as ordered:

14. Interventions help maintain ICP at a level consistent with optimal CPP.

• corticosteroids, usually dexamethasone (Decadron)

• Although the value of corticosteroids in reducing ICP is controversial, clinicians usually consider them effective in reducing cerebral edema in some clinical problems, such as tumors. Their exact mechanism of action is unknown.

• diuretics: see the "Potential fluid volume excess" nursing diagnosis in this care plan.

• Diuretics limit cerebral intracellular and extracellular swelling and CSF volume.

• CSF drainage, via an intraventricular drain

• Draining CSF helps control erratic ICP increases and is most helpful when decreased CSF absorption is causing increased ICP.

• barbiturate coma, typically with pentobarbital (Nembutal) or thiopental (Pentothal Sodium), for severe, persistent, refractory increased ICP in adults

• Barbiturates induce cerebral vasoconstriction and decrease cerebral metabolism, thus lowering ICP, preserving ischemic cells, and preventing irreversible damage. Because barbiturate coma requires complete life support and extensive nursing supervision, it is used for management of uncontrolled intracranial hypertension unresponsive to conventional treatment.

15. When noninvasive therapeutic interventions do not control ICP, prepare the patient and family for surgical intervention. (See the "Craniotomy" care plan, page 66.)

15. Surgical intervention may be necessary to control the cause, such as intracranial hematoma, or to "buy time" to prevent herniation while slower therapies reduce swelling. The latter is achieved by removing a bone flap to allow brain expansion.

16. Additional individualized interventions: ____________

16. Rationales: ____________

Target outcome criteria

Within 72 hours, the patient will:
• have ICP of 0 to 15 mm Hg and CPP >50 mm Hg
• have MAP >70 mm Hg
• display no clinical signs of increased ICP and herniation.

Within 1 week, the patient will demonstrate improved neurologic status.

Nursing diagnosis: *Potential for infection related to invasive techniques, immunosuppression, and/or surgical or other trauma*

NURSING PRIORITIES: (a) Prevent infection and (b) monitor for signs and symptoms of infection.

Interventions	Rationales
1. Maintain strict sterile or aseptic technique as appropriate: sterile catheterizations and endotracheal tube care, and aseptic technique care of closed intracranial drainage systems.	1. Sepsis is the primary concern with any invasive equipment or procedure. Using the appropriate technique will help prevent infection.
2. Change dressings as ordered, using sterile technique. Usually, change the dressing at the intracranial monitoring device site every 24 to 48 hours. Apply gentamicin or other ointment around the insertion site, only as ordered.	2. Preventing infection and sepsis is of primary importance, particularly at sites that have direct access to the brain. Cerebral infection increases the cerebral metabolic rate and CBF, thus increasing ICP. Practices regarding use of antibiotic ointment around the insertion site vary among doctors.
3. Maintain ICP and hemodynamic monitoring devices as closed systems. Do not flush the system routinely. Instill antibiotic solutions (such as bacitracin or gentamicin) via the ICP monitoring line every 24 to 48 hours, followed by flushing with normal saline solution, only as ordered.	3. Many studies suggest that a closed system is a critical factor in preventing infections in the cerebrospinal fluid. Flushing the line of an intracranial pressure monitor is not a routine procedure and is not considered a safe practice by many clinicians, so it should be done only on specific orders. Prophylactic instillation of antibiotics may be effective in helping control infection but is highly controversial.
4. Assess periodically for signs and symptoms of infection: • redness, tenderness, or warmth around all insertion sites or wounds (check daily) • cloudy or foul-smelling drainage (check daily) • fever (check every 4 hours) • elevated white blood cell (WBC) count (monitor as ordered) • positive urine, sputum, blood, or wound cultures (monitor as ordered) • infiltrates on chest X-ray (monitor as ordered).	4. Early detection of infection allows for prompt and appropriate intervention. An elevated WBC count may confirm an infection; however, the value may be elevated if the patient is on steroids.
5. Administer antibiotics, as ordered, typically if the patient has an ICP monitoring or ventricular drainage system, or if signs and symptoms of infection are present. Document administration and monitor for effectiveness and adverse reactions.	5. Broad-spectrum antibiotics may be ordered prophylactically if a direct access route to the brain exists. Once infection has been documented, selecting appropriate antibiotics is guided by culture results.
6. Additional individualized interventions: ______________	6. Rationales: ______________

Target outcome criteria

Within 48 to 72 hours, the patient will:
- have normal body temperature
- have WBC count within normal limits.

By transfer, the patient will display no indicators of infection.

Collaborative problem: *Potential for increased cerebral metabolism related to temperature elevations caused by infection and hypothalamic injury*

NURSING PRIORITY: Maintain normothermia.

Interventions	Rationales
1. Monitor and document temperature every 4 hours and as needed.	1. In the later stages of increased ICP, pressure on the hypothalamus may cause hypothalamic injury and disrupt thermoregulatory mechanisms normally controlled by the hypothalamus. Extremely elevated temperatures may result. Because an elevated temperature increases systemic and cerebral blood flow and contributes to increased ICP, it should be controlled as soon as possible.
2. Administer antipyretics, as ordered, typically acetaminophen (Tylenol). Administer tepid sponge baths, as ordered.	2. With infection, the temperature will rise because interleukin 1 (IL-1) may act as a pyrogen. Both IL-1 and the fever it triggers activate the body's defense mechanisms. These measures along with antibiotic administration (discussed previously) may be sufficient to control an elevated temperature caused by infection.
3. Apply a cooling (hypothermia) blanket, as ordered, for an elevated temperature that does not respond to more conservative measures.	3. Temperature elevation from hypothalamic injury and loss of autoregulatory control usually requires more aggressive intervention to reduce the temperature to normothermic levels.
4. Maintain appropriate precautions while the patient is on the hypothermia blanket:	4. Hypothermia has numerous physiologic effects that may result in injury.
• Cover the hypothermia blanket with a sheet or bath blanket.	• Direct contact between the patient's skin and the hypothermia blanket can cause skin damage similar to that caused by frostbite.
• Check the rectal temperature every 30 minutes (or use a rectal probe).	• The degree of hypothermia must be controlled carefully to prevent adverse reactions. A rectal thermometer or probe accurately measures body temperature.
• Turn the blanket off when the rectal temperature reaches 99.8° F. (37.7° C.).	• The patient's temperature will continue to "drift" lower as much as 10° C. and will return only gradually to room temperature because the solution inside the blanket is still cold.
• Control shivering by administering medication, as ordered, usually chlorpromazine hydrochloride (Thorazine).	• As mentioned earlier, shivering is a form of isometric contraction which results in increased ICP.
5. Remove excess bed clothes, and allow for adequate ventilation in the patient's room.	5. Inadequate ventilation and excess bed clothes maintain body temperature and increase the time needed to reduce the patient's temperature to normal.
6. Additional individualized interventions: ____________	6. Rationales: ____________

Target outcome criteria

By transfer, the patient will maintain a temperature within normal limits without the aid of a hypothermia blanket.

Collaborative problem: *Potential respiratory failure related to increased ICP, cerebral dysfunction, obstructed airway, absence of spontaneous respirations and gag or cough reflex, aspiration, atelectasis, ventilation/perfusion abnormalities, alteration in level of consciousness, or neurogenic pulmonary edema*

NURSING PRIORITY: Maintain effective gas exchange.

Interventions	Rationales
1. Assess and document the respiratory rate, depth, and pattern every 15 to 60 minutes. Notify the doctor of rate <14 or >24, shallow respirations, or changes in the respiratory pattern. Assist with intubation if the patient cannot maintain adequate airway, respiratory depth, or respiratory pattern.	1. Respiratory status is the result of a complex interplay of factors including airway patency and medullary and pontine control mechanisms. The respiratory rate is a sensitive indicator of airway patency and increasing ICP, whereas respiratory patterns may correlate with the level of brain-stem dysfunction. If the patient cannot maintain adequate gas exchange, intubation and sometimes mechanical ventilation are necessary to avert cardiopulmonary arrest.
2. Auscultate breath sounds every 2 hours and as needed to determine adequacy of aeration and presence of adventitious sounds. Observe for restlessness and tachycardia. Assess for cyanosis around the mouth, in nail beds, and in earlobes.	2. Normal breath sounds indicate proper lung expansion. Adventitious sounds may require therapeutic intervention. Restlessness and tachycardia are key findings in early hypoxemia. Cyanosis indicates inadequate gas exchange, although it is a late finding.
3. Assess the color, amount, and consistency of respiratory secretions. Culture as needed.	3. Secretions may indicate infection or the need for hydration to facilitate clearance.
4. Monitor ABG levels, as ordered. Keep ABG levels within prescribed parameters, as previously described under the "Potential cerebral ischemia" diagnosis above. Obtain chest X-rays, as ordered. Correlate the findings with clinical observations.	4. Objective documentation on the status of the pulmonary system is a valuable adjunct to clinical observations.
5. Position the patient with the head of bed elevated to the prescribed height and the patient's waist at the break in the bed.	5. Proper positioning allows for complete lung expansion.
6. Turn the patient every 2 hours, if ICP levels allow.	6. Dependent lung lobes are not fully expanded, thus compromising gas exchange. Turning allows for full expansion of all lobes and aids in preventing atelectasis and pneumonia, which interfere with gas exchange. However, turning may increase ICP levels, as described earlier, so its benefits must be weighed against its risk.
7. Suction as needed, hyperventilating with 100% oxygen before and after suctioning and limiting suctioning to <15 seconds.	7. Suctioning-induced hypoxemia contributes to increased ICP and compromised CPP. Suctioning can raise ICP to levels as high as 100 mm Hg.
8. Implement care related to mechanical ventilation, if used. See the "Mechanical Ventilation" care plan, page 108.	8. CO_2 and oxygen levels are more precisely controlled when the patient is intubated and ventilated mechanically. The "Mechanical Ventilation" care plan contains detailed information about this intervention.
9. Additional individualized interventions: ______________	9. Rationales: ______________

Target outcome criteria

Within 24 hours, the patient will:
- have an airway free of secretions
- have ABG levels within desired limits
- have a clear chest X-ray.

By transfer, the patient will:
- have a normal respiratory rate and pattern
- have normal ABG levels.

Nursing diagnosis: *Potential for fluid volume deficit related to diuretic therapy, fluid restriction, diabetes insipidus (DI), hyperthermia, and/or GI suction*

NURSING PRIORITY: Maintain fluid volume within prescribed limits.

Interventions	Rationales
1. See Appendix C, "Fluid-Electrolyte Imbalances".	1. The "Fluid-Electrolyte Imbalances" appendix contains general information on these problems. This plan focuses on problems specific to increased ICP.
2. Monitor and correlate intake and output, on both an hourly and cumulative basis. Measure and document specific gravity. Report the following:	2. Diuretic therapy, hyperthermia, a restricted fluid intake, and DI (explained below) may produce an overwhelming fluid deficit. Hourly and cumulative correlation of values aids in prompt deficit detection.
• output >200 ml/hour for 2 hours, with specific gravity 1.001 to 1.005	• Urine output >200 ml/hour usually indicates DI. In patients with increased ICP, DI results from failure of the pituitary gland to secrete antidiuretic hormone (ADH) because of damage to the hypothalamus, the supraopticohypophyseal tract, or the posterior lobe of the pituitary gland. The most common clinical setting of DI in this case is after neurosurgery, but it can also occur secondary to vascular lesions or severe head injury. Because ADH is absent, the renal tubules fail to conserve water, resulting in the excretion of large volumes of dilute urine. The low specific gravity reflects the dilute urine. Urine output of this magnitude can rapidly create a fluid volume deficit.
• output <30 ml/hour for 2 hours, with specific gravity >1.030.	• A urine output of <30 ml/hour for 2 hours with a high specific gravity indicates that a fluid volume deficit already exists.
3. Monitor laboratory values, as ordered. Report the following: • urine osmolality, usually <200 mOsm/kg • serum osmolality, usually >300 mOsm/kg • serum sodium, usually >145 mEq/L • hematocrit and BUN, usually elevated.	3. Laboratory values provide objective evidence of an imbalance. The low urine osmolality reflects the diuresis occurring, whereas the elevated serum osmolality, serum sodium, and hematocrit reflect hemoconcentration.
4. Monitor the EKG and hemodynamic pressures continuously. Report promptly:	4. Continuous monitoring provides prompt warning of potentially fatal conditions.
• the appearance of U waves, prolonged QT interval, depressed ST segment, and low T waves	• EKG signs reflect cardiac cells' decreased responsiveness to stimuli, which results from hypokalemia secondary to renal potassium washout.
• dysrhythmias, particularly bradycardia, first and second degree heart block, atrial dysrhythmias, and premature ventricular contractions (PVCs)	• Bradycardia, heart blocks, atrial dysrhythmias, and PVCs reflect hypokalemia. Prompt treatment is necessary to prevent hypokalemic arrest.
• low hemodynamic pressures and cardiac output.	• Low pressures reflect hypovolemia, whereas decreased cardiac output indicates insufficient preload.

Interventions	Rationales
5. Administer replacement therapy, as ordered, usually isotonic solution with potassium chloride (KCl) added if serum potassium is low. Monitor the I.V. flow rate closely. Anticipate increased fluid requirements if hyperthermia or infection is present.	5. Isotonic solution is the replacement fluid of choice for loss of body fluids. Close monitoring is essential to prevent fluid volume overload. Solutions with potassium should be carefully monitored because potassium is very irritating to the vein, and hyperkalemia can be easily produced by potassium rapid infusion. Hyperkalemia can result in complete heart block, ventricular fibrillation, and ventricular standstill. Hyperthermia and infection accelerate fluid loss via an increased metabolic rate and increased skin and respiratory fluid excretion.
6. Additional individualized interventions: ________	6. Rationales: ________

Target outcome criteria

By transfer, the patient will:

- maintain a urine output within normal limits
- have electrolytes, hematocrit, BUN, and serum osmolality within normal limits
- maintain hemodynamic values within normal limits.

Nursing diagnosis: *Potential fluid volume excess related to stress, steroid therapy, or syndrome of inappropriate antidiuretic hormone (SIADH) secretion*

NURSING PRIORITY: Maintain fluid volume within prescribed limits.

Interventions	Rationales
1. See Appendix C, "Fluid-Electrolyte Imbalances".	1. The "Fluid-Electrolyte Imbalances" appendix contains general information on fluid and electrolyte problems. This plan focuses on problems specific to increased ICP.
2. Monitor and correlate intake and output hourly. Report a urine output <30 ml/hour for 2 hours with specific gravity >1.030. Insert an indwelling urinary catheter, if necessary and as ordered.	2. Carefully monitoring fluid intake and urinary output helps detect potential problems that increase ICP. Decreased urinary output may reflect a fluid volume deficit (see the previous diagnosis) or SIADH, whereas high specific gravity reflects avid water reabsorption. SIADH is characterized by abnormally high levels or continuous secretion of ADH, resulting in water being continually reabsorbed from the kidney tubules. Increased ADH secretion is caused by several factors present in patients with increased ICP, including hyperthermia, hypotension, trauma, stress response, and administration of drugs, such as chlorpromazine hydrochloride (Thorazine), barbiturates, and acetaminophen (Tylenol). Sodium and water retention also are caused by corticosteroids and the physiologic response to stress. Awareness of water retention may prevent further complications, such as pulmonary edema.
3. Monitor electrolytes, BUN level, creatinine, osmolality, and hematocrit daily or as ordered. Report the following: • urine osmolality, usually high • serum osmolality, usually <280 mOsm/kg • serum sodium, usually <126 mEq/L • hematocrit and BUN levels, usually low.	3. High urine osmolality reflects water retention. Low serum osmolality, sodium, hematocrit, and BUN levels reflect hemodilution.

(continued)

Interventions	Rationales
4. Monitor the EKG and hemodynamic pressures continuously. Report promptly:	4. Constant monitoring provides early warning of impending problems.
• the appearance of U waves, prolonged QT interval, depressed ST segment, or low T waves	• The EKG reflects a dilutional hypokalemia.
• dysrhythmias, particularly bradycardia, first- and second-degree heart block, atrial dysrhythmias, and premature ventricular contractions	• The rhythms listed are those precipitated commonly by hypokalemia.
• elevated hemodynamic pressures and decreased cardiac output.	• Hemodynamic pressures indicate fluid overload, whereas decreased cardiac output results from the heart's inability to handle the excessive preload.
5. Institute therapy, as ordered.	5. An increase in cerebral blood volume increases ICP.
• fluid restriction	• Fluid restriction aids in decreasing extracellular fluid in the body. Patients usually are maintained in a slightly dehydrated state.
• diuretics, generally mannitol and furosemide (Lasix).	• Mannitol is an osmotic diuretic that moves water from the brain and CSF into plasma by an osmotic gradient, thus decreasing ICP. Furosemide, a loop diuretic, inhibits distal tubular reabsorption, promoting diuresis. Additionally, furosemide appears to selectively dehydrate injured cerebral tissue, thus reducing cerebral edema and ICP.
6. Additional individualized interventions: ______________	6. Rationales: ______________

Target outcome criteria

By transfer, the patient will:

- display electrolyte levels, BUN, hematocrit, and serum osmolality within normal limits
- have a urine output within normal limits
- manifest hemodynamic values within normal limits.

Nursing diagnosis: *Potential for injury related to decreased level of consciousness, seizure activity, and drug therapy*

NURSING PRIORITY: Maintain patient safety.

Interventions	Rationales
1. Observe the patient closely at all times. Keep side rails up at all times, except for periods of direct nursing care.	1. Decreased level of consciousness is one of the earliest indications of increased ICP. The patient may not be alert and aware of surroundings and possible danger, for example, falling out of bed.
2. Assess for seizure activity. Implement seizure precautions, such as padded side rails. Administer and document anticonvulsant medication, as ordered, generally phenytoin (Dilantin).	2. Seizure activity may be precipitated by the altered neuronal function caused by increased ICP. If the patient does have a seizure, padded side rails lessen the potential for physical injury such as cuts, abrasions, and fractures.
3. Assess for gastric bleeding. Administer medications, as ordered, usually antacids, such as Maalox, or cimetidine (Tagamet).	3. Gastric irritation and GI bleeding are major adverse reactions of corticosteroid therapy. Also, gastric bleeding occurs with increased ICP, although the exact mechanism is unknown. Increased ICP hypothetically stimulates the vagal nuclei directly, resulting in hypersecretion of gastric acid and hyperacidity. Patients with increased ICP are usually placed on prophylactic antacid and cimetidine therapy to decrease the risk of bleeding.

Interventions	Rationales
4. Assess for an absent corneal reflex and apply artificial tears and eye patches, as needed.	4. During the later stages of increased ICP, brain-stem dysfunction results in the loss of the corneal reflex. Artificial tears lubricate the eyes, whereas both the tears and patches prevent injury to the cornea.
5. Additional individualized interventions: ____________	5. Rationales: ____________

Target outcome criteria
During the unit stay, the patient will remain free of injury.

Transfer planning

NURSING TRANSFER CRITERIA

Upon transfer, documentation shows evidence of:
- stable ICP within normal limits
- stable vital signs
- absence of pulmonary or cardiovascular complications
- absence of gastrointestinal bleeding
- normal fluid and electrolyte balance
- ABG levels within normal limits
- stable temperature
- stable neurologic function
- removal of ICP monitoring line.

PATIENT-FAMILY TEACHING CHECKLIST

Document evidence that patient and family demonstrate understanding of:

___ nature of causative factors for increased ICP
___ extent of neurologic deficits, if present
___ need for continued family support
___ requirements for rehabilitation program, if known.

DOCUMENTATION CHECKLIST

Using outcome criteria as a guide, document:

___ clinical status on admission
___ significant changes in status
___ pertinent laboratory/diagnostic test findings
___ fluid intake and output
___ neurologic status
___ neurologic deficits, if present
___ GI bleeding, if any
___ seizure activity, if any.

ASSOCIATED CARE PLANS

Acute Pain
Impaired Physical Mobility
Ineffective Coping
Knowledge Deficit
Nutritional Deficit
Sensory-Perceptual Alteration

REFERENCES

Boortz-Marx, R. "Factors Affecting Intracranial Pressure: A Descriptive Study," *Journal of Neurosurgical Nursing* 17(2):89-94, April 1985.

Caine, R.M., and Bufalina, P.M., eds. *Nursing Care Planning Guides for Adults.* Baltimore: Williams and Wilkins, 1987.

Gordon, M. *Nursing Diagnosis, Process and Application,* 2nd ed. New York: McGraw-Hill Book Co., 1987.

Habermann-Little, B. "Increased Intracranial Pressure and Herniation Syndromes," in *Acute Neuroscience Nursing Concepts and Care.* Edited by Lundgren, J. Boston: Jones and Bartlett Publishers, Inc., 1986.

Hickey, J.V. *The Clinical Practice of Neurological and Neurosurgical Nursing,* 2nd ed. Philadelphia: J.B. Lippincott Co., 1986.

Jimm-Zegeer, L. "Brain Edema: Concepts and Nursing Care," in *Acute Neuroscience Nursing Concepts and Care.* Edited by Lundgren, J. Boston: Jones and Bartlett Publishers, Inc., 1986.

Kee, J.L. *Laboratory and Diagnostic Tests with Nursing Implications,* 2nd ed. East Norwalk, Conn.: Appleton & Lange, 1987.

Kenner, C.V., et al. *Critical Care Nursing, Body, Mind, Spirit,* 2nd ed. Boston: Little, Brown & Co., 1985.

Lewis, S.M., and Collier, I.C. *Medical-Surgical Nursing Assessment and Management of Clinical Problems,* 2nd ed. New York: McGraw-Hill Book Co., 1987.

Nikas, D.L. "Critical Aspects of Head Trauma," *Critical Care Nursing Quarterly* 10(1):19-40, June 1987.

Nikas, D.L., ed. *The Critically Ill Neurosurgical Patient.* New York: Churchill Livingstone, 1982.

Ricci, M., ed. *American Association of Neuroscience Nurses Core Curriculum for Neuroscience Nursing,* vol. 1. Park Ridge, Ill.: American Association of Neuroscience Nurses, 1984.

Robinet, K. "Increased Intracranial Pressure: Management with an Intraventricular Catheter," *Journal of Neurosurgical Nursing* 17(2):95-104, April 1985.

Walleck, C.A. "Intracranial Hypertension: Interventions and Outcomes," *Critical Care Nursing Quarterly* 101:45-54, June 1987.

Seizures

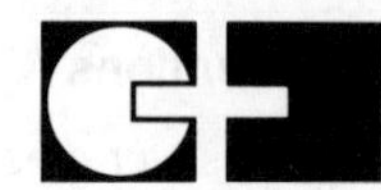

DRG information

DRG 024 Seizure and Headache. Age over 17.
With Complications or Comorbidity (CC).
Mean LOS = 5.2 days
Principal diagnoses include:
• cerebral arteritis
• convulsions or epilepsy (seizures)
• benign intracranial hypertension (increased intracranial pressure)
• reaction to spinal or lumbar puncture
• postconcussion syndrome.

DRG 025 Seizure and Headache. Age over 17.
Without CC.
Mean LOS = 3.6 days
Principal diagnoses include selected principal diagnoses listed under DRG 024.

DRG 026 Seizure and Headache. Age 0 to 17.
Mean LOS = 2.5 days
Principal diagnoses include selected principal diagnoses listed under DRG 024.

Introduction

DEFINITION AND TIME FOCUS

A seizure represents uncontrolled, paroxysmal, abnormal electrical discharge in the central nervous system (CNS). The precise mechanism involved is not known, but a decreased neuronal firing threshold or excessive irritability is suspected.

Seizures are described as primary or secondary, depending on whether the cause can be identified. Primary (idiopathic) seizures appear without any identifiable cause, commonly arising in childhood, and may result from a congenital tendency. Secondary seizures are triggered by specific metabolic, structural, chemical, or physical abnormalities. Diagnostically, seizures are classified into two broad groups: partial and generalized. Partial seizures involve localized areas of brain irritability and are characterized by physical activity that corresponds to the affected area of the brain. Loss of consciousness may not occur. Generalized seizures involve both brain hemispheres and, usually, major bilateral muscle activity and loss of consciousness.

In the critical care setting, seizures are seen commonly as a sign of underlying abnormality, and any seizure, even in a patient with a preexisting seizure history, must be evaluated within the context of the patient's overall condition. In some patients, a single, brief seizure episode may be of minimal concern; in others, it may represent grave deterioration in the patient's neurologic status. Persistent or recurrent generalized seizures warrant immediate pharmacologic control and prompt identification and treatment of the underlying cause. Because seizures present such a wide range of physical manifestations, this care plan focuses on the patient exhibiting generalized tonic-clonic seizures; you should, however, be knowledgeable about and alert for more subtle types of seizure activity as well.

ETIOLOGY AND PRECIPITATING FACTORS

• metabolic conditions—hyperpyrexia, hypoxia, hypoglycemia, hyperglycemia, electrolyte imbalances, uremia, fluid overload
• chemical or pharmacologic conditions—inadequate serum anticonvulsant levels, alcohol or drug overdose or toxicity, alcohol or drug withdrawal
• infections— meningitis and encephalitis
• structural or physical conditions—increased intracranial pressure (ICP), cerebral edema, cerebral or subdural hematoma, cerebral hemorrhage, eclampsia, malignant hypertension, tumor, congenital malformations
• degenerative conditions—Alzheimer's disease, multiple sclerosis, systemic lupus erythematosus
• reduced cardiac output—Stokes-Adams syncope, other dysrhythmias
• idiopathic origin

Focused assessment guidelines

Note: The patient exhibiting generalized seizure activity in the critical care setting usually cannot provide relevant historical information, so the nursing history (functional health patterns) section of this care plan has been omitted. Instead, guidelines for observing and documenting the seizure activity are presented as an essential aid to accurate diagnosis and effective intervention. Attempt to describe findings with precision and accuracy, as follows:

Preictal phase

• Did an aura or warning precede seizure onset? What was the patient doing when the seizure began (or when the aura was noted)?

Tonic-clonic phases

• Did the patient give a shrill cry?
• Did the patient fall?
• What kind of movement was noted first?
• Where did it begin?
• Were other areas progressively involved? If so, in what pattern?
• If a tonic (rigid) phase occurred, how long did it last?
• If a clonic (jerking) phase occurred, how long did it last?
• How long did the entire seizure last?
• Was the patient incontinent?

• During the phases of the seizure, did the pupils react? Deviate?
• Did the patient lose consciousness? If so, when?

Postictal phase

• What was the patient's level of consciousness after the seizure?
• Did the patient exhibit amnesia, confusion, disorientation, or agitation when he regained consciousness?
• Did the patient have any motor, sensory, or perceptual deficits after the seizure?
• How long did the postictal phase last?

PHYSICAL FINDINGS

Note: Physical findings vary widely, depending on the type of seizure activity, the area of brain tissue involved, and the phase of the seizure. All findings have a neurologic origin, but they have been grouped by body systems here to help in the organization of the assessment. This list is only partial; the range of physical manifestations is almost limitless.

General appearance

• tonic—shrill cry
• clonic—facial grimacing
• clonic—excessive salivation

Neurologic

• tonic and clonic—loss of consciousness
• tonic and clonic—dilated fixed pupils, possibly deviating laterally
• postictal—confusion, disorientation, amnesia

Musculoskeletal

• tonic—opisthotonos
• tonic—rigidity
• tonic—jaw clenching
• tonic—extension of extremities
• tonic—clenched fists
• clonic—bilateral, rhythmic, jerking motions
• postictal—flaccidity

Pulmonary

• tonic—apneic period, usually lasting 10 to 30 seconds, occasionally as long as 60 seconds
• clonic—stertorous respirations

Renal

• clonic—urinary incontinence

Gastrointestinal

• clonic—fecal incontinence

Integumentary

• tonic—cyanosis
• clonic—diaphoresis
• clonic—flushing

Cardiovascular

• tonic—bradycardia (slowed heart rate)
• clonic—bradycardia or tachycardia
• clonic—initially, elevated blood pressure; after 30 minutes, blood pressure may fall as autonomic mechanisms fail

DIAGNOSTIC STUDIES

Because a seizure represents a clinical sign, not a diagnosis, testing is usually done to determine the seizure's cause. The following tests are a partial list of possible studies that may be ordered for this purpose.
• serum glucose tests—may be ordered to rule out hypoglycemia or hyperglycemia as a cause of seizure
• serum phenytoin or serum phenobarbital levels—may be obtained to evaluate sufficient dosage of anticonvulsant in patients with known seizure history
• blood urea nitrogen, creatinine studies—may be obtained to evaluate renal function because uremia may precipitate seizures
• serum electrolytes—may be ordered because electrolyte imbalances, particularly calcium deficit, may precipitate seizure activity
• arterial blood gas values—may be obtained because hypoxia may precipitate seizures or result from prolonged seizure activity or associated respiratory depression
• toxicology screens—may be ordered if drug ingestion is suspected as a causative factor
• blood cultures—may be obtained to rule out sepsis as a cause of seizures
• computed tomography (CT) scan—may identify cerebral abnormality, such as tumor, arteriovenous malformation, hemorrhage, or edema
• lumbar puncture—may identify infection, indicated by bacteria, increased white blood cell count, and decreased glucose level in cerebrospinal fluid. Increased pressure may indicate a space-occupying lesion, or bleeding may indicate hemorrhage
• EEG—may identify the lesion area. Increased electrical activity and spikes are characteristically seen with generalized motor seizures. Repeated studies may be necessary to record actual seizure activity
• magnetic resonance imaging (MRI)—may reveal intracerebral abnormality
• skull X-rays—may indicate fractures or areas of calcification
• cerebral angiography—evaluates cerebral circulatory status and identifies vascular abnormalities
• ICP monitoring—may be instituted to monitor for possible increased ICP as cause of seizure

POTENTIAL COMPLICATIONS

• status epilepticus
• airway obstruction
• respiratory arrest
• aspiration pneumonia
• hyperthermia
• hypoglycemia
• renal failure
• cerebral ischemia

Nursing diagnosis: *Ineffective airway clearance related to loss of consciousness, apnea, excessive secretions, jaw clenching, and/or airway occlusion by tongue or foreign body*

NURSING PRIORITIES: (a) Maintain patent airway and (b) promote adequate oxygenation.

Interventions	Rationales
1. If an aura or warning phase occurs, clear the patient's mouth of any foreign bodies and insert a soft cloth or gauze pad at the corner of the mouth. Never try to force the jaw open or insert an oral airway during the seizure. Turn the patient to the side and use the chin lift or jaw thrust maneuver as needed to maintain an open airway.	1. Insertion of a soft airway protector may help keep the tongue from occluding the airway and reduce the risk of trauma to the tongue and teeth. Attempts to force the jaw open or insert objects during actual seizure activity may cause damage to the teeth or injury to the caregiver. Turning the patient to the side promotes drainage of saliva from the mouth and reduces the risk of aspiration. An apneic period of up to 60 seconds is usually followed by resumption of spontaneous respiration. If the airway becomes occluded during the tonic phase, significant hypoxia may ensue, so maintenance of an open airway is essential.
2. Suction the oropharynx, as needed. Provide supplemental oxygen via nasal cannula.	2. During the clonic and postictal phases, the obtunded patient is at risk for aspirating saliva that has accumulated during the tonic phase. Vomiting may also occur. Supplemental oxygen is indicated because seizure activity causes increased oxygen demands. Also, some degree of respiratory depression commonly follows generalized seizure activity. A cannula is preferred because a mask may hamper airway clearance if vomiting occurs.
3. If seizure activity is persistent (unresponsive to drug therapy) or frequently recurring, notify the doctor immediately and anticipate the need for endotracheal intubation and mechanical ventilation. See the "Mechanical Ventilation" care plan, page 108.	3. Status epilepticus, in which seizure activity persists or recurs without the patient regaining consciousness, is a medical emergency. Irreversible brain damage may result from the prolonged apnea that occurs. Mechanical ventilation may be necessary to ensure adequate oxygenation while attempting to stop the seizures. The "Mechanical Ventilation" care plan contains detailed interventions for the care of the patient on a ventilator.
4. Insert a nasogastric tube and connect it to low suction, as ordered.	4. Emptying the stomach of gastric contents prevents accidental aspiration should vomiting occur.
5. Additional individualized interventions: ______________	5. Rationales: ______________

Target outcome criteria

Throughout seizure duration, the patient will maintain clear airway.

Collaborative problem: *Potential status epilepticus related to inadequate pharmacologic control or misidentification of underlying cause*

NURSING PRIORITIES: (a) Stop seizure activity and (b) treat underlying cause(s).

Interventions	Rationales
1. Administer I.V. anticonvulsant medication, as ordered. Commonly ordered medications for acute seizure activity include the following:	1. Prolonged seizure activity may result in respiratory depression or arrest, cardiovascular insufficiency, or cerebral edema. Anticonvulsant medications suppress the ectopic focus.
• diazepam (Valium), 5 to 10 mg, I.V. push. Observe the patient closely for respiratory depression. Monitor for undesirable drug interactions, especially if the patient is also taking phenothiazines, barbiturates, narcotics, or monoamine oxidase inhibitors.	• Diazepam is the initial drug of choice for generalized motor status epilepticus, although it is neither recommended nor sufficient for ongoing seizure control. It appears to act on the limbic system, thalamus, and hypothalamus to stop seizure activity. Respiratory depression is a common adverse reaction. The medications listed may potentiate the actions of diazepam and increase the risk of respiratory compromise.
• phenobarbital (Luminal) and other barbiturate anticonvulsants. The usual dose of phenobarbital ranges from 60 to 400 mg/day. Observe the patient closely for respiratory depression, especially if the patient also received diazepam. Monitor carefully for undesirable drug interactions, especially if the patient is on phenothiazines, warfarin, digoxin, or disulfiram (Antabuse).	• Like diazepam, phenobarbital depresses the central nervous system. Its precise action is unclear, but it appears to reduce cerebral oxygen consumption and may help decrease intracranial pressure. It also potentiates phenothiazines. Phenobarbital may decrease warfarin absorption and digoxin metabolism. Antabuse may increase the likelihood of toxicity.
• phenytoin (Dilantin). Usual loading dose is 10 to 15 mg/kg, followed by 100 mg every 6 to 8 hours. Administer phenytoin slowly in normal saline solution, giving no more than 50 mg/minute. Observe the patient's EKG during phenytoin administration. Monitor closely for adverse reactions or indications of possible toxicity, such as anemia, elevated serum glucose levels, GI upset, and diplopia with nystagmus.	• Phenytoin appears to act on the motor cortex to stabilize the threshold against neuronal hyperexcitability, possibly by aiding the efflux of sodium from neurons. Phenytoin must be administered in saline solutions because it precipitates in glucose-containing solutions. EKG monitoring is essential; giving phenytoin too rapidly may cause dysrhythmias or cardiac arrest.
• Monitor therapeutic blood levels, as ordered.	• Assessing serum phenytoin levels is essential to achieve the optimum dosage and minimize the risk of toxicity.
• Monitor carefully for possible drug interactions. Drugs that may increase serum phenytoin levels include chloramphenicol, isoniazid, salicylates, sulfonamides, cimetidine, warfarin, and benzodiazepines; acute alcohol ingestion also may increase serum phenytoin levels. Phenytoin may increase metabolism of warfarin and digitoxin. Digitoxin, reserpine, prednisone, phenobarbital, and chronic alcoholism may decrease phenytoin levels.	• Phenytoin reacts with many other medications. Achieving seizure control may involve careful balancing of several pharmacologic parameters. Be aware of the possibility of untoward reactions to avert possible toxicity or inadequate therapeutic effect.
2. Consider possible underlying causes. Assist with identification and treatment.	2. In a patient without a history of seizures, treating the underlying cause is paramount to seizure control.
• head trauma	• Secondary seizures are caused most commonly by head trauma. If the patient was admitted after an acute traumatic event, this link may be obvious. However, seizures may occur months or even years after head injury, as scar tissue creates a focus for abnormal neuronal activity, so careful history-taking is indicated.
• electrolyte imbalance	• Electrolyte imbalances may precipitate seizures by altering cell membrane permeability, thus interfering with normal neuronal electrical conduction.
• hypoxia	• Sufficient oxygen is essential for maintaining the normal neuronal ionic gradient. Any condition that lowers the level of oxygen delivered to sensitive brain tissue may contribute to seizure activity.

(continued)

Interventions	Rationales
• hypoglycemia or hyperglycemia	• Cerebral neurons are exquisitely sensitive to decreased glucose levels because glucose is their primary substrate. A sudden drop in blood glucose appears more likely to precipitate neurologic problems than a gradual decline. Hyperglycemia may contribute to a hyperosmolar crenation of brain cells, with resultant irritability and altered conduction pathways. Also, seizure activity increases cerebral metabolic needs and depletes stores of glucose and energy.
• brain tumors	• Seizures are the major initial sign in as many as 18% of patients with undetected brain tumors. Tissue compression from tumor growth is the likely precipitating mechanism.
• infections	• Infections may contribute to seizures for several possible reasons: scarring in response to inflammatory changes, cerebral edema in acute infections, hyperpyrexia, abscesses, or autoimmune demyelinization, as in encephalomyelitis.
• cerebral hemorrhage	• Localized ischemic damage to brain tissue may cause seizures.
• toxins.	• Toxins may cause seizures by interfering with the cell's metabolic processes, altering cell membrane function and integrity. Some hydrocarbons, lead, mercury, and arsenic may cause seizures in high concentrations. Hypersensitive persons may develop seizures in response to certain medications, such as phenothiazines. Withdrawal from alcohol or barbiturates is a common cause of seizures because abrupt withdrawal from the CNS-depressant effects of either appears to increase neuronal irritability.
3. If seizures are refractory to drug therapy, anticipate possible preparation for neuromuscular blockade or general anesthesia, with mechanical ventilation.	3. Status epilepticus has a mortality of about 10% and causes one third of all seizure-related deaths. As seizure activity persists, cerebral vasodilation occurs, perfusion pressure drops, and irreversible cell damage follows from nutritional depletion and neuronal exhaustion. Neuromuscular blockade stops motor activity but does not directly interrupt brain electrical activity. General anesthesia causes global depression of cerebral function, interrupting the cycle of hyperexcitability at its source.
4. Additional individualized interventions: ______________________	4. Rationales: ______________________

Target outcome criteria

Following onset of seizure activity, the patient will:
- be recognized as being at risk for status epilepticus
- receive appropriate anticonvulsants promptly
- have underlying causes identified and treated.

During the critical care unit stay, the patient will:
- maintain therapeutic drug levels
- receive appropriate therapy for underlying cause of seizures.

Nursing diagnosis: *Potential for injury: trauma or myoglobinuria related to excessive uncontrolled muscle activity*

NURSING PRIORITY: Prevent injury.

Interventions	Rationales
1. At the seizure's onset, ensure safe patient positioning. Place pillows or padding around the patient and raise and pad the bed side rails. Do not restrain arms and legs.	1. Violent muscle contractions may cause injury unless protective measures are instituted. Padded side rails help prevent injury if the patient strikes the rails during the seizure. Restraining arms and legs may result in fractures during the clonic phase.
2. During the seizure, stay with the patient. Provide privacy, as possible.	2. The seizing patient is extremely vulnerable to injury because he cannot control muscle activity. Patients are commonly embarrassed and ashamed of the loss of control. Providing privacy helps protect the patient's dignity.
3. After motor activity stops, perform a neurologic evaluation, noting pupil size and reactivity, level of consciousness, responsiveness to stimuli, and respiratory status. Repeat the evaluation every 15 to 30 minutes until condition stabilizes. Inspect the oropharynx, tongue, and teeth for seizure-related injury.	3. Careful monitoring of status during the postictal period is essential because respiratory depression is common. Violent seizure activity may result in mouth injury. Oropharyngeal bleeding or loose teeth may be aspirated.
4. Avoid excessive environmental stimulation during the postictal period.	4. Environmental stimulation, such as bright lights; loud, sudden noises; or abrupt movement, may reactivate neuronal irritability and stimulate further seizure activity.
5. If seizure activity was prolonged, monitor urine for possible myoglobinuria, indicated by a red or cola color. Send urine sample for myoglobin testing. Report findings to the doctor promptly.	5. Repeated, vigorous muscle contraction releases excess amounts of myoglobin into the bloodstream from muscle cell breakdown. If the quantity is sufficient, the accumulated myoglobin may occlude the kidneys and cause renal failure. Treatment involves flushing the renal system, using fluids and diuretics.
6. Additional individualized interventions: ______	6. Rationales: ______

Target outcome criteria
During and after the seizure episode, the patient will experience no injury from muscular contractions.

Transfer planning

NURSING TRANSFER CRITERIA

Upon transfer, documentation shows evidence of:
- cause of seizure activity identified and treated
- seizure activity controlled
- respiratory status stable
- neurologic status stable.

PATIENT-FAMILY TEACHING CHECKLIST

Document evidence that patient and family demonstrate understanding of:
__ cause and implications of seizure activity
__ treatment modalities instituted
__ signs of possible recurrence
__ safety precautions.

DOCUMENTATION CHECKLIST

Using outcome criteria as a guide, document:
__ clinical status on admission
__ significant changes in status
__ pertinent diagnostic test findings
__ episodes of seizure activity
__ safety precautions instituted
__ pharmacologic interventions
__ patient and family teaching
__ transfer planning.

ASSOCIATED CARE PLANS

Craniotomy
Diabetes Ketoacidosis
Drug Overdose
Hyperglycemic Hyperosmolar Nonketosis
Increased Intracranial Pressure
Mechanical Ventilation
Multiple Trauma
Sensory-Perceptual Alteration

REFERENCES

Alspach, J., and Williams, S. *Core Curriculum for Critical Care Nursing,* 3rd ed. Philadelphia: W.B. Saunders Co., 1983.

Burrell, L., and Burrell, Z. *Critical Care,* 4th ed. St. Louis: C.V. Mosby Co., 1982.

Henneman, E. "Brain Resuscitation," *Heart & Lung* 151:3-11, January 1986.

Hudak, C., et al. *Critical Care Nursing: A Holistic Approach,* 4th ed. Philadelphia: J.B. Lippincott Co., 1986.

Kneisl, C., and Ames, S. *Adult Health Nursing: A Biopsychosocial Approach.* Menlo Park, Calif.: Addison-Wesley Publishing Co., 1986.

Rudy, E. *Advanced Neurological and Neurosurgical Nursing.* St. Louis: C.V. Mosby Co., 1984.

Thompson, J., et al. *Clinical Nursing.* St. Louis: C.V. Mosby Co., 1986.

RESPIRATORY SYSTEM

Adult Respiratory Distress Syndrome

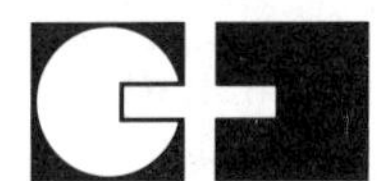

DRG information

DRG 099 Respiratory Signs and Symptoms.
With Complications or Cormorbidity (CC).
Mean LOS = 4.2 days
Principal diagnoses include:
- adult respiratory distress syndrome(ARDS)
- dyspnea and other respiratory abnormalities
- hemoptysis
- cough.

DRG 100 Respiratory Signs and Symptoms.
Without CC.
Mean LOS = 2.9 days
Principal diagnoses include selected principal diagnoses listed under DRG 099. The distinction is that DRG 100 excludes CC.

DRG 087 Pulmonary Edema and Respiratory Failure.
Mean LOS = 6.1 days
Principal diagnoses include:
- ARDS caused by trauma or after surgery
- respiratory failure
- pulmonary edema.

DRG 475 Respiratory System Diagnosis With Ventilator Support.
Mean LOS = 8.8 days
Principal diagnoses include:
- respiratory failure
- chronic obstructive pulmonary disease
- acute or chronic bronchitis
- pneumonia of various etiologies
- ARDS.

Additional DRG information: ARDS is rarely a principal diagnosis. It is most often seen as a CC to other diseases, trauma, or surgery. Used as a secondary diagnosis, it can increase the weight of a particular DRG because it qualiifies as a CC. The above DRGs, however, are calculated with ARDS as a principal diagnosis.

Introduction

DEFINITION AND TIME FOCUS

ARDS is a complex, poorly understood syndrome of diffuse damage to the alveolar-capillary membrane. The most common cause of respiratory failure in the critical care unit, ARDS may represent the ultimate manifestation of several unrelated physiologic insults that produce direct or indirect pulmonary injury. Key clinical features necessary for its diagnosis include a history consistent with ARDS, moderate to severe hypoxemia, bilateral diffuse infiltrates on chest X-ray, and exclusion of other causes of pulmonary congestion, specifically left heart failure.

Known by many other names (such as noncardiogenic pulmonary edema, shock lung, and postpump lung), ARDS is characterized by interstitial and alveolar pulmonary edema resulting from increased permeability of the pulmonary microvasculature. Other key pathophysiologic features include a massive pulmonary shunt, decreased lung compliance, and increased alveolar dead space. On autopsy, lungs are heavy and wet, demonstrating congestive atelectasis, and marked by hyaline membrane formation and pulmonary fibrosis.

The chemical mediators involved in ARDS are complex and poorly understood. One interesting theory is that in sepsis, bacteria stimulate granulocytes lodged in the lung. The resulting oxidative burst involves the release of toxic metabolites (such as free radicals) and proteolytic enzymes, both of which can cause severe pulmonary injury. Other chemical mediators implicated in ARDS include histamine, serotonin, and prostaglandins. This care plan focuses on the patient newly diagnosed with ARDS.

ETIOLOGY AND PRECIPITATING FACTORS

- gram-negative sepsis, *Pneumocystis carinii* pneumonia, bacterial or viral pneumonia, or other infections
- aspiration of gastric contents, fresh or salt water (near drowning), or other liquids
- pulmonary contusion, nonthoracic trauma, burns, or other types of trauma
- inhalation of smoke, toxic levels of oxygen, corrosive chemicals, or other toxins
- shock of any etiology
- fat embolism, cardiopulmonary bypass, massive transfusions, disseminated intravascular coagulation, transfusion reaction, or other hematologic causes
- drug overdose, particularly heroin, methadone, and propoxyphene (Darvon).

Focused assessment guidelines

NURSING HISTORY (Functional health pattern findings)

Health perception–health management pattern

- demonstrates a history of catastrophic pulmonary insult followed by a lag time of several hours to several days and then progressive dyspnea

PHYSICAL FINDINGS

General appearance

- restlessness

Pulmonary
- tachypnea
- hyperventilation
- progressive dyspnea
- fine, diffuse crackles
- increased peak inspiratory pressure (if on ventilator)

Neurologic
- deteriorating level of consciousness

Integumentary
- cyanosis

DIAGNOSTIC STUDIES
No single diagnostic test exists for ARDS.
- arterial blood gas (ABG) values—reveal moderate to severe hypoxemia ($PaO_2 < 50$ mm Hg), even when the inspired oxygen concentration is > 60%, and hypercarbia ($PaCO_2 > 50$ mm Hg)
- alveolar-arterial gradient—reveals increased gradient (>15 mm Hg on room air or > 50 mm Hg on 100% oxygen)
- shunt calculation—reveals pulmonary shunt in excess of 5%, typically 20% to 30%
- bronchial fluid protein to serum protein ratio— >0.5, indicating unusually high concentration of protein in bronchial fluid (implying that a damaged alveolar-capillary membrane is allowing proteins to leak through capillary walls)
- chest X-ray—reveals bilateral diffuse infiltrates
- lung compliance—reduced below 50 ml/cm H_2O, typically to the range of 20 to 30 ml/cm
- pulmonary capillary wedge pressure—normal or only slightly elevated (<15 mm Hg), indicating that left heart failure is not the cause of the pulmonary congestion
- functional residual capacity—reduced.

POTENTIAL COMPLICATIONS
- respiratory arrest
- respiratory failure
- pulmonary fibrosis
- disseminated intravascular coagulation
- persistent pulmonary function abnormalities after recovery (such as mild restrictive disease, impaired gas transfer, or expiratory small airway obstruction)

Collaborative problem: *Hypoxemia related to pulmonary shunt, interstitial edema, and alveolar edema*

NURSING PRIORITIES: (a) Prevent further deterioration of lung function, (b) support the lung during healing, and (c) maintain oxygenation.

Interventions	Rationales
1. Monitor for clinical signs and symptoms:	1. Clinical signs and symptoms, when correlated with ABG values and chest X-ray results, indicate progression of the syndrome.
• initial insult period: persistent unexplained mild tachypnea, breathlessness, air hunger, and normal breath sounds	• The catastrophic insult is followed by a variable lag period of several hours to several days before the onset of clear clinical signs and symptoms. About 60% of patients develop clinical indicators within the first 24 hours, 30% within 24 to 72 hours, and 10% after more than 72 hours. During the initial insult period, signs and symptoms are mild and nonspecific. Tachypnea, despite a normal PaO_2, the most characteristic finding, probably results from stimulation of juxtacapillary receptors in the alveolar interstitium.
• latent period: persistent moderate tachypnea; increasing dyspnea; neck, chest, or abdominal muscle use; fatigue; restlessness; confusion; and crackles	• Signs and symptoms during the latent phase reflect borderline hypoxemia and interstitial edema.
• progressive pulmonary insufficiency: severe tachypnea and hyperventilation, progressive dyspnea, rhonchi, and deteriorating level of consciousness	• As the syndrome worsens, respiratory distress becomes marked. Increased dead space causes a need for high minute volumes whereas decreasing compliance causes a need for high inspiratory pressures. The continuing capillary leak produces frank alveolar edema, whereas the massive pulmonary shunt produces hypoxemia.
• terminal stage: depressed level of consciousness, dysrhythmias, and profound shock leading to asystole.	• In the terminal stage, hypoxemia refractory to therapy produces profound dysfunction of the brain and heart, terminating in cardiopulmonary arrest.

Interventions	Rationales
2. Obtain chest X-ray daily, as ordered, and monitor serial findings. Be alert for reports indicating patchy infiltrates or "white out." Also note any other abnormal findings.	2. Chest X-rays are used to monitor the degree of edema and the development of complications. During the period of initial insult, the X-ray typically is normal. Patchy infiltrates appear during the latent period, worsen during pulmonary insufficiency, and culminate in a complete "white out" in the terminal stage.
3. Obtain ABG values at least every 4 hours, as ordered. Note degree of hypoxemia and any acid-base imbalance, typically:	3. ABG values provide a way to assess and document gas exchange abnormalities.
• normal PaO_2, mild hypocapnia, and respiratory alkalosis during the insult period	• During the insult period, tachypnea maintains a normal PaO_2, but the accompanying CO_2 blow-off produces hypocapnia and respiratory alkalosis.
• borderline hypoxemia during the latent period	• Borderline hypoxemia reflects early impairment of gas diffusion.
• progressive hypoxemia, increasing hypercapnia, and worsening respiratory and metabolic acidosis as pulmonary insufficiency becomes more pronounced	• Hypercapnia develops later because CO_2 is much more diffusible than oxygen. CO_2 retention produces respiratory acidosis. The worsening oxygen deprivation causes cells to switch from aerobic to anaerobic metabolism, resulting in lactic acidosis.
• refractory hypoxemia, hypercapnia, and severe respiratory and metabolic acidosis during the terminal stage.	• Refractory hypoxemia results from a massive pulmonary shunt. Interstitial edema compresses alveoli, whereas alveolar edema fills them with fluid. In either case, they cannot oxygenate capillary blood flowing past them. The resulting perfusion without ventilation converts the alveolar-capillary units to shunt units. Without open alveoli, supplemental oxygen cannot physically reach capillary blood, rendering such treatment ineffective.
4. Continuously monitor gas exchange status, as ordered, by monitoring arterial hemoglobin saturation (SaO_2) with an ear oximeter or monitoring mixed venous oxygen saturation ($S\bar{v}O_2$) with an $S\bar{v}O_2$ catheter.	4. Conventional ABG sampling provides only an intermittent indicator of gas exchange, and a lag time occurs between the time the sample is obtained and the time results are available. Continuous monitoring provides constant, real-time data useful to detect impending deterioration, monitor the effects of nursing interventions, and titrate the effects of multiple interventions that may have opposing effects on oxygenation and cardiac output, such as administration of dopamine and nitroprusside to a patient on positive-pressure ventilation and positive end-expiratory pressure (PEEP). Ear oximetry monitors oxygen supplied to tissues, whereas SvO_2 monitoring provides an indication of tissue oxygen consumption.
5. Prepare for endotracheal intubation if the patient has a respiratory rate exceeding 30 breaths/minute and is: • elderly, chronically ill, or suffering from preexisting pulmonary disease • fatigued • exhibiting an increasing $PaCO_2$.	5. Endotracheal intubation is usually necessary to protect the airway and allow for delivery of high levels of oxygen and PEEP. Advanced age, chronic illness, or preexisting pulmonary disease increase the likelihood the patient will be unable to tolerate the rapid respiratory rate. Fatigue and increasing $PaCO_2$ are ominous signs indicating that the patient is failing to maintain adequate spontaneous ventilation.

(continued)

Interventions

6. Implement mechanical ventilation, as ordered. See the "Mechanical Ventilation" care plan, page 108, for specifics.

Rationales

6. The widespread pulmonary congestion impairs alveolar expansion. Without alveolar distension, surfactant production decreases, making alveoli even more difficult to expand. The high inspiratory pressures required to expand alveoli and the high minute volume needed to compensate for increased physiologic dead space increase the work of breathing so markedly that patients become exhausted and incapable of maintaining spontaneous ventilation. In addition, hypoxemia makes the patient prone to respiratory arrest. Mechanical ventilation conserves the patient's energy, prevents respiratory arrest, and allows time for the lung injury to heal.

7. Implement PEEP, as ordered, typically if an inspired oxygen concentration >50% is needed for more than 24 hours or if PaO_2 falls below 50 mm Hg even though oxygen concentration exceeds 60%.

7. PEEP, a mainstay in the treatment of ARDS, is believed to increase alveolar size and convert shunt units (those with perfusion but without ventilation) to normal ones. It thus increases functional residual capacity, decreases shunt, improves ventilation-perfusion matching, and improves compliance.

8. Monitor compliance, as described in the "Mechanical Ventilation" care plan, page 108.

8. Compliance is an objective measure of the ease with which lung expansion can occur. Decreasing compliance, implying increasing lung stiffness, indicates that ARDS is worsening. Details of calculating compliance are covered in the "Mechanical Ventilation" care plan.

9. Administer medications, as ordered. Document effectiveness and observe for adverse reactions.

9. Medications are of limited effectiveness in ARDS but may be prescribed empirically.

• corticosteroids, typically methylprednisolone (Solu-Medrol)

• Administration of corticosteroids in ARDS is controversial. Although anecdotal reports and limited clinical and animal studies suggest possible effectiveness in certain types of ARDS, such as radiation pneumonitis, no randomized, controlled study in humans has demonstrated their effectiveness.

• antibiotics.

• Antibiotics are usually prescribed for suspected or documented infection. Although many doctors prescribe them prophylactically in ARDS, such use has not been proven effective.

10. Additional individualized interventions: ____________

10. Rationales: ____________

Target outcome criteria

Within 5 days of the initial insult and continuously thereafter, the patient will:

• display eupnea
• have a respiratory rate of 12 to 20 breaths/minute
• have clear lung sounds
• display a level of consciousness equal to or better than on admission
• have a chest X-ray returning to normal
• manifest ABG values returning to normal limits for the patient
• record an SaO_2 of 95% or better and an SvO_2 of 60% to 80%, if oximetry is being used.

Nursing diagnosis: *Potential for injury: complications related to additional lung insults stemming from dysfunction of other organ systems*

NURSING PRIORITY: Prevent additional insults to the lung.

Interventions	Rationales
1. Maintain adequate cardiac output. Assist with insertion of a pulmonary artery (PA) catheter, if indicated. Monitor PA pressures, vital signs, EKG, and urinary output according to Appendix A "Monitoring Standards".	1. Arterial oxygen transport (the amount delivered to the tissues) depends on cardiac output and oxygen content. Close monitoring of hemodynamics is essential because optimal fluid management is difficult to achieve in these patients. Enough fluid must be given to maintain cardiac output, yet too much fluid worsens the pulmonary capillary leak. A PA catheter is also helpful in differentiating cardiac from noncardiac pulmonary edema.
2. Administer packed red blood cells, as ordered, to maintain the hemoglobin level at 12 to 15 g/dl.	2. Oxygen content depends on the hemoglobin level, hemoglobin saturation, and PaO_2. This hemoglobin level is optimum for maintaining normal oxygen transport.
3. Administer crystalloid or colloid I.V. fluids, as ordered. Monitor fluid administration meticulously.	3. The choice of appropriate fluid in ARDS remains controversial. Crystalloids readily cross from the vascular to the interstitial space, potentially worsening edema. Colloids also cross the leaky capillary membrane, move into the interstitial space, and draw water to them via an osmotic pull, which also worsens edema. Factors affecting the choice of fluid in a particular patient include doctor preference, cost, and availability. Meticulous monitoring helps minimize development of two risk factors for ARDS: shock and fluid overload.
4. If the patient has gastric distension, a decreased level of consciousness, or impaired airway protection reflexes, obtain an order to institute gastric drainage.	4. Aspiration of gastric contents is a risk factor for ARDS. Gastric drainage, when properly maintained, prevents such aspiration.
5. Provide nutritional support, as ordered. See the "Nutritional Deficit" care plan, page 53.	5. The protracted period of mechanical ventilation necessary for most ARDS patients requires total parenteral nutrition to maintain pulmonary muscle strength and immunologic defense mechanisms. The "Nutritional Deficit" care plan covers nutritional support in detail.
6. Maintain strict asepsis. Monitor for signs and symptoms of infection, and document and report them promptly to the doctor. Institute aggressive treatment measures, as ordered.	6. Because sepsis is a common precursor to ARDS, identification of a septic focus can prove instrumental in combating ARDS. Development of major infections in an ARDS patient is an ominous sign. If the source cannot be identified, the patient is very likely to die. Identification of the source and prompt, aggressive therapy may improve the possibility for survival.
7. Observe for signs of single or multiple organ failure, especially central nervous system failure, renal failure, and GI dysfunction.	7. Failure or dysfunction of additional organ systems appears to be associated with increased mortality in ARDS.
8. Implement general supportive nursing measures to prevent the complications of immobility. See the "Impaired Physical Mobility" care plan, page 33.	8. Patients on prolonged bed rest are at risk for many complications that worsen lung function, such as pneumonia, atelectasis, and pulmonary embolism. The "Impaired Physical Mobility" care plan contains detailed interventions for these and other potential complications of immobility.

(continued)

Interventions

9. Additional individualized interventions: ____________

Rationales

9. Rationales: ____________

Target outcome criteria

Within 24 hours of the initial insult and then continuously, the patient will:

- have a heart rate, blood pressure, and pulmonary artery and wedge pressures within normal limits for the patient
- display normal sinus rhythm
- produce an hourly urine output >30 ml
- show no signs of infection.

Nursing diagnosis: *Potential ineffective coping related to abrupt onset of life-threatening illness*

NURSING PRIORITY: Maximize coping skills of patient and family.

Interventions

1. Implement the measures outlined in the "Ineffective Coping" care plan, page 26.

2. Additional individualized interventions: ____________

Rationales

1. Whether ARDS occurs after a catastrophic incident, such as trauma, or complicates an already critical illness, its onset can be a cruel blow to hope. The stress of the disease is exacerbated by its treatment, particularly mechanical ventilation, which precludes oral communication at the time when the patient and family most need it. Using the measures detailed in the "Ineffective Coping" care plan to provide sensitive emotional support not only makes the ordeal more bearable, but also lessens anxiety-induced oxygen requirements.

2. Rationales: ____________

Target outcome criteria

See the "Ineffective Coping" care plan.

Transfer planning

NURSING TRANSFER CRITERIA

Upon transfer, documentation shows evidence of:

- stable vital signs within normal limits for the patient
- spontaneous respiratory rate of 12 to 24 breaths/minute
- patent airway without endotracheal intubation
- discontinuation of PA catheter.

PATIENT-FAMILY TEACHING CHECKLIST

Document evidence that patient and family demonstrate understanding of:

__ definition and pathophysiology of ARDS
__ probable precipitator(s) for this patient
__ prognosis
__ rationale for mechanical ventilation, PEEP, and other therapies.

DOCUMENTATION CHECKLIST

Using outcome criteria as a guide, document:

__ clinical status on admission
__ significant changes in status
__ pertinent diagnostic test findings
__ airway care
__ tolerance of ventilator and PEEP
__ response to medications
__ fluid therapy
__ nutritional support
__ nursing care to combat effects of immobility
__ psychological coping
__ patient/family teaching
__ transfer planning.

ASSOCIATED CARE PLANS

Disseminated Intravascular Coagulation
Grieving and Dying
Impaired Physical Mobility
Ineffective Coping
Mechanical Ventilation
Multiple Trauma
Nutritional Deficit
Sensory-Perceptual Alteration

REFERENCES

Bernard, G.R., and Bradley, R.B. "Adult Respiratory Distress Syndrome: Diagnosis and Management," *Heart & Lung* 15(3):250-55, May 1986.

Brandstetter, R.D. "The Adult Respiratory Distress Syndrome—1986," *Heart & Lung* 15(2):155-64, 1986.

Celentano-Norton, L. "Mechanical Ventilation Strategies in Adult Respiratory Distress Syndrome," *Critical Care Nurse* 6(4):71-83, 1986.

Elliott, C.G., et al. "Prediction of Pulmonary Function Abnormalities after Adult Respiratory Distress Syndrome (ARDS)," *American Review of Respiratory Disorders* 135:634-38, 1987.

Karnes, N. "Don't Let ARDS Catch You Off Guard." *Nursing87* 17(5):34-38, 1987.

Mechanical Ventilation

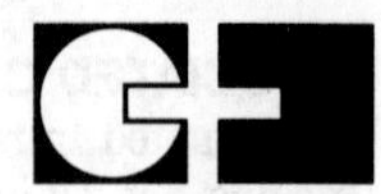

DRG information

DRG 475 Respiratory System Diagnosis With Ventilator Support.
Mean LOS = 8.8 days
Principal diagnoses include:
- respiratory failure
- chronic obstructive pulmonary disease
- acute or chronic bronchitis
- pneumonia of various etiologies
- adult respiratory distress syndrome.

Additional DRG information: To use DRG 475, one of the above diagnoses must appear as the principal diagnosis. A patient with Guillain-Barré syndrome complicated by respiratory failure will not be assigned DRG 475 because the respiratory failure is a secondary diagnosis. Besides the respiratory principal diagnosis, both mechanical ventilator assistance and insertion of endotracheal tube must be coded.

Introduction

DEFINITION AND TIME FOCUS

Mechanical ventilation, the artificial provision of gas volumes sufficient to maintain alveolar ventilation, commonly is required for patients with significant ventilatory abnormalities that lead to apnea or actual or impending respiratory failure. This care plan focuses on the patient receiving positive pressure ventilation, the most common type in critical care.

ETIOLOGY AND PRECIPITATING FACTORS

- central respiratory depression, such as from drug overdose, head trauma, cerebrovascular accident, anesthesia, or cardiac arrest
- airway diseases, such as asthma or bronchitis
- parenchymal diseases, such as adult respiratory distress syndrome (ARDS), pulmonary edema, pneumonia, or emphysema
- neuromuscular disorders, such as myasthenia gravis and Guillain-Barré syndrome
- chest wall injury, such as pneumothorax, flail chest, and major thoracic surgery

Focused assessment guidelines

NURSING HISTORY (Functional health pattern findings)

Health perception–health management pattern

- manifests sudden or progressive onset of abnormal ventilatory patterns or airway obstruction
- if able to speak, reports severe dyspnea or air hunger
- may have history of motor vehicle accident, assault, or other type of head, chest, or orthopedic trauma
- may be under treatment for long-standing chronic respiratory disease
- may have had recent major surgical procedure involving the thorax or upper abdomen
- may have history of drug or alcohol abuse

PHYSICAL FINDINGS

Pulmonary

- labored breathing
- shallow breathing
- absent breath sounds
- agonal breathing or other abnormal breathing pattern
- tachypnea
- retractions
- nasal flaring
- accessory muscle use
- decreased or absent breath sounds
- crackles, rhonchi, or wheezes

Neurologic

- restlessness
- confusion
- agitation
- somnolence
- unconsciousness

Cardiovascular

- tachycardia (early), bradycardia (late)
- dysrhythmias
- hypertension or hypotension

Integumentary

- diaphoresis
- cyanosis

DIAGNOSTIC STUDIES

- arterial blood gas (ABG) levels—reveal hypercapnia or hypoxemia, manifested by $Paco_2$ >50 mm Hg in previously eucapnic patient (or >10 mm Hg increase above usual value in chronic obstructive pulmonary disease [COPD] patient) or Pao_2 <50 mm Hg on supplemental oxygen
- alveolar-arterial (A-a) gradient—may be >300 mm Hg on 100% oxygen
- shunt—may be >30%
- minute ventilation (spontaneous)—may be <5 liters/minute, indicating too low a ventilation to remove CO_2 adequately, or >10 liters/minute, indicating excessive work of breathing
- vital capacity (VC)—may be <15 ml/kg body weight, indicating poor ventilatory reserve

• maximum inspiratory force (MIF)—may be <20 cmH_2O, indicating weak respiratory drive or respiratory musculature
• dead space/tidal volume (V_D/V_T) ratio—may be >0.6, indicating excessive wasted ventilation

POTENTIAL COMPLICATIONS
• tension pneumothorax
• GI hemorrhage
• shock
• pneumonia
• ventilator malfunction

Collaborative problem: *Ineffective alveolar ventilation related to failure to maintain prescribed ventilator settings*

NURSING PRIORITY: Maintain settings as ordered.

Interventions	Rationales
1. Confirm orders for mechanical ventilation, particularly:	1. Mechanical ventilation may be achieved with many combined modes and settings.
• type of ventilator (pressure- or volume-cycled)	• Positive-pressure ventilators may be pressure-cycled or volume-cycled. Pressure-cycled ventilators (such as Bennett PR-II) deliver a preset inspiratory pressure and then end inspiration. If the patient's airflow resistance or lung compliance varies, the tidal volume will fluctuate—sometimes dramatically. Volume-cycled ventilators (such as Bennett 7200) deliver a preset tidal volume and end inspiration. Even if the patient's airway resistance or lung compliance varies, a consistent tidal volume (V_T) is delivered (although inspiratory pressure fluctuates). Some ventilators (such as Servo) can be used as either pressure-cycled ventilators or volume-cycled ventilators. The type of ventilator selected for a particular patient depends on the patient's needs. Pressure ventilators are appropriate for patients with normal lung compliance; when the relationship between the inspiratory pressure and tidal volume is relatively predictable and constant, as in such patients, one can be reasonably sure that the preset pressure will deliver a sufficient V_T. Volume-cycled ventilators are best for patients with poor or variable compliance, in whom a given pressure may or may not deliver the desired V_T.
• inspiratory mode:	• Inspiratory modes determine the type and degree of control over inspiration.
□ control	□ The control mode provides complete ventilatory support by delivering a set number of breaths per minute, regardless of the patient's inspiratory efforts. The least-used mode, it is appropriate only for apneic or paralyzed patients (such as those with central nervous system dysfunction or drug-induced paralysis), or chest trauma patients in whom negative inspiratory pressure would be detrimental (such as with flail chest).
□ assist-control	□ Assist-control is suitable for the patient with a weak respiratory drive or weak respiratory musculature. This mode assures delivery of a preset minimum number of breaths per minute but allows the patient to initiate the breath and to to breathe more rapidly if desired. If the patient initiates a breath, the machine delivers the desired volume; if the patient does not breathe, the machine supplies the breath. Because the ventilator delivers a preset volume even on patient-initiated breaths, it lessens the work of breathing, yet improves alveolar ventilation.

(continued)

Interventions

□ intermittent mandatory ventilation (IMV)

Rationales

□ IMV, once used only for difficult-to-wean patients, is now considered a standard ventilatory mode in widespread use for full or partial ventilatory support. The machine delivers a preset number of breaths. In between, the patient can breathe spontaneously through the ventilator circuit without any assistance from the machine. Because these spontaneous breaths depend on the negative pressure the patient can generate, their V_T may vary significantly from the ventilator V_T. Advantages of IMV include the rare need for sedation to synchronize spontaneous and ventilator breaths, lower mean airway pressures (thus reduced risk of barotrauma—lung damage from excessive pressure—and less depression on cardiac output), less risk of hyperventilation, maintenance of respiratory muscle strength, and more even distribution of ventilation throughout the lung.

• expiratory maneuvers:

• Expiratory maneuvers determine the degree of resistance to expiration.

□ positive end-expiratory pressure (PEEP)

□ PEEP is used commonly with positive-pressure ventilation of patients with alveolar collapse (from loss of surfactant, early small airway closure, or atelectasis) or those with alveolar filling (for example, with pulmonary edema). In such patients, nonfunctioning alveoli, unable to oxygenate blood flowing through pulmonary capillaries, produce an abnormal pulmonary shunt and hypoxemia refractory to oxygen therapy. PEEP helps reexpand collapsed alveoli, increase functional residual capacity (FRC) and recruit shunt units. Because it improves ventilation-perfusion matching, oxygenation improves. PEEP commonly allows lowering of inspired oxygen concentration, a valuable consideration in preventing lung damage from excessive oxygen exposure.

□ continuous positive airway pressure (CPAP)

□ CPAP is similar to PEEP but is used for spontaneously breathing patients. It maintains positive airway pressure throughout the respiratory cycle. Benefits are similar to PEEP. It can be applied through a ventilator (for non-IMV breaths), through various devices for the intubated patient off a ventilator, or via a special mask for the nonintubated patient.

□ expiratory retard.

□ This maneuver is infrequently used to improve lung emptying when FRC is increased. Like pursed-lip breathing used by COPD patients, it involves adding resistance to the ventilator's expiratory line. It slows the expiratory phase but does not increase airway pressure.

2. Collaborate with the respiratory therapist to monitor prescribed settings: when settings are changed; when arterial blood is drawn for ABG measurements, routinely every 1 to 4 hours; and as needed for unstable patients.

2. Depending on the unit protocol, either you or the respiratory therapist may be responsible for performing the ventilator checks. If the respiratory therapist performs the checks, you should confirm that ventilator settings are as ordered when you first assume responsibility for nursing the patient. Close collaboration between you and the respiratory therapist is essential for optimal patient care. Checks at the times indicated ensure accuracy of the prescribed settings.

Interventions	Rationales
• respiratory rate: count the machine rate and the patient's rate for one minute each and compare	• With all ventilatory modes, the ventilator may not actually deliver the number of breaths set. In addition, with assist-control or IMV, the patient can breathe above the set rate. With most volume ventilators, the rate is set with a knob. With pressure ventilators, the rate is a by-product of the speed of gas flow, controlled by the inspiratory time flow-rate control. The faster the flow, the faster inspiration, so the faster the respiratory rate. The slower the flow, the lower the respiratory rate. Slower rates are preferred generally because they cause better gas flow characteristics—less turbulence, lower mean airway pressure, and better gas distribution within the lungs.
• tidal volume: Compare delivered V_T with desired V_T, typically 10 to 15 ml/kg. On newer models, read inspired V_T from the digital readout. On older models lacking a readout, measure exhaled V_T with a Wright respirometer.	• V_T is the amount of air inspired or expired. V_T is set with a dial on volume ventilators or determined by the inspiratory time flow-rate control on pressure ventilators. Measuring exhaled V_T indicates the amount actually received. Decreasing V_T may signify decreased compliance, whereas increasing V_T may reflect increased compliance, resolution of the disease process, or a machine, cuff, or patient leak.
• minute ventilation (MV): If the patient is on assist-control or IMV, compare actual and desired MV. If the patient is on IMV, also compare total and non-IMV MV.	• MV, the product of the respiratory rate and the V_T, determines alveolar ventilation. MV is related inversely to $PaCO_2$: as MV increases, $PaCO_2$ decreases, and vice versa. Decreased MV is associated with CO_2 retention and respiratory acidosis, whereas increased MV is associated with CO_2 blow-off and respiratory alkalosis. Comparing actual and desired MVs indicates how well the machine is meeting the patient's ventilatory needs. Comparing total and non-IMV MVs indicates what amount the patient's spontaneous breaths are contributing to total MV; monitoring this amount can assist the doctor or therapist in evaluating the patient's readiness for weaning.
• inspiratory flow rate	• This rate is the speed of airflow per unit of time. In the volume-cycled ventilator, it is set with a knob. In the pressure-cycled ventilator, it is determined by the inspiratory time flow-rate control. Older models dump air to the atmosphere at the set peak flow rate; if the patient needs a faster flow, he can become quite uncomfortable. In that case, you may find it necessary to increase the flow rate so that the patient has time for exhalation before the next breath is triggered. Newer models contain demand valves so the patient can receive the flow needed.
• inspiratory expiratory (I/E) ratio, typically 1:2 or greater	• Expiration must be longer than inspiration to avoid air trapping.
• airway pressure, normally 20 to 40 cmH_2O and relatively constant. Monitor both peak inspiratory pressure and inspiratory plateau pressure, noting sudden changes in airway pressures or a trend of increasing pressures.	• Peak inspiratory pressure is the pressure at peak inspiration. It reflects the maximum pressure necessary to overcome resistance to flow and to lung and chest wall expansion. Increased peak inspiratory pressure implies increased airway resistance, such as from secretions or bronchospasm. Plateau pressure is the pressure at end-inspiration. It reflects the pressure necessary to hold the airways open and deliver the volume of gas. Increased plateau pressure implies stiffness of lung tissue.

(continued)

Interventions	Rationales
• pressure limit (on volume-cycled ventilators)	• This setting limits the amount of pressure that the machine can exert when delivering volume in order to prevent barotrauma. Once this level is reached, inspiration is ended even if the desired V_T has not been delivered. The pressure limit may be reached occasionally if the patient is coughing, has excessive airway secretions, or the ventilator tubing is kinked. Consistently reaching the pressure limit suggests decreased compliance or a pneumothorax.
• sensitivity (typically -2 cmH_2O)	• The sensitivity knob controls the amount of negative inspiratory pressure the patient must generate in order to trigger an inspiration.
• sigh, typically 1½ to 2 times V_T at a rate of 6 to 10 breaths/hour.	• A sigh is a periodic, "deep breath" delivered by the ventilator. Thought to prevent atelectasis, sighing was popular when patients were ventilated with smaller tidal volumes than at present. With the move toward ventilation with high V_T, sighing has become less popular, although it still may be used for persistent atelectasis.
3. In collaboration with the respiratory therapist, monitor compliance every 8 hours:	3. Compliance is a measure of the resistance to expansion. It is determined by the amount of change in volume that results from a given change in pressure (volume in ml divided by pressure in cmH_2O equals compliance in ml/cmH_2O). Decreased lung compliance signifies that the lungs are requiring more pressure to ventilate; they are stiffer than usual, for example in ARDS. Increased compliance, rarely a clinical problem, indicates the lungs are easier than usual to ventilate. For example, in emphysema where elasticity is lost, lung compliance increases, though airway obstruction still may render the patient difficult to ventilate.
• Determine static compliance (V_T divided by end-inspiratory [plateau] pressure) or dynamic compliance (V_T divided by peak inspiratory pressure). If PEEP is used, subtract PEEP value from pressure before dividing.	• Static compliance indicates compliance when the lungs are at rest, whereas dynamic compliance indicates compliance when airflow is occurring. Static compliance values reflect lung compliance, whereas dynamic compliance reflects airway resistance as well.
• Compare the patient's values to normal values (static: 100 ml/cmH_2O; dynamic: 50 ml/cmH_2O). Monitor compliance curves or note trend of values.	• Comparing static and dynamic values can help identify the source of difficulty in ventilating a patient. For example, a near-normal static compliance with a low dynamic compliance suggests the problem is increased airway resistance, whereas both low static and low dynamic compliances suggest the problem is the lung itself, such as occurs with ARDS. Compliance curves—serial plotting of pressure changes compared to volume changes—indicate trends graphically and may help to determine the best combination of pressure and volume for a patient.
4. Evaluate pulmonary status at least every 2 hours. Note particularly the symmetry of chest excursion, bilateral breath sounds, and any adventitious sounds.	4. These factors provide data about adequacy of airflow throughout the pulmonary tree and about secretions or obstructions to flow.
5. Additional individualized interventions: ______	5. Rationales: ______

Target outcome criteria

Upon institution of mechanical ventilation and continuously thereafter, the patient will:

- have bilaterally equal chest excursion and breath sounds
- manifest compliance values within usual limits for the underlying disorder
- have ABG levels within expected limits for the underlying disorder.

Collaborative problem: *Potential hypoxemia related to insufficient oxygen delivery or inadequate level of PEEP*

NURSING PRIORITY: Maintain optimal oxygenation.

Interventions	Rationales
1. Compare delivered oxygen percentage to that desired, typically 100% initially and thereafter adjusted according to PaO_2. With newer models, read delivered oxygen percentage from the digital readout reflecting the built-in oxygen analyzer. With older models, use a hand-held oxygen analyzer.	1. The machine may or may not deliver the set oxygen percentage. Using the oxygen analyzer evaluates the accuracy of oxygen delivery. Too low a percentage promotes hypoxemia, whereas too high a percentage promotes oxygen toxicity (see the "Potential for injury" collaborative problem on page 115).
2. Be aware if the fraction of inspired oxygen (FIO_2) is >50%.	2. Prolonged exposure to high alveolar oxygen tension promotes potential oxygen toxicity. Although an FIO_2 >60% does not cause clinically significant parenchymal abnormalities in normal lungs, an FIO_2 >50% may cause serious lung dysfunction in previously damaged or susceptible lung tissue.
• Consider, with the doctor, the risk of exposure in relation to the need for oxygen therapy. If possible, implement ways to lower the oxygen dose, as ordered.	• Lowering the oxygen dose, as may be achieved through the application of PEEP, helps to lower the risk of toxicity. However, the need for relief of hypoxemia takes precedence over the potential danger of oxygen toxicity.
• If it is not possible to lower the oxygen dose, observe the patient for, document, and promptly notify the doctor about: sharp, pleuritic chest pain (typically after about 6 hours on 100% O_2), decreased vital capacity and decreased compliance (typically after 18 hours), or signs and symptoms of ARDS (typically after 24 to 48 hours).	• Signs and symptoms of oxygen toxicity reflect the progression from the initial phase of tracheobronchitis through the exudative phase of alveolar-capillary membrane damage. If unchecked, the syndrome progresses to a proliferative stage resulting in pulmonary fibrosis. To assess for chest pain in an intubated patient, observe for indications of pain, such as grimacing, and analyze pain characteristics by asking the patient questions that can be answered with a "yes" or "no" signal.
3. Note PEEP, typically ordered if the patient cannot maintain PaO_2 >60 mm Hg on <50% oxygen.	3. By increasing FRC and recruiting shunt units, PEEP improves oxygen transport and allows use of a lower inspired oxygen concentration.
• Visually monitor the PEEP level (usually 5 to 15 cmH_2O) on the PEEP gauge or inspiratory pressure gauge (instead of dropping to zero at end-expiration, the needle drops to the PEEP level).	• Visual monitoring confirms that the prescribed level of PEEP is being maintained.
• Assist the doctor with titration of PEEP by correlating PEEP level with inspired oxygen percentage, resulting PaO_2, and hemodynamic values. Typically, apply PEEP in increments of 3 to 5 cmH_2O to reach a maintenance level of 5 to 15 cm H_2O, as ordered.	• The optimal PEEP level for a given patient is a medical judgment based on numerous factors, including shunt reduction, lung compliance, and cardiac output. The desired goal is maintenance of an adequate PaO_2 on less than 60% oxygen. Levels of PEEP above 15 cm are associated with increased barotrauma and depression of cardiac output.
4. Additional individualized interventions: ______________	4. Rationales: ______________

Target outcome criteria
Within 24 hours of onset of mechanical ventilation and then continuously, the patient will:
- maintain a PaO_2 >50 mm Hg
- display no signs or symptoms of oxygen toxicity.

Nursing diagnosis: *Ineffective airway clearance related to endotracheal tube, increased secretions, and underlying pathology*

NURSING PRIORITY: Maintain airway patency.

Interventions	Rationales
1. Provide artificial airway care according to unit protocol or as ordered, including the following:	1. Meticulous airway care can prevent numerous potential complications associated with endotracheal intubation.
• Support the ventilator tubing so the tube does not press on the edge of the patient's nose or mouth.	• Maintaining proper alignment prevents accidental extubation, tube advancement, or nasotracheal or orotracheal erosion.
• Measure cuff pressures and volumes every 8 hours; report to the doctor pressures over 20 mm Hg or a trend of increasing pressures or cuff volumes.	• Monitoring cuff pressures and volumes provides for early detection of pressures high enough to cause tracheal ischemia and necrosis.
• Use minimal occluding volume or minimal leak technique for inflating the balloon.	• These techniques help prevent tracheal erosion, tracheal stenosis, and tracheoesophageal fistula.
2. Monitor endotracheal tube position. Check tube placement every 8 hours by noting the relationship between the patient's lip and the centimeter marks on the tube. Compare with previous measurements and alert the doctor if movement has occurred.	2. An endotracheal tube can migrate downward to rest against the carina, obstructing airflow and causing increased coughing and fighting the ventilator, or to enter one of the bronchi (usually the right main stem), preventing ventilation of the opposite lung. It also can migrate upward, increasing the risk of unintended extubation. Monitoring tube position provides adequate warning of tube movement to take corrective action.
3. Keep a manual self-inflating bag and mask at the bedside, connected to 100% oxygen. If accidental extubation occurs, open the airway and ventilate with the bag and mask. Summon medical assistance.	3. Using the bag and mask provides emergency support of ventilation in the event of accidental extubation. Reintubation will need to be performed by someone skilled in the technique.
4. Change the patient's position every 1 to 2 hours. Provide chest physiotherapy (PT) as indicated.	4. Position changes help drain secretions and promote ventilation of all lung areas. Chest PT promotes secretion drainage.
5. Suction when needed, as indicated by dyspnea, coughing, rhonchi, secretions visible in the tube, or a high-pressure alarm. Observe these guidelines for suctioning:	5. Intubation prevents an effective cough reflex to clear the airway. Routine suctioning is inadvisable because of the risks of suction-induced hypoxemia, dysrhythmias, bronchospasm, and loss of PEEP.
• If the patient's PaO_2 is normal or low, oxygenate before and after suctioning with 100% oxygen. For suctioning, use a catheter with a diameter <50% of endotracheal tube diameter. Suction for <15 seconds. Always reset the oxygen to its previous level after hyperoxygenation.	• Suctioning causes arterial oxygen desaturation, the degree of which depends on presuctioning PaO_2, catheter size in relation to endotracheal tube size, duration of suctioning, and other factors. Following the recommended guidelines helps minimize hypoxemia. Resetting the oxygen level minimizes the risk of oxygen toxicity.
• If the patient is on PEEP, use a manual self-inflating bag with a PEEP valve when suctioning.	• Use of a bag modified with a PEEP valve minimizes loss of PEEP support.

Interventions	Rationales
• Monitor blood pressure, heart rate, and EKG pattern during suctioning. If adverse reactions such as bradycardia, hypotension, or dysrhythmias occur, immediately remove the suctioning catheter and ventilate the patient with 100% oxygen.	• Bradycardia, hypotension, and dysrhythmias may result from stimulation of vagal fibers at the carina, hyperinflation, or hypoxemia.
• While suctioning, observe for paroxysmal coughing without deep breaths; remove the catheter if it occurs.	• Paroxysmal coughing is analogous to a sustained Valsalva's maneuver at pressures high enough to cause bradycardia and hypotension. Removing the catheter reduces airway obstruction.
• If the patient reacts adversely to traditional suctioning, consult with the doctor about:	• Because suctioning is still necessary, adverse reactions should be forestalled when possible.
□ administering an anticholinergic agent, such as atropine, or an anesthetic, such as lidocaine, before suctioning	□ An anticholinergic agent will prevent bradycardia caused by vagal stimulation. Lidocaine decreases coughing and, in patients with increased intracranial pressure (ICP), helps prevent further pressure increases.
□ using a closed airway system with a suctioning adapter. Note the patient's reaction to this method of suctioning; if signs and symptoms of hypoxemia occur, discontinue the method.	□ A closed suctioning system maintains the ventilator connection, including PEEP, and may minimize hypoxemia. However, if suction flow is greater than the volume delivered by the ventilator's delivery of volume, alveolar collapse may occur, producing arterial desaturation.
6. Additional individualized interventions: ____________	6. Rationales: ____________

Target outcome criteria

Continuously during mechanical ventilation, the patient will:

• have a patent airway

• have clear breath sounds bilaterally, as underlying condition allows.

Collaborative problem: *Potential for injury: complications related to patient deterioration, mechanical breakdown, increased intrathoracic pressure, and/or bypassed defense mechanisms*

NURSING PRIORITIES: (a) Prevent complications when possible and (b) respond appropriately if complications occur.

Interventions	Rationales
ABRUPT RESPIRATORY DISTRESS	
1. Keep ventilator alarms turned on at all times.	1. The patient's life depends on maintenance of this therapy. Alarms can warn of various potentially fatal problems associated with this complex intervention. Turning them off places the patient at risk for an unobserved disconnection, cardiac arrest, or other catastrophe.
2. Familiarize yourself with troubleshooting techniques in advance of any possible need. Take advantage of technical training provided by the manufacturer and your institution; read the Grossbach articles listed in the references, page 121.	2. Troubleshooting techniques are complex and vary somewhat among ventilators. The Grossbach articles contain detailed information on 15 common problems. Learning troubleshooting techniques in advance of need will reduce your anxiety and improve the likelihood of prompt, successful resolution of a problem.

(continued)

Interventions	Rationales
3. Continuously observe whether the patient is breathing in synchrony with the ventilator. If the patient develops sudden respiratory distress or the ventilator fails abruptly:	3. Breathing out of synchrony (sometimes called "fighting the ventilator" or "breathing out of phase with the ventilator") markedly increases intrathoracic pressure, whereas failure of mechanical ventilation places the patient's life in jeopardy.
• Immediately disconnect the ventilator, open the airway if necessary, and ventilate the patient using a manual self-inflating bag and 100% oxygen.	• Determining whether the cause of the respiratory distress is patient-related or ventilator-related is crucial. Patient-related problems (such as airway obstruction or tension pneumothorax) require immediate intervention, whereas distress from ventilator malfunction can be relieved by ventilating the patient manually until the exact cause of the problem can be evaluated. Manually ventilating the patient provides a quick way to distinguish the two categories, supplies adequate emergency ventilation, and allows rapid detection of the patient problems of increased airway resistance or decreased compliance.
• Once ventilation is established, reevaluate the patient. If the distress has cleared, check the ventilator settings. Obtain ABG levels immediately or evaluate oximetric monitoring data.	• If the respiratory distress has cleared, the problem is with the ventilator. ABG levels or oximetric data may reveal hypoxemia or hypercapnia, indicators of possible inadequate mechanical ventilation. The ventilator may need to be replaced or adjusted to better meet the patient's needs.
• If the distress continues, perform a rapid cardiopulmonary assessment, suction the airway if indicated, or obtain medical assistance.	• This examination may reveal the cause of the distress, such as airway obstruction or tension pneumothorax.
• Evaluate for signs and symptoms of tension pneumothorax, such as a sudden unexplained increase in inspiratory pressure, shock, decreased or absent breath sounds on affected side, tracheal deviation away from affected side, air hunger, or intense anxiety. If present, anticipate needle thoracentesis or chest tube insertion.	• Positive pressure ventilation increases the risk of barotrauma. Tension pneumothorax, a life-threatening emergency, may result from such factors as rupture of lung blebs, friable tissue, suture disruption, or central line insertion. Immediate chest decompression is necessary to prevent cardiopulmonary arrest from mediastinal shift.
• If an objective source of the problem cannot be identified and patient panic is suspected, hand-ventilate the patient at a rate faster than his own, gradually slow down to the ventilator rate, and then reconnect the ventilator, coaching the patient in a calm, reassuring tone to breathe in synchrony with the ventilator.	• The patient may panic about the need for mechanical ventilation or the sensations associated with the procedure. Hyperventilation may worsen the panic. Adjusting the ventilatory rate as described gains control over hyperventilation. Conveying calmness while coaching the patient in specific maneuvers helps build a sense of trust and provides reassurance that the situation is under control.
• If the problem persists, implement changes in ventilator settings, sedate the patient (usually with morphine sulfate), or paralyze the patient, for example, with pancuronium bromide (Pavulon), as ordered. If paralysis is prescribed, be sure that sedation with an amnesic agent, such as diazepam (Valium) or midazolam (Versed) also is prescribed.	• Persistent struggling may indicate the need for ventilator adjustments or pharmacologic support. Morphine reduces anxiety and respiratory drive. Pavulon induces apnea, eliminating the problem of "fighting" the ventilator, but does not blunt consciousness. Because paralysis can be terrifying for the fully conscious patient, sedation with an amnesic agent is indicated.
4. Monitor patients on PEEP closely for barotrauma, decreased cardiac output, water retention, and, if the patient has an ICP monitor, increased ICP.	4. Because PEEP is superimposed on intrathoracic pressure already increased from mechanical ventilation, it further increases the risks of barotrauma and cardiovascular deterioration. The mechanism by which PEEP alters fluid imbalance is unclear, but it may be mediated by antidiuretic hormone (ADH), baroreceptors, renin production, or stimulation of the sympathetic nervous system. PEEP may increase pressure in the superior vena cava, thereby impeding cerebral venous drainage and raising ICP.

Interventions	Rationales
5. Additional individualized interventions: ____________	5. Rationales: ____________
DECREASED CARDIAC OUTPUT	
1. Monitor the patient for signs and symptoms of decreased cardiac output, such as hypotension, tachycardia, deteriorating mental status, and dysrhythmias. Report findings promptly to the doctor. Administer I.V. fluid or vasopressors, as ordered.	1. The increased intrathoracic pressure associated with mechanical ventilation diminishes venous return and may cause a right-to-left shift of the interventricular septum that impinges on left ventricular filling. Also, reducing the work required for breathing and adminstering oxygen, sedation, or other therapies, such as vasodilators, can cause abrupt significant decreases in the level of sympathetic tone previously supporting blood pressure. Most patients placed on mechanical ventilation develop hypotension, but it usually responds well to fluid and vasopressor support.
2. Read pulmonary artery (PA) and wedge pressures at end-expiration.	2. PA waveforms reflect fluctuations in intrathoracic pressure. Positive pressure ventilation causes the waveforms to rise during inspiration and drop during expiration. Reading pressures at end-expiration minimizes the effects of respiratory variation.
3. If the patient is on PEEP, consult the doctor about the specific technique for reading wedge pressures. In general, leave the patient on the ventilator, and do not make any adjustments to the readings; instead, monitor the trend of values over time.	3. Controversy exists over the extent to which PEEP affects wedge pressures. Usually, wedge pressures obtained on the ventilator are similar to those obtained with the ventilator disconnected, so the benefit of maintaining PEEP argues in favor of reading pressures on the ventilator. (The lack of effect is thought to occur because poorly compliant lungs do not transmit airway pressures well to the heart and pulmonary capillary bed.) If a discrepancy is present, the doctor may wish to confirm by X-ray that the tip of the catheter lies in the basal third of the lung, where pulmonary vascular pressures are believed to be least affected by alveolar pressure.
4. Additional individualized interventions: ____________	4. Rationales: ____________
PULMONARY INFECTION	
1. Monitor the humidifier's water level and temperature, usually set at body temperature.	1. Artificial airways bypass the upper-airway mechanisms for warming, humidifying, and purifying inspired air. Humidification is added to the ventilator to prevent mucosal dehydration and inspissated secretions. The temperature is controlled to prevent loss of body heat or tracheal burns.
2. Drain condensed fluid in the ventilator tubing into a basin rather than back into the humidifier.	2. This condensation, from humidified air passed through the ventilator, is considered contaminated and must be discarded because it increases expiratory pressure and resistance in the ventilatory circuit. It also could be aspirated by the patient.
3. Observe for signs and symptoms of pulmonary infection, such as fever, purulent secretions, or elevated white blood cell count.	3. Artificial airways provide a direct access by which contaminants may enter the lungs.
4. If signs and symptoms of infection are present, consult with the doctor.	4. Pulmonary infections are a major contributor to mortality from mechanical ventilation. Because they usually occur in debilitated patients and are caused by virulent pathogens, they require prompt, aggressive therapy.

(continued)

Interventions	Rationales
5. Additional individualized interventions: ___________	5. Rationales: ___________
GASTROINTESTINAL BLEEDING	
1. Insert a nasogastric tube, as ordered.	1. Nasogastric intubation helps prevent gastric dilatation and reduces risk of aspiration.
2. Administer antacids, ranitidine, or cimetidine, as ordered, spacing doses. Implement additional measures from the "Gastrointestinal Hemorrhage" care plan, page 191, as appropriate.	2. GI hemorrhage may result from the development of a stress ulcer, a complication of prolonged mechanical ventilation. Although its exact cause is not well understood, it is thought to result from excess gastric acid secretion and decreased gastric mucosal resistance. Antacids neutralize gastric acid; cimetidine and ranitidine decrease gastric acid secretion. Antacids should not be given concurrently with cimetidine because they may impair its absorption. The "Gastrointestinal Bleeding" care plan contains detailed interventions for ulcer-related bleeding.
3. Additional individualized interventions: ___________	3. Rationales: ___________
FLUID RETENTION	
1. Monitor for signs and symptoms of fluid retention. If present, consult with the doctor about treatment.	1. Fluid retention may result from the humidifier's interference with insensible water loss via the lungs, decreased lymphatic flow, or altered secretion of ADH.
2. Additional individualized interventions: ___________	2. Rationales: ___________

Target outcome criteria

Throughout the period of mechanical ventilation, the patient will:

- have vital signs within acceptable limits
- maintain a cardiac index of 2.5 to 4.0 liters/minute/m^2
- remain free of pulmonary infection
- display no signs of GI bleeding.

Nursing diagnosis: *Fear related to inability to speak and dependence on a machine for life support*

NURSING PRIORITY: Promote acceptance of mechanical ventilation.

Interventions	Rationales
1. Implement the general measures in the "Ineffective Coping" care plan, page 26, as appropriate.	1. Mechanical ventilation is an extremely stressful experience for most patients. The "Ineffective Coping" care plan contains comprehensive information on ways to decrease the stress of critical illness and facilitate positive coping.
2. Establish a communication method, such as eye blinks, magic slate, or paper and pencil. Be sure the call light is always within reach.	2. Intubation prevents use of the vocal cords. Needing to communicate and being unable to do so is extremely stressful. Provision of alternate methods increases security and promotes patient safety.

Interventions

3. Reduce the patient's need for verbal communication by anticipating needs, providing consistency in staffing and routines, using frequent eye contact, and reassuring the patient that his condition is monitored constantly. Emphasize that a nurse is immediately available if needed.

Rationales

3. Although alternate communication methods do work, they are cumbersome and fatiguing. Reducing the need for verbal communication helps reduce the patient's fatigue and frustration, whereas reassurance helps reduce fear.

4. Explain the reason for mechanical ventilation. Briefly orient the patient and family to the ventilator's features, if appropriate, stressing features (such as alarms) which may be important to them. Encourage questions. Stress the temporary nature of ventilation, if applicable.

4. Mechanical ventilation commonly is instituted under crisis conditions, and explanation and emotional preparation may not have been possible initially. Even if they were provided, stress may have caused blocking or selective filtering of information. Briefly reviewing the procedure and encouraging questions may relieve unstated anxiety about the device.

5. Additional individualized interventions: ____________

5. Rationales: ____________

Target outcome criteria
Within 2 hours of the onset of mechanical ventilation and then continuously, the patient will:
- be able to communicate needs, if conscious
- appear relaxed.

Collaborative problem: *Potential ineffective weaning related to lack of physiologic or psychological readiness*

NURSING PRIORITY: Promote a smooth transition to spontaneous ventilation.

Interventions

1. Anticipate weaning when the patient meets these criteria: improvement in underlying disease process (as manifested by A-a gradient <300 mm Hg on 100% oxygen, shunt $<20\%$, $V_D/V_T < 0.6$, RR <24/minute, MV 5 to 10 liters), stable hemodynamic status, and adequate muscle strength (as manifested by VC >10 to 15 ml/kg and MIF > -20 cmH_2O).

Rationales

1. Many factors affect the success of weaning attempts. Premature attempts to wean impose unnecessary physiologic stress on the patient, jeopardizing recovery. Meeting the listed criteria increases the likelihood that weaning will be accomplished with few or no setbacks.

2. Ascertain that the patient is rested, well-nourished, oriented, able to follow commands, and not receiving any respiratory depressants.

2. Reestablishing spontaneous ventilation is physically demanding, and the patient must have adequate energy reserves to succeed. The ability to take a deep breath and cough on command helps prevent atelectasis and airway obstruction. A strong respiratory drive is essential to resume spontaneous breathing.

3. Explain the weaning process to the patient and family. Mention that the patient may feel short of breath initially. Stress that the patient will be attended closely during the trial of spontaneous breathing and that if it is not successful, it will be tried again later.

3. Weaning is stressful psychologically. Thorough emotional preparation promotes a sense of security. Preparing the patient for the possibility of "trying again later" may reduce the sense of failure if the weaning attempt is unsuccessful.

4. Obtain baseline vital signs, ABG levels, and pulmonary function measurements. Suction the airway.

4. These measurements provide a basis for comparison with later ones used to evaluate the appropriateness of weaning. Suctioning the airway reduces the risk of aspiration because secretions may have accumulated above the cuff.

(continued)

Interventions

5. Implement the weaning method ordered: CPAP, IMV, or T-piece.

Rationales

5. CPAP may facilitate weaning for the patient on PEEP by maintaining some positive pressure during the trial of spontaneous breathing. IMV supplies periodic mandatory deep breaths; the rate can be decreased by 2 breaths at a time until the patient's breathing is completely spontaneous. A T-piece provides supplemental oxygen during weaning.

6. Monitor the blood pressure, heart rate, EKG rhythm, respiratory rate, ease of breathing, level of consciousness, and level of fatigue constantly for the first 20 to 30 minutes and every 5 minutes thereafter until weaning is complete.

6. Frequent monitoring of the indicated parameters provides ongoing indications of the success or failure of the weaning attempt.

7. In collaboration with the doctor, terminate weaning if adverse reactions occur, such as heart rate increase >20 beats/minute, systolic blood pressure increase >20 mm Hg, respiratory rate <8 or >24 breaths/minute, ventricular dysrhythmias, labored or erratic breathing, fatigue, or panic.

7. Attempts to persist in weaning an unstable patient may precipitate cardiorespiratory arrest from hypoxia or dysrhythmogenesis.

8. If weaning continues, measure the V_T, MV, and ABG levels in 20 to 30 minutes. Compare to desired values for this patient, determined in collaboration with the doctor, typically V_T 300 to 700 ml, MV 5 to 10 liters, pH 7.35 to 7.45, PaO_2 >70 mm Hg, and $PaCO_2$ 35 to 45 mm Hg.

8. Values at this point help determine the appropriateness of weaning.

9. If physiologic parameters indicate weaning is feasible, but the patient resists, consider the possibility of psychological dependence on the ventilator. Consult with the doctor, pulmonary nurse specialist, or psychiatric nurse clinician, as appropriate.

9. Psychological dependence on the ventilator is a common problem for patients following prolonged periods of mechanical ventilation. Possible causes for dependency include fear of dying, depression from chronic illness, and secondary gains from illness role. Consultation with other professionals may help to uncover causes and formulate appropriate intervention to resolve underlying fears or conflicts.

10. Assist with extubation, when ordered. Confirm that someone qualified to reintubate is present when extubation is performed.

10. The same criteria used to evaluate readiness for weaning are used to determine readiness for extubation. Patients ventilated for short periods (24 to 48 hours) commonly are ready for extubation after a 30-minute trial of spontaneous breathing, whereas those ventilated for longer periods may require days to weeks of gradual weaning. Availability of immediate reintubation is critical because postextubation airway obstruction can be sudden and fatal.

11. Additional individualized interventions: ______________

11. Rationales: ______________

Target outcome criteria
During the weaning process and continuously thereafter, the patient will:
- maintain a clear airway
- maintain a spontaneous RR of 12 to 24 breaths/minute
- manifest ABG levels within normal limits
- display pulmonary function measurements within normal limits
- display normal sinus rhythm (NSR) with no ectopic beats, or a benign variant such as sinus arrhythmia or an NSR with <4 PVCs/minute
- remain alert and oriented.

Transfer planning

NURSING TRANSFER CRITERIA

Upon transfer, documentation shows evidence of:
- respiratory status (after extubation) stable for >12 hours
- absence of significant dysrhythmias (without I.V. antiarrhythmic drugs) for >12 hours
- level of consciousness stable for >12 hours
- vital signs within normal limits.

PATIENT-FAMILY TEACHING CHECKLIST

Document evidence that patient and family demonstrate understanding of:
__ reason for instituting mechanical ventilation
__ communication measures
__ alarms
__ weaning process.

DOCUMENTATION CHECKLIST

Using outcome criteria as a guide, document:
__ clinical status on admission
__ significant changes in status
__ pertinent diagnostic test findings
__ ventilator and patient checks
__ ventilator alarm status
__ airway care
__ measures to prevent or detect and treat complications
__ communication measures
__ emotional support
__ sedative or paralyzing pharmacologic agents, if used
__ weaning process
__ patient/family teaching
__ transfer planning.

ASSOCIATED CARE PLANS

Adult Respiratory Distress Syndrome
Impaired Physical Mobility
Ineffective Coping
Nutritional Deficit
Sensory-Perceptual Alteration

REFERENCES

Bernard, G., and Bradley, R. "Adult Respiratory Distress Syndrome: Diagnosis and Management," *Heart & Lung* 15:250-55, May/June 1986.

Brent-Hemman, E. "Ventilatory Support," in *Critical Care Nursing,* 4th ed. Edited by Hudak, C., et al. Philadelphia: J.B. Lippincott Co., 1986.

Celentano-Norton, L. "Mechanical Ventilation Strategies in Adult Respiratory Distress Syndrome," *Critical Care Nurse* 6:71-83, July/August 1986.

Chalkian, J., and Weaver, T. "Mechanical Ventilation: Where It's At, Where It's Going," *American Journal of Nursing* 84:1373-79, November 1984.

Grossbach, I. "Troubleshooting Ventilator- and Patient-Related Problems, Part I," *Critical Care Nurse* 6:58-70, July/August 1986.

Grossbach, I. "Troubleshooting Ventilator- and Patient-Related Problems, Part II," *Critical Care Nurse* 6:64-79, September/October 1986.

Holloway, N., and Jacobs, S. "Aeration Treatment Disorders," in *Nursing the Critically Ill Adult,* 3rd ed. Edited by Holloway, N. Menlo Park, Calif.: Addison-Wesley Publishing Co., 1988.

Shapiro, B., et al. *Clinical Application of Respiratory Care,* 3rd ed. Chicago: Yearbook Medical Publishers, 1985.

Pulmonary Embolism

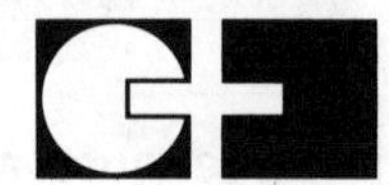

DRG information

DRG 078 Pulmonary Embolism.
Mean LOS = 9.0 days
Principal diagnoses include:
- pulmonary embolism and/or infarction
- air or fat embolism.

Introduction

DEFINITION AND TIME FOCUS

A pulmonary embolus (PE) is an undissolved mass deposited in a branch of the pulmonary artery that obstructs blood flow partially or completely. The severity of the associated signs and symptoms depends on the amount of lung involved and the embolus size. The episode may be massive or submassive.

In submassive embolism, numerous small emboli may occur. They usually lodge in the periphery of the pulmonary arterial bed and may or may not cause cardiopulmonary decompensation. A massive pulmonary embolus, on the other hand, obstructs more the 50% of the pulmonary arterial circulation and leads to severe, commonly life-threatening cardiopulmonary sequelae. Venous thromboemboli are the most common cause of obstruction, accounting for approximately 95% of cases; the vast majority of these arise from deep venous thrombosis in the legs. Bone fragments, air emboli, amniotic fluid, fat emboli, and septic emboli also may occur. This clinical plan focuses on the immediate care of the symptomatic, newly diagnosed thromboembolic patient in a critical care setting.

ETIOLOGY AND PRECIPITATING FACTORS

- venous stasis, such as with deep venous thrombosis, elderly population, postpartum, immobility, burns, varicose veins, congestive heart failure, atrial fibrillation, or right ventricular infarction
- injury of vascular endothelium, such as with venipuncture of the legs, surgery (especially abdominal, pelvic, or hip), I.V. drug abuse, or trauma (particularly long bone fractures or myocardial injury)
- hypercoagulability, such as with dehydration, cancer (especially of lung, pancreas, or stomach), oral contraceptive use, blood dyscrasias, or pregnancy

Focused assessment guidelines

NURSING HISTORY (Functional health pattern findings)

Health perception–health management pattern

- reports sudden shortness of breath (most common symptom)

Cognitive-perceptual pattern

- complains of chest pain, similar to angina but worsened by inspiration
- may report apprehension or a sense of impending doom
- may report headache

Coping–stress tolerance pattern

- may report anxiety or fear

PHYSICAL FINDINGS

General appearance

- in acute distress

Cardiovascular

- tachycardia (in 60% to 75% of patients)
- accentuated P_2 (in massive PE)
- neck vein distention (in massive PE)
- syncope
- murmur
- hypotension
- S_3 gallop (rare)

Pulmonary

- tachypnea
- crackles
- wheezes
- decreased breath sounds
- pleural friction rub
- cough (usually seen with concurrent pulmonary infarction)
- hemoptysis (usually seen with concurrent pulmonary infarction)

Neurologic

- decreased level of consciousness
- confusion
- restlessness
- hallucinations
- euphoria (rare)

Integumentary

- pallor
- cyanosis
- diaphoresis

Musculoskeletal

Note: More than half of all patients with deep venous thrombosis in the leg have no signs or symptoms of phlebitis. If present, they include:
- swelling
- pain
- warmth
- redness

Renal

• oliguria

DIAGNOSTIC STUDIES

Note: No diagnostic laboratory test exists for PE; laboratory data are used to rule out other conditions or provide general confirming evidence.

• arterial blood gas (ABG) levels—may reveal PaO_2 <80 mm Hg and $PaCO_2$ <35 mm Hg, indicating respiratory alkalosis and increasing the likelihood of a PE

• sedimentation rate—increased (a nonspecific response)

• serum bilirubin—increased if right heart failure is present

• pulmonary angiogram—considered the diagnostic standard for detecting and confirming pulmonary emboli; it reveals constant intraluminal filling defect(s) on multiple films and sharp cutoff in vessels >2.5 mm in diameter

• 12-lead EKG—used to rule out myocardial infarction; it commonly reveals various dysrhythmias, especially paroxysmal atrial tachycardia and, in massive PE, right bundle branch block; if right heart failure is present, it may reveal typical changes such as predominantly negative QRS complexes in leads 1 to 3 and inverted T waves in V_1 and V_2

• chest X-ray—may be normal, or it may reveal:
  - □ infiltration
  - □ pleural effusion
  - □ atelectasis
  - □ elevated diaphragm on affected side
  - □ enlarged pulmonary arteries
  - □ sudden cut-off of a pulmonary shadow
  - □ cardiac enlargement with prominent right atrial border, right ventricular dilatation, and dilated superior vena cava
  - □ a hump-shaped shadow on the affected side, if infarction is present.

• impedance plethysmography—performed commonly because 85% of pulmonary emboli arise from deep leg veins; it reveals increased pressure in veins distal to obstruction

• ventilation-perfusion lung scan—may reveal area of normal ventilation with decreased or absent perfusion

POTENTIAL COMPLICATIONS

• recurrent embolism
• atelectasis
• right ventricular failure
• shock
• cardiopulmonary arrest
• dysrhythmias
• pulmonary hemorrhage (rare)
• pulmonary infarction (rare)

Collaborative problem: *Hypoxemia related to ventilation-perfusion mismatch*

NURSING PRIORITY: Maintain adequate ventilation.

Interventions	Rationales
1. Assess pulmonary status at least every 4 hours. Note the presence of:	1. Serial assessments indicate the severity of the disorder and effectiveness of interventions.
• tachypnea and dyspnea	• Tachypnea, a cardinal sign, is a compensatory measure to increase oxygenation. The tachypneic breathing pattern is attributed to stimulation of intrapulmonary receptors in the alveolar-capillary wall. Dyspnea results from apprehension or the sudden increase in alveolar dead space from alveoli that are ventilated but not perfused. The mismatch of ventilation and perfusion causes impaired gas exchange.
• wheezing	• Wheezing results from pneumoconstriction following hypocapnia and platelet degranulation. Local hypocapnia constricts bronchial smooth muscle, increasing airway resistance, and redirecting ventilation to better perfused areas; the resulting reduction in wasted ventilation is a protective mechanism. The thromboembolus consists of fibrin, red blood cells, and platelets; platelet degranulation releases substances that provoke bronchoconstriction and vasoconstriction.
• decreased or absent breath sounds	• Normally, surfactant reduces surface tension as alveoli deflate, preventing alveolar collapse and lessening the work of breathing necessary to reinflate alveoli. Decreased surfactant production leads to atelectasis.

(continued)

Interventions	Rationales
• crackles and rhonchi	• Normally, surfactant also minimizes transudation of capillary fluid into alveoli by controlling alveolar surface tension. Decreased surfactant increases surface tension and allows fluid transudation, resulting in interstitial edema.
• mentation changes.	• Mentation changes reflect cerebral hypoxemia.
2. Monitor ABG levels, as ordered.	2. ABG levels provide objective evidence of the degree of hypoxemia, useful in evaluating the severity of the PE and effectiveness of interventions.
3. Administer supplemental oxygen, as ordered.	3. Supplemental oxygen administration prevents the immediate sequelae of hypoxemia, which may include dysrhythmias, cerebral ischemia, and myocardial infarction.
4. Elevate the head of the bed 30 to 45 degrees. Use pillows to support the patient in a comfortable position.	4. This position promotes respiratory excursion and reduces the cardiopulmonary work load.
5. Maintain strict bed rest. Assist with bathing, eating, and other activities that increase dyspnea.	5. Rest conserves energy needed for the work of breathing.
6. Implement a program of vigorous pulmonary hygiene, including deep-breathing exercises and frequent repositioning. Suction as necessary.	6. Elevated $PaCO_2$ levels can be reduced by adequate alveolar ventilation. Restoring effective aeration may prevent the onset of pneumonia from retention of secretions in the atelectatic area.
7. Assist with intubation and mechanical ventilation with positive end-expiratory pressure (PEEP), as needed. Refer to the "Mechanical Ventilation" care plan, page 108, for guidelines.	7. If the above measures are ineffective at controlling hypoxemia, intubation and mechanical ventilation with PEEP may reopen collapsed alveoli. The "Mechanical Ventilation" care plan details the care involved in this therapeutic modality.
8. Additional individualized interventions: ____________	8. Rationales: ____________

Target outcome criteria

Within 48 hours of onset, the patient will:

- have ABG levels returning to normal limits
- have clear breath sounds bilaterally
- display no dyspnea.

Collaborative problem: *Potential decreased cardiac output related to pulmonary arterial hypertension and right heart failure*

NURSING PRIORITY: Support adequate cardiac output.

Interventions	Rationales
1. Institute constant EKG monitoring, if not already present. Observe for dysrhythmias, particularly paroxysmal atrial tachycardia (PAT) or right bundle-branch block.	1. The right ventricle may decompensate in response to the sudden elevation in pulmonary pressure. PAT or other atrial dysrhythmias reflect atrial stretching from volume overload, whereas bundle branch block probably reflects right ventricular strain. Other dysrhythmias may result from cardiac ischemia or hypoxemia; and cardiopulmonary arrest may occur in massive embolism.
2. Maintain patency of an I.V. line and administer fluids, as ordered.	2. Although the PE patient is not volume depleted, I.V. access is critical for medication administration.

Interventions	Rationales
3. Assist with insertion of a pulmonary artery (PA) catheter, as ordered. Monitor pulmonary artery pressure (PAP) and pulmonary capillary wedge pressure (PCWP), as ordered, typically every hour until stable and then every 4 hours.	3. A PA catheter facilitates monitoring of objective data useful in assessing hemodynamic function of the left and right sides of the heart.
4. Monitor for signs and symptoms of right heart failure, such as neck vein distention and elevated central venous pressure readings. If any are present, notify the doctor and implement measures in the "Acute Heart Failure" care plan, page 140, as appropriate.	4. Mechanical obstruction from the embolus and release of vasoconstrictor substances, previously described, elevate pulmonary vascular resistance. The increased resistance to right ventricular ejection may precipitate right heart failure. The "Acute Heart Failure" care plan contains comprehensive information on this potential problem.
5. Monitor for signs and symptoms of cardiogenic shock, such as severe hypotension and elevated PCWP. If present, notify the doctor and implement measures in the "Shock" care plan, page 173, as appropriate.	5. Major obstruction to ventricular ejection produces cardiogenic shock. The "Shock" care plan presents detailed assessment and interventions for cardiogenic shock.
6. If above measures are ineffective or the PE is life-threatening, prepare the patient for emergency surgery, if ordered.	6. Pulmonary embolectomy may be a life-saving operation.
7. Additional individualized interventions: ____________	7. Rationales: ____________

Target outcome criteria

Within 48 hours of onset, the patient will have:
- blood pressure within normal limits
- cardiac rhythm within normal limits
- PAP and PCWP within normal limits
- warm and dry skin
- urine output >60 ml/hour.

Nursing diagnosis: *Potential for injury: complications related to recurrent emboli, anticoagulant therapy, or thrombolytic therapy*

NURSING PRIORITY: Prevent or minimize complications.

Interventions	Rationales
1. Provide standard nursing care to prevent thromboemboli, such as applying antiembolic stockings; performing active or passive leg exercises; ensuring adequate fluid intake; and avoiding high Fowler's position, knee gatching, and leg massage.	1. These measures help maintain peripheral venous blood flow by preventing stasis, hypercoagulability, and dislodgment of any clots present. They also minimize additional clot formation.
2. Administer heparin, as ordered, typically by continuous low dose infusion. Monitor the partial thromboplastin time daily and maintain within prescribed therapeutic range, typically twice the control value.	2. Heparin is a potent anticoagulant that inactivates thrombin and blocks further clot formation. It also inhibits platelet degranulation around the thrombus and limits the release of vasoconstricting substances. Subtherapeutic values indicate the person is not fully anticoagulated and therefore still at risk for recurrent emboli. Values beyond the therapeutic range indicate the patient is excressively anticoagulated and at risk for bleeding episodes.

(continued)

Interventions	Rationales
3. Administer streptokinase or urokinase therapy, according to unit protocol, as ordered. Protocols vary but generally include: • contraindications: recent surgery or cerebral vascular accident; active bleeding; and severe hypertension • administration via a pulmonary artery catheter or systemic infusion • a loading dose followed by constant infusion for several hours • maintenance of thrombin time at 2 to 5 times normal • monitoring for bleeding episodes.	3. Streptokinase or urokinase therapy may be ordered for the unstable patient with massive embolism. These thrombolytic agents dissolve already formed clots, resulting in decreased symptomatology. Streptokinase, the enzyme from beta-hemolytic streptococcus, converts plasminogen to plasmin, producing fibrinolysis, and resulting in decreased blood viscosity, improved microcirculation, and improved oxygen delivery. Urokinase also converts plasminogen to plasmin, degrading fibrin clots, fibrinogen, and other plasma proteins. Unit protocols vary regarding details of administration and monitoring for side effects, the most significant of which is bleeding.
4. Minimize the risk of bleeding, for example, avoid intramuscular injections when possible and collaborate with the doctor or clinical pharmacist to limit interactions between anticoagulants or thrombolytic agents and other medications the patient is receiving. Monitor for both apparent and occult bleeding, for example, by observing for hematomas and by guaiac-testing gastric contents and stool.	4. Anticoagulation and thrombolytic therapy increase the risk of bleeding. Early detection provides time for adjusting doses before massive hemorrhage occurs.
5. If emboli recur despite above measures, prepare the patient for surgery, as ordered.	5. Vena cava ligation or insertion of a vena cava umbrella can trap recurrent emboli, which fibrinolysis then can dissolve.
6. Additional individualized interventions: ____________	6. Rationales: ____________

Target outcome criteria

Throughout the unit stay, the patient will:

- experience minor bleeding only
- display no signs of recurrent emboli.

Nursing diagnosis: *Ineffective coping related to potentially life-threatening situation*

NURSING PRIORITY: Provide emotional support to the patient and family.

Interventions	Rationales
1. Implement measures in the "Ineffective Coping" care plan, page 26, as appropriate. If death is imminent, implement measures in the "Grieving and Dying" care plan, page 15, as appropriate.	1. Pulmonary embolism is a major psychological threat, acknowledged in the classic finding of a sense of impending doom. The "Ineffective Coping" care plan contains measures to help the patient and family deal with the emotional aftermath of a PE. If therapeutic measures are ineffective and the patient's condition continues deteriorating, measures contained in the "Grieving and Dying" care plan may help the patient and family cope with approaching death.
2. Additional individualized interventions: ____________	2. Rationales: ____________

Target outcome criteria
By the time of transfer, the patient and family will meet the outcome criteria identified in the "Ineffective Coping" care plan.

Otherwise, by the time of death, the patient and family will meet the outcome criteria identified in the"Grieving and Dying" care plan.

Transfer planning

NURSING TRANSFER CRITERIA

Upon transfer, documentation shows evidence of:
- stable blood pressure, pulse, and respiratory rate
- removal of PA catheter.

PATIENT-FAMILY TEACHING CHECKLIST

Document evidence that patient and family demonstrate understanding of:
__ underlying reasons for clot development
__ rationale for therapy
__ measures to prevent recurrence.

DOCUMENTATION CHECKLIST

Using outcome criteria as a guide, document:
__ clinical status on admission
__ significant changes in status
__ pertinent diagnostic test findings
__ oxygen therapy
__ heparin therapy
__ thrombolytic therapy
__ patient/family teaching
__ transfer planning.

ASSOCIATED CARE PLANS

Acute Heart Failure
Acute Pain
Grieving and Dying
Ineffective Coping
Shock

REFERENCES

Burke, C., and Morris, A. "Perfusion Scans and Pulmonary Angiography," *Heart & Lung* 15(4):357-60, 1986.

Fahey, A. "Life-Threatening Pulmonary Embolism," *Critical Care Quarterly* 8:81-88, September 1985.

Hall, J., et al. "Urokinase Therapy for Massive Pulmonary Embolism," *Critical Care Quarterly* 8:69-72, March 1985.

Hamer, S., and Lemberg, L. "A Complication Commonly Overlooked," *Heart & Lung* 11:588-92, 1982.

Holloway, N., and Jacobs, S. "Pulmonary Embolus," in *Nursing the Critically Ill Adult,* 3rd ed. Edited by Holloway, N. Menlo Park, Calif.: Addison-Wesley Publishing, Co. 1988.

Woodruff, M. "Pulmonary Thromboembolism: Risk Factors, Pathophysiology and Management," *Critical Care Nurse* 4:52-63, July/August 1984.

Thoracotomy

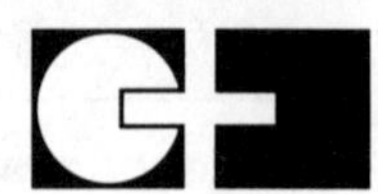

DRG information

DRG 075 Major Chest Procedures.
Mean LOS = 12.3 days
Principal procedures include:
- exploratory thoracotomy
- biopsy of diaphragm, pericardium, thymus, bronchus, or lung
- surgical collapse of lung
- incision of lung, bronchus, or thoracic vessels
- reopening of recent thoracotomy site
- pleurectomy and/or repair of pleura
- repair of diaphragmatic hernia, abdominal or thoracic approach.

Additional DRG information: Thoracotomy as an operative approach for other procedures may or may not be classified under DRG 075, depending on the definitive procedure accomplished.

Introduction

DEFINITION AND TIME FOCUS

A thoracotomy is an incision into the chest wall (thorax), whose location depends on the purpose of the surgery. A posterolateral or anterolateral approach (through the ribs) is common with general thoracic surgery, whereas a median sternotomy (through the sternum) is used commonly for cardiothoracic surgical procedures. The ribs or sternal halves are spread to gain access to the operative area within the pleural cavities or the mediastinum. Common thoracotomy procedures on the lungs include exploratory thoracotomy, pneumonectomy (removal of a lung), lobectomy (removal of a lobe), segmental resection (removal of one or several lung segments), wedge resection (removal of part of a lung segment), decortication (removal of scarred, fibrous tissue over the pleura), or thoracoplasty (removal of ribs). Thoracotomies are also used to perform esophageal, diaphragmatic, aortic, or open heart procedures. A thoracotomy is a major surgical procedure that requires careful preoperative and postoperative patient management and may require the use of mechanical ventilation and closed chest drainage. This care plan focuses on preoperative care, postoperative stabilization, and initial recovery of the thoracotomy patient.

ETIOLOGY AND PRECIPITATING FACTORS

- pulmonary conditions, such as cancer, benign tumors, tuberculosis, abscesses or infection, bronchiectasis, blebs or bullae caused by emphysema, or empyema
- cardiac conditions, such as arteriosclerotic coronary arteries, valvular disease, mural wall defects, aortic aneurysm, cardiomyopathy, or congenital heart disease
- hiatal hernias or esophageal problems
- chest trauma involving one or more of the vital chest structures (lungs, heart, aorta, trachea, esophagus, or superior or inferior vena cava)

Focused assessment guidelines

NURSING HISTORY (Functional health pattern findings)

Health perception–health management pattern

- may report shortness of breath or labored breathing on exertion
- may report bloody or excessive sputum
- may report feeling more tired and having less exercise tolerance than usual
- may report swelling of feet and ankles
- may report family history of heart disease or lung conditions, such as asthma
- may report high risk cardiac and respiratory health patterns, such as sedentary life-style, overeating, lack of exercise, stress, smoking, or exposure to respiratory toxins
- may have experienced a major traumatic accident with a blow to the chest

Nutritional-metabolic pattern

- may report a loss of appetite with either a respiratory or cardiac problem
- may report a weight gain with a cardiac problem
- may report a weight loss with a respiratory problem

Activity-exercise pattern

- may report difficulty in breathing at rest and during exercise
- may report weakness and fatigue

Cognitive-perceptual pattern

- may express fear about serious nature of illness and impending major surgery
- may report periods of dizziness

Self-perception–self-concept pattern

- may report fear of disfigurement and scarring

Role-relationship pattern

- may report fear of inability to return to work after surgical procedure
- may have a high-risk job with excessive stress or exposure to respiratory toxins

Sexuality-reproductive pattern

- may report fatigue and inability to sustain sexual activity

PHYSICAL FINDINGS

Note: Physical findings may vary depending on the nature of the condition requiring the thoracotomy.

General appearance

- if a cardiac condition, may present with typical signs and symptoms of angina, acute myocardial infarction, or heart failure. See the "Acute Myocardial Infarction" care plan, page 150, and the "Acute Heart Failure" care plan, page 140, for the general appearance of patients with these problems.
- if a pulmonary condition, may present with respiratory distress or general debilitation depending on whether the condition is rapidly progressing or more chronic in nature
- if chest trauma, may present with respiratory and cardiac distress and obvious crushing or penetrating injuries to the chest

Cardiovascular

- dysrhythmias
- classic angina (substernal pain radiating to left shoulder and arm that is relieved by nitroglycerin or rest)
- unstable angina (substernal and radiating pain that is not relieved by nitroglycerin or rest and that is more serious, prolonged, and unpredictable)
- noncardiac chest pain
- hypotension
- tachycardia

Pulmonary

- dyspnea
- shortness of breath
- tachypnea
- use of accessory muscles
- rhonchi, wheezes, crackles
- if chest trauma, possible open, sucking wound, flail chest, paradoxical asymmetric chest movements, or orthopnea

Gastrointestinal

- if a hiatal hernia or esophageal problem, may have regurgitation, heartburn 30 to 60 minutes after meals, substernal pain, dysphagia, or feelings of fullness
- if a cardiac problem, may have nausea and vomiting

Integumentary

- cyanosis
- pallor
- if chest trauma, abrasions or open wounds

DIAGNOSTIC STUDIES

Because of the various conditions for which thoracotomy may be performed, no typical laboratory data exist. This section instead presents tests used to monitor the patient.

- arterial blood gas (ABG) levels—monitor oxygenation, ventilation, and acid-base status
- cardiac enzymes, creatine phosphokinase, lactic acid dehydrogenase—may reveal cardiac tissue damage
- complete blood count—monitors red blood cell count, white blood cell (WBC) count, and platelets. Altered hemoglobin and hematocrit levels reflect any potential blood loss and the oxygen-carrying ability of the blood. An elevated WBC count and an elevated sedimentation rate may reflect an inflammatory response.
- serum creatinine, blood urea nitrogen levels—monitor the adequacy of renal function
- serum electrolyte panel—monitors fluid, electrolyte, and acid-base status
- urinalysis—monitors the renal status including renal secretion and concentration abilities
- sputum assessment—monitors for potential infection
- blood coagulation studies—monitor clotting
- *For all etiologies:*
  - □ chest X-ray—may reveal abnormalities of the chest structures and heart and lung tissues
  - □ EKG—may reveal changes associated with ischemia
  - □ fluoroscopy—may reveal mobility abnormalities of the intrathoracic structures
  - □ magnetic resonance imaging—may reveal abnormalities of the thoracic structures and organs
- *For cardiac or pulmonary etiologies:*
  - □ computed tomography—may reveal abnormalities of the lung, such as tumors, calcium deposits, or cavities; and abnormalities of the heart, such as an enlarged heart
  - □ biopsy—may aid in definitive diagnosis of lung or heart problems
  - □ gallium scan—may reveal inflammation or tumors of the heart or lungs
- *For pulmonary etiologies:*
  - □ ventilation-perfusion pulmonary scan—may reveal areas of nonventilation and nonperfusion
  - □ pulmonary function tests—monitor static and dynamic lung volumes and capacities
  - □ bronchoscopy—may reveal abnormalities of the pulmonary tree
  - □ sonogram of the lung—may reveal collections of fluid and may be used postoperatively to locate the best site for thoracentesis
  - □ thoracentesis—may reveal abnormalities of fluid or tissue specimens
  - □ bronchograms—may reveal abnormalities of the airway structures or the presence of tumor
- *For cardiac etiologies:*
  - □ cardiac radionuclide imaging—may reveal areas of ischemia and necrosis in the heart tissue
  - □ echocardiography—may reveal structural and motion abnormalities of the heart
  - □ cardiac catheterization—may reveal abnormalities of the coronary arteries (during left heart catheterization) or pulmonary artery vasculature (during right heart catheterization)

- *For esophageal problems:*
  - □ barium swallow, esophagoscopy, motility studies—may reveal abnormalities of the esophagus

POTENTIAL COMPLICATIONS

- cardiac dysrhythmias
- atelectasis
- pleural effusion
- pericardial effusion
- tension pneumothorax
- hemothorax
- infection
- pulmonary edema
- pulmonary embolism
- hemorrhage
- cardiac arrest
- shock
- cardiac tamponade

Nursing diagnosis: *Knowledge deficit: preoperative and postoperative care related to impending thoracotomy*

NURSING PRIORITY: Prepare the patient and family preoperatively for surgery and postoperative care.

Interventions	Rationales
1. Refer to the "Knowledge Deficit" care plan, page 45.	1. The "Knowledge Deficit" care plan contains general assessments and interventions for teaching and learning. This plan focuses on specifics for thoracotomy.
2. Provide information about the surgery. Document teaching and the patient's and family's response. Include the following points:	2. Preoperative teaching may allay fears and anxiety about the "unknown" and allow the patient to cooperate with care and to summon energy for healing.
• purpose, goal, and general procedure	• A general understanding of the purpose, goal, and procedure will help orient the patient to the care he or she will receive.
• type of incision	• Preoperative knowledge about the length and nature of the incision may reduce anxiety.
• usual scar	• Knowledge that the surgical incision scar will heal to a thin, white line may reduce fear of major disfigurement.
• preoperative medication	• Knowledge of the availability of preoperative sedation may reduce anxiety.
• anesthesia	• Knowledge about the methods and effects of anesthesia may prepare the patient for the postoperative side effects.
• expected location for recovery in the immediate postoperative period	• Knowledge of the location for recovery may reduce postoperative disorientation.
• I.V. and other lines	• Postoperative thoracotomy patients may have many lines, including peripheral I.V., central I.V., and monitoring lines. The necessary tubing and equipment could be frightening without preoperative preparation.
• oxygen therapy	• All thoracotomy patients require oxygen therapy postoperatively because of the atelectasis and hypoxemia produced by opening the chest and by anesthesia. The specific type of oxygen therapy varies depending on the surgery. Preoperative preparation about the oxygen therapy to be used with the patient may increase postoperative cooperation, particularly with patients who will be intubated and placed on mechanical ventilation.
• chest tubes and drainage system	• Explanations of the need for chest tubes and a drainage system to help re-expand the lungs and hasten recovery may allay anxiety about the invasive appearance of these tubes.
• nasogastric (NG) tube	• Explanation about the use of the NG tube to reduce abdominal discomfort until the GI tract resumes function may increase patient tolerance for this tube.

Interventions

• Foley catheter.

Rationales

• Explanation about the need to closely monitor intake and output, including urine, in the postoperative period may reduce anxiety about the catheter.

3. Describe the use of endotracheal intubation and the use of a mechanical ventilator, if appropriate. See the "Mechanical Ventilation" care plan, page 108. Document.

3. Explanation about intubation and mechanical ventilation, including the prevention of speech, may allay anxiety about this treatment. The "Mechanical Ventilation" care plan includes detailed information about caring for a mechanically ventilated patient.

4. Explain the surgery's general effects on the lungs and describe re-expansion methods. Provide practice on deep breathing, coughing, the use of incentive inspirometers, if ordered, and procedures for the measurement of vital capacity and maximum inspiratory pressures. Observe return demonstrations. Document teaching and response.

4. Explaining the effect that opening the chest wall has on the lungs and describing re-expansion methods provide an incentive for active patient involvement postoperatively. The patient's postoperative efforts to re-expand lungs, remove secretions, and participate in respiratory function measurements may be more successful if practice has been provided preoperatively, during a less stressful and pain-free time.

5. Discuss and document methods to relieve postoperative pain, including pain medication and the use of a pillow to splint the incision during deep breathing and coughing.

5. Thoracotomy pain is described as severe by most patients. Patients may be reassured to learn that adequate pain relief is an important part of therapy. Explanations about the timely use of pain medication and pillow splinting during coughing and deep breathing may increase the patient's willingness to initiate and perform such maneuvers as coughing and deep breathing.

6. Describe and document the expected levels of postoperative activity, including turning from side to side, as allowed, every 2 hours during the day of surgery, sitting in a semi-Fowler's position and sitting on the bedside with his legs dangling the first day after surgery, getting into a chair with assistance the first or second day after surgery, and ambulating in the room and hallway the second or third day after surgery. Emphasize the importance of activity despite postoperative discomfort.

6. Thoracotomy patients commonly resist activity because of pain, fatigue, and weakness. Knowledge of expected activity levels and importance of activity provide a foundation on which the nurse can capitalize postoperatively when implementing the activity schedule.

7. Explain and demonstrate the use of antiembolism stockings. Document.

7. Antiembolism stockings aid venous return and prevent the formation of thrombus in the lower extremities.

8. Additional individualized interventions: ____________

____

8. Rationales: ____________

____

Target outcome criteria

Within 2 hours after preoperative teaching, the patient, on request, will:

• explain the purpose, goal, and general procedure for a thoracotomy and specific points covered during teaching

• demonstrate deep breathing, coughing, the use of an inspirometer, pillow splinting, and range-of-motion (ROM) and other exercises.

Collaborative problem: *Hypoxemia related to hypoventilation from anesthesia, pain, and analgesic medications as well as dysrhythmias, atelectasis, and inspissated secretions*

NURSING PRIORITY: Optimize ventilation and oxygenation.

Interventions	Rationales
1. Postoperatively, assess the following every 15 minutes until stable, every 30 minutes for 2 hours, then every 1 to 2 hours and as needed. Document and notify the doctor of abnormal findings.	1. The patient usually returns from surgery with a pulmonary artery catheter, arterial line, peripheral I.V. lines, and pleural or mediastinal chest tubes, or both. Frequent assessments of the cardiorespiratory system may reveal problems and allow timely interventions.
• respiratory rate, depth, and pattern; pulse rate; and blood pressure	• Hypoxemia of any cause is reflected in vital sign changes.
• level of consciousness	• Decreased oxygen delivery to the brain is reflected in changing level of consciousness and mentation changes.
• bilateral breath sounds and bilateral chest movements	• Commonly, after thoracotomy, sounds and chest movements may be diminished over the operative area. These findings usually lessen and then disappear as recovery progresses. Adventitious sounds or persistence or worsening of the above findings may reflect fluid accumulation, atelectasis, or other respiratory problems.
• use of accessory muscles	• Use of accessory muscles may reflect dyspnea.
• tracheal position	• Tracheal deviation from midline may indicate increased intrathoracic pressures on the opposite side of the deviation or lung collapse on the same side as the deviation.
• color of mucous membranes, circumoral skin, and earlobes.	• Cyanotic mucous membranes, circumoral skin, and earlobes may indicate hypoxemia.
2. Assess the percussion notes and vocal fremitus as well as the amount, color, and consistency of sputum every 1 to 2 hours and as needed.	2. Dullness to percussion and decreased vocal fremitus are common postoperatively and reflect consolidation from atelectatic areas. Resonance to percussion and normal vocal fremitus should return gradually as recovery progresses, except in pneumonectomy. Sputum characteristics may reflect hydration status, bleeding or infection, or pulmonary edema.
3. Palpate the chest wall every 1 to 2 hours and as needed. Note the presence of tenderness, pain, or subcutaneous emphysema.	3. Areas of increasing tenderness or pain imply infection or another complication. Subcutaneous emphysema may occur when an air leak increases intrapleural pressure and eventually results in air spreading throughout the surrounding tissues. Subcutaneous emphysema is usually self-limiting and will reabsorb in several days, but may indicate a need for increased pleural suction pressures.
4. Monitor cardiac rhythm constantly. Note and report to the doctor atrial fibrillation, premature ventricular contractions (PVCs), or other cardiac dysrhythmias. Refer to Appendix A, "Monitoring Standards".	4. Cardiac dysrhythmias, including atrial fibrillation and PVCs, are common after a thoracotomy, particularly after open heart surgery. The "Monitoring Standards" appendix includes specific assessments and interventions for dysrhythmias.
5. Monitor ABG levels every shift and as needed for suspected changes in respiratory status, as ordered. Notify the doctor and document results.	5. ABG levels reflect general oxygenation levels. Low PaO_2 levels may indicate a need for increased oxygen therapy and more vigorous pulmonary hygiene.
6. Monitor and document arterial oxygen levels using ear or pulse oximetry twice a shift and as needed, as ordered.	6. Oximetry monitors arterial oxygen levels without the need for invasive needle sticks.

Interventions	Rationales
7. Provide humidified oxygen for the first 1 to 2 days and as needed for respiratory distress. Document.	7. Oxygen therapy may be required until the lungs are fully re-expanded and the breathing pattern and airway clearance are more effective.
8. Medicate with analgesics for pain every 1 to 4 hours and as needed, as ordered. Monitor respiratory status to prevent respiratory depression. Document. Refer to the "Acute Pain" care plan, page 10, for further details.	8. Pain relief promotes effective deep breathing and coughing. Respiratory depressants such as morphine sulfate must be used cautiously to prevent inadequate ventilation, which would be counterproductive to the effects of deep breathing and coughing. The "Acute Pain" care plan contains general assessments and interventions for pain.
9. Provide incisional support with hands or a small, hard pillow as needed during deep breathing and coughing efforts. Teach the patient to hug a small pillow against the incision during coughing efforts. Encourage deep breathing and coughing two to three times every hour while awake.	9. Support over the incisional area may decrease the pain by limiting rapid and jerky chest motion in that area during deep breathing and coughing. Regular deep breathing and coughing promotes reexpansion of the lungs, mobilizes secretions, and prevents atelectasis.
10. Promote and document the use of an incentive inspirometer, as ordered, several times an hour while awake.	10. Inspirometers encourage deep inspiratory efforts, which are more effective in re-expanding alveoli than forceful expiratory efforts.
11. Provide adequate hydration. Document.	11. Adequate hydration promotes liquidity of lung secretions and ease of removal. The use of other means of humidification, such as intermittent positive pressure breathing, may be undesirable for humidification because of the danger of a pneumothorax with some chest surgery.
12. Provide an overhead trapeze bar or hand pulls attached to the end of the bedframe to assist the patient to the upright position for deep-breathing and coughing efforts.	12. An upright position promotes lung expansion by gravity pull. These devices provide better mobility during independent deep-breathing and coughing efforts than do weak attempts to sit upright by pushing against the bed.
13. Implement and document a progressive activity program, as allowed, typically:	13. Progressive activity is important to restore optimal cardiopulmonary function.
• turning from side to side every 2 hours during the day of surgery, sitting in a semi-Fowler's position and sitting on the bedside with legs dangling on the first postoperative day	• Frequent changes of position re-expand the lungs and prevent atelectasis and pooling of secretions. A patient who has had a pneumonectomy can be turned slightly toward the operative side or onto the back. Turning toward the non-operative side could collapse the remaining lung, drain secretions into that lung, or cause a dangerous mediastinal shift. A semi-Fowler's position may aid re-expansion of the lungs by gravity, whereas having the patient sit on the edge of the bed with legs dangling provides time for neurovascular reflexes to adjust to the upright position after surgery.
• getting into a chair with assistance on the first or second postoperative day, and ambulating in the room or hallway on the second or third postoperative day.	• Early chair-sitting and ambulation may prevent the development of thrombus in the lower extremities and aid reflexes to adjust to the upright position after surgery.
14. Additional individualized interventions: ______	14. Rationales: ______

Target outcome criteria

Within 2 to 4 hours postoperatively, the patient will:
- perform deep breathing and coughing
- use the incentive inspirometer
- request pain medication when needed.

Within 8 hours postoperatively, the patient will:
- manifest normal vital signs
- display his or her usual level of consciousness
- display minimally diminished breath sounds and chest movements
- display absent deviated trachea
- have pink mucous membranes
- display minimal dullness to percussion over operative side, except for pneumonectomy
- display absent subcutaneous emphysema
- display absent PVCs or other dysrhythmias
- turn every 2 hours with assistance.

Within 1 to 2 days postoperatively, the patient will:
- use an inspirometer 2 to 3 times an hour while awake
- display minimal or absent crackles, rhonchi, or wheezes
- manifest normal ABG levels and oximetry levels
- display minimal pain
- sit up in a chair.

Within 3 days postoperatively, the patient will:
- have nearly equal bilateral breath sounds, chest expansion, and resonance to percussion, as appropriate for type of surgery
- begin to ambulate.

Collaborative problem: *Potential respiratory distress related to pneumothorax, hemothorax, or mediastinal shift secondary to malfunction or removal of chest drainage system*

NURSING PRIORITIES: (a) Maintain patency of chest drainage system, and (b) after chest tube removal, observe for complications.

Interventions	Rationales
1. Maintain an intact waterseal drainage system, if used. In the event of a disconnection or a broken chamber, reattach or submerge the tube in water while the patient exhales. If reattachment is not possible or water is unavailable, leave the chest tube open to air until a new system can be attached. Notify the doctor and document occurrence. Arrange for a chest X-ray.	1. Although most thoracotomy patients have chest tubes, chest tubes are not usually used for a patient who has had a pneumonectomy because the collection of serous fluid promotes the development of fibrotic tissue in the empty space. If chest tubes are present, a disconnected system may allow air to enter the pleural space and cause a pneumothorax. Exhalation during reattachment may force excess air from the pleural space. Leaving the tube open to air, with a potential for a small open pneumothorax, may be less harmful than clamping the tube and potentially causing a tension pneumothorax, especially with a patient who has an air leak. A chest X-ray may be necessary to assess the respiratory status.
2. Observe the chest tube insertion site every 2 hours and as needed for the presence of:	2. Frequent observations may reveal problems and allow for timely interventions.
• intact occlusive dressings	• Occlusive dressings are used to prevent air from entering the pleural space around the chest tube insertion site and to prevent accidental dislodgment of the tubes.
• absence of blood or drainage on the dressing	• Blood or drainage on the dressing may indicate fresh bleeding or infection.
• proper position of the chest tubes within the chest and attachment to the chest wall.	• Regular assessment may reveal accidental dislodgment of the tubes and prevent a dangerous increase of air or drainage within the pleural space, which could cause a collapsed lung.

Interventions	**Rationales**
3. Observe the drainage tubing and connectors every 1 to 2 hours for proper connection and taping of connectors. Coil the tubing to prevent dependent loops.	3. The closed drainage system must be airtight to prevent atmospheric air from entering the pleural space. Taped connectors prevent accidental disconnections and air leaks. Improperly looped tubing may inhibit the gravity flow of the drainage.
4. Milk and strip the tubing every 1 to 2 hours and as needed, as ordered, during the first postoperative day. Document.	4. This procedure assists drainage by creating negative pressure and preventing clotting and plugging of the tubes.
5. Assess the drainage receptacle every 1 to 2 hours and as needed for secure attachment to the drainage tubing. Maintain the end of the tube in the waterseal chamber 2 cm below the water level.	5. The secure attachment of the drainage tubing to the drainage receptacle and the placement of the end of the waterseal tube below the water level prevent the entrance of atmospheric air into the drainage system and the pleural space.
6. Observe and document tidalling (fluctuation during respirations) in the submerged waterseal tube every 2 hours. To do this, temporarily turn off the suction or pinch the suction tubing.	6. Tidalling during respiration indicates a functioning and airtight system between the pleura and the drainage receptacle. During spontaneous ventilation, inspiration creates negative pressure in the pleura and the system, which pulls the water level upward in the tubing. The level moves downward on expiration. Fluctuations are opposite for a patient on mechanical ventilation: the positive pressure applied during inspiration pushes the water level downward, whereas termination of the positive pressure on expiration allows the water level to move upward. Absence of tidalling may indicate a blocked chest tube or complete lung expansion.
7. Observe the waterseal chamber for intermittent bubbling during respiration every 2 hours and as needed. Document the amount of bubbling and when it occurs during the respiratory cycle.	7. Intermittent bubbling represents drainage of air from within the pleural spaces. Bubbling normally will occur during expiration with spontaneous ventilation or during inspiration if a patient is on mechanical ventilation.
8. If continuous bubbling occurs in the waterseal, briefly clamp consecutive parts of the system, beginning at the chest wall, until the bubbling stops. If the bubbling stops when the clamp is proximal to the chest wall, notify the doctor. If the bubbling stops as a part of the system distal to the chest wall is clamped, replace the system beyond that point.	8. Continuous bubbling may indicate an air leak within the patient or the system itself. Clamping as described allows isolation of the leak. Bubbling that stops when the clamp is proximal to the chest wall indicates an air leak within the patient, which requires medical evaluation. Bubbling that stops with distal clamping isolates the source of the leak as the drainage system, which requires replacement of the system.
9. Maintain and document the ordered amount of suction, if used. With Emerson suction, check the pressure set on the dial and the pressure registering on the gauge. With a Pleurevac or other type of multiple-chamber system, check the level of water in the suction control chamber to ensure that it equals the amount of negative pressure ordered.	9. Negative pressure may be required to remove secretions and air from the intrapleural space. Inadequate negative pressure may prevent drainage and re-expansion of the lungs, whereas excessive pressure may damage pleural tissue.
10. Monitor the amount, color and consistency of the chest tube drainage every 30 minutes for 2 hours, every hour for 6 hours, and then every 2 hours and as needed. Notify the doctor if large continuing amounts of drainage occur, typically if >200 ml/hr for 3 hours. Document.	10. Large amounts of drainage may indicate bleeding and require immediate intervention to prevent shock. Absence of drainage, particularly in the immediate postoperative period, may indicate a plugged chest tube which could cause a dangerous increase in intrapleural pressure. Chest tubes commonly drain up to 500 ml in the first 8 hours, decreasing to zero drainage 3 to 4 days postoperatively as the pleura become realigned and the lungs reexpanded.
11. Assist with removal of chest tubes 3 to 4 days postoperatively:	11. Chest tubes are removed when the lungs have reexpanded.

(continued)

Interventions	Rationales
• Before removal, note absence of chest tube drainage and absence of tidalling with respiration as well as the return of breath sounds in the affected area.	• These signs indicate lung re-expansion, which allows tube removal.
• Medicate with an analgesic before removal, as ordered.	• An analgesic may decrease pain during the procedure.
• Place the patient in a high Fowler's position. Have the patient take a deep breath and cough vigorously. At maximum inspiration, assist in removing the tube and tightening the purse string skin suture.	• A high Fowler's position, deep breath, and vigorous cough may prevent a pneumothorax during tube removal and suture tightening by providing maximum lung expansion and positive intrapleural pressure.
• Apply a sterile occlusive dressing.	• A sterile occlusive dressing may prevent infection and air entrance into the pleural space.
• After removal, assess for signs and symptoms of respiratory distress, including dyspnea, pain, absent breath sounds, uneven chest movement, dull percussion sounds, cardiac dysrhythmias, or anxiety.	• Rarely, the patient may develop the complications of pneumothorax, hemothorax, or mediastinal shift, which may compromise the respiratory and cardiac systems. Careful assessment allows early identification and interventions for these complications.
12. If necessary, assist the doctor with reinsertion of the chest tubes or thoracentesis. Document.	12. Rarely, the patient may have reaccumulation of fluid or air and may require reinsertion of chest tubes or thoracentesis.
13. Additional individualized interventions: ___________	13. Rationales: ___________

Target outcome criteria

On admission and continuously, the patient will have a properly functioning chest drainage system.

Within 3 to 4 days postoperatively, the patient will:

- have fully expanded lungs
- display absent air or fluid in pleural space
- have chest tubes removed.

Within one week postoperatively, the patient will:

- display absent dyspnea
- have normal respiratory status.

Nursing diagnosis: *Potential for injury: complications related to surgical procedure*

NURSING PRIORITY: Promptly detect complications.

Interventions	Rationales
1. See Appendix F, "Postoperative Considerations".	1. The "Postoperative Considerations" appendix covers general postoperative problems and interventions. This problem focuses on information specific to thoracotomy.
2. Monitor for signs and symptoms of hemorrhage. If present, alert the doctor immediately and document. Observe for:	2. Hemorrhage may result from surgical trauma, inadequate hemostasis, or other factors. It always requires immediate medical evaluation and intervention.
• tachycardia, hypotension, low hemodynamic measurements, and excessive chest drainage	• These signs may indicate hemorrhage and require a return to surgery for ligation of bleeding vessels or re-exploration.
• decreasing or absent breath sounds, increasing dullness to percussion, or decreased or absent fremitus	• These signs may reflect a hemothorax. A thoracentesis or reinsertion of chest tubes may be necessary.
• decreased heart sounds, paradoxical pulse >10 mm Hg on inspiration, or high central venous pressure.	• These signs and symptoms may indicate a cardiac tamponade, which requires an immediate pericardiocentesis.
3. Monitor for signs and symptoms of pneumothorax, including tachypnea, dyspnea, decreased or absent breath sounds, absent vocal fremitus, and hyperresonance. Notify the doctor and document.	3. A pneumothorax prevents re-expansion of the lungs and may require reinserting chest tubes.

Interventions	Rationales
4. Monitor for signs and symptoms of pleural effusion, including decreased or absent breath sounds, decreased vocal fremitus, increased dullness, and tachypnea. Notify the doctor and document.	4. A pleural effusion may compress the lungs, causing hypoxemia. Chest tube reinsertion may be necessary to remove the fluid and re-expand the lungs. Failure to remove the fluid may result in an empyema.
5. Monitor for signs and symptoms of increasing atelectasis, including fever, tachypnea, tachycardia, increasing dullness, increased vocal fremitus, and bronchial or bronchovesicular breath sounds in the lung periphery. Notify the doctor and document.	5. Atelectasis (collapsed alveoli), commonly caused by poor bronchial hygiene, produces hypoxemia, reflected in tachypnea and tachycardia. The dullness, increased fremitus, and abnormal breath sounds all result from consolidation.
6. Monitor for signs and symptoms of pulmonary edema, including tachypnea; tachycardia; dyspnea; shortness of breath; cough; crackles; wheezing; pink, frothy sputum; and anxiety. Notify the doctor and document.	6. Pulmonary edema is a life-threatening condition that requires immediate intervention, which may include diuretics, inotropic agents, rotating tourniquets, and positive-pressure breathing. A patient with other problems, particularly cardiac problems, may be at high risk for this complication.
7. Continuously monitor a pneumonectomy patient for the following complications:	7. A pneumonectomy, a more traumatic surgery than others, has a high incidence of complications.
• hemorrhage: if a patient has a sudden, large hemoptysis, place the patient in a high Fowler's position, turned toward the operative side; summon immediate medical assistance	• Hemorrhage may result from inadequate surgical hemostasis, development of a bronchopleural fistula, or other factors. Placement in a high Fowler's position toward the operative side may prevent drainage into the remaining lung.
• bronchopleural fistula: observe for hemoptysis, an extensive air leak, subcutaneous emphysema, or fever	• A bronchopleural fistula may develop after surgery, most commonly during the first week, causing bleeding, air leaks, or infection. Depending on the size and location of the fistula, it may require surgery to close the bronchial stump and antibiotics.
• subcutaneous emphysema: observe for swelling, puffiness, or crepitation of skin	• A bronchial stump leak may cause a large amount of subcutaneous emphysema. An air leak usually resolves over 3 days to a week but may require surgery.
• excessive mediastinal shift: observe for excessive deviation of trachea at sternal notch, hypotension, tachycardia, weak peripheral pulses, or other signs of decreased cardiac output.	• After lung removal, the mediastinum is unsupported on one side and may shift. The residual pleural space should fill after surgery by a combination of mediastinal shift, diaphragm elevation, coagulation of serous drainage, and development of fibrotic tissue. If mediastinal shift is excessive, decreased cardiac output may occur, requiring mediastinal stabilization by fluid or air injection or thoracentesis.
8. Monitor for signs and symptoms of pulmonary embolism, including chest pain, dyspnea, fever, hemoptysis, changes in vital signs, and increased central venous pressure. Notify the doctor and document. Refer to the "Pulmonary Embolism" care plan, page 122, for further information.	8. Pulmonary embolism, a serious complication, may result from deep vein thrombosis and cause varying signs and symptoms depending on the size of the embolism. Prompt medical treatment is required to prevent further pulmonary tissue damage. The "Pulmonary Embolism" care plan covers this disorder in detail.
9. Additional individualized interventions: ________	9. Rationales: ________

Target outcome criteria

By 3 to 7 days postoperatively, the patient will display no signs of complications, such as hemorrhage, cardiac dysrhythmias, hemothorax, cardiac tamponade, pneumothorax, pleural effusion, atelectasis, subcutaneous emphysema, bronchopleural fistula, or mediastinal shift.

Nursing diagnosis: *Potential for infection related to surgical incision and endotracheal intubation*

NURSING PRIORITY: Prevent infection.

Interventions	Rationales
1. Monitor for signs and symptoms of pneumonia, including fever, tachypnea, bronchial or bronchovesicular breath sounds in the periphery, increased vocal fremitus, increased dullness, and dyspnea. Notify the doctor and document.	1. Patients with invasive chest surgery and endotracheal intubation are at high risk for pneumonia. Treatment may require aggressive pulmonary hygiene, antibiotics, and positive-pressure treatments.
2. Assess for signs and symptoms of wound infection every 2 to 4 hours and as needed, including elevated temperature, increased vital signs, odor, drainage, and pain around incisions. When the incision can be seen directly, observe for redness and swelling. Monitor for elevated WBC or sedimentation rate, as ordered.	2. Regular assessments may provide early warning of infection. Occlusive dressings may remain over the incision sites for 1 to 3 days, making visualization of the sites difficult.
3. Monitor cultures and sensitivities of wound drainage, as ordered.	3. Cultures and sensitivities provide information about the type of infective microorganisms and the most effective antibiotic treatment.
4. Reinforce or change dressings as needed, using aseptic technique.	4. A thoracotomy incision is extensive and may have moderate amounts of serosanguineous drainage. The dressing is usually reinforced during the first 1 to 2 days postoperatively to maintain its occlusiveness.
5. Additional individualized interventions: ____________	5. Rationales: ____________

Target outcome criteria

Within 3 days postoperatively, the patient will:
- have a clean, dry, and healing wound
- display a normal temperature and vital signs
- display a normal WBC and sedimentation rate.

By transfer, the patient will have clear breath sounds, normal fremitus, and normal resonance to percussion, as appropriate to type of surgery.

Transfer planning

NURSING TRANSFER CRITERIA

Upon transfer, documentation shows evidence of:
- stable vital signs and monitoring parameters
- clear breath sounds, bilateral lung expansion, and bilateral resonance to percussion, as appropriate to type of surgery
- absence of subcutaneous emphysema, infection, pneumothorax, hemothorax, or other major complications
- healing surgical incision(s).

PATIENT-FAMILY TEACHING CHECKLIST

Document evidence that patient and family demonstrate understanding of:

__ surgical procedure, including expected postoperative course
__ deep breathing, coughing, and inspirometer use
__ comfort measures, including pain medication and incisional splinting
__ ROM and other exercises
__ purpose and mechanism of chest drainage system.

DOCUMENTATION CHECKLIST

Using outcome criteria as a guide, document:

__ clinical status on admission
__ significant changes in status
__ pertinent diagnostic test findings
__ chest drainage (amount, consistency, and color)
__ functioning of chest drainage equipment
__ complications, such as subcutaneous emphysema
__ deep breathing, coughing, and inspirometer efforts
__ oxygen therapy
__ pain and effects of medication
__ activity levels, ROM, and other exercises
__ patient/family teaching
__ transfer planning.

ASSOCIATED CARE PLANS

Acute Pain
Grieving and Dying
Knowledge Deficit
Mechanical Ventilation
Pulmonary Embolism

REFERENCES

Allan, D. "Chest Tube Patients," *Nursing Times* 24-25, January 30, 1985.

Kniesl, C., and Ames, S. *Adult Health Nursing.* Menlo Park, Calif.: Addison-Wesley Publishing, Co., 1986.

Lewis, S.M., and Collier, I.C. *Medical-Surgical Nursing: Assessment and Management of Clinical Problems,* 2nd ed. New York: McGraw-Hill Book Co., 1987.

Luckmann, J., and Sorensen, K. *Medical-Surgical Nursing: A Psychophysiological Approach,* 3rd ed. Philadelphia: W. B. Saunders Co., 1987.

Mims, B. "Helping Your Patient Breathe Easier After Chest Surgery," *RN* 25-29, December 1984.

Mims, B. "You Can Manage Chest Tubes Confidently," *RN* 39-42, January 1985.

O'Byrne, C. "Postoperative Care and Complications in the Thoracotomy Patient," *Critical Care Quarterly* 7(4):53-58, 1985.

Palau, D., and Jones, S. "Test Your Skill at Troubleshooting Chest Tubes," *RN* 43-45, October 1986.

Pfister, S., and Bullas, J. "Caring for a Patient with a Chest Tube Connected to the Emerson Pump," *Critical Care Nurse* 5:26-32, 1985.

Acute Heart Failure

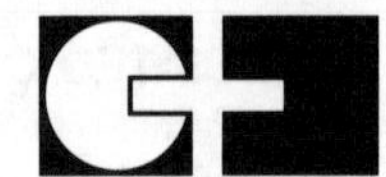

DRG information

DRG 127 Heart Failure and Shock.
Mean LOS = 6.2 days
Principal diagnoses include:
- benign, malignant, or unspecified hypertensive heart disease with congestive heart failure
- heart failure
- congestive heart failure
- shock without trauma.

Introduction

DEFINITION AND TIME FOCUS

Heart failure (HF) is the heart's inability to produce a cardiac output (CO) sufficient to meet the body's metabolic demands. A major problem in critical care, acute HF may appear in many guises: pulmonary congestion, pulmonary edema, or cardiogenic shock. The symptoms may range from mild to severe, and CO itself may be low, normal, or high. The left ventricle (LV) or right ventricle (RV) may fail independently, or biventricular failure may occur. CO depends on a complex interplay of preload, contractility, afterload, and heart rate, and abnormalities of any of these factors may produce acute HF. Signs and symptoms may result from the backup of fluid behind the failing ventricle ("backward failure") or from decreased stroke volume ("forward failure"). This plan focuses on the patient with acute heart failure producing pulmonary congestion or peripheral hypoperfusion.

ETIOLOGY AND PRECIPITATING FACTORS

- increased preload, such as in fluid volume overload, valvular stenosis or insufficiency, intracardiac shunt, papillary muscle dysfunction, or rupture of chordae tendineae
- decreased myocardial contractility, such as in myocardial ischemia or infarction, cardiomyopathy, ventricular aneurysm, myocarditis, atherosclerotic heart disease, constrictive pericarditis, or cardiac tamponade
- increased afterload, such as in systemic hypertension, pulmonary hypertension, or massive pulmonary embolism
- severely abnormal heart rate, such as in severe tachycardia, bradycardia, or conduction disturbances
- high output states, such as in anemia, fever, septic shock, or hyperthyroidism

Focused assessment guidelines

NURSING HISTORY (Functional health pattern findings)

Health perception–health management pattern

- may report fatigue, weakness, shortness of breath, or tightness of shoes or belt
- if under treatment for chronic congestive heart failure, may report nonadherence to prescribed low-salt diet or medication regimen

Nutritional-metabolic pattern

- may report anorexia, nausea, or vomiting
- may report recent weight gain

Activity-exercise pattern

- may report dyspnea on exertion or at rest
- may report palpitations
- may report dizziness or fainting (syncope)

Sleep-rest pattern

- may complain of insomnia, paroxysmal nocturnal dyspnea, or nocturia
- may report using several pillows to elevate head (orthopnea)

Coping–stress tolerance pattern

- may report marked anxiety, apprehension, or sense of impending doom

PHYSICAL FINDINGS

Cardiovascular

- tachycardia or other dysrhythmias
- S_3 or S_4 heart sounds or both
- jugular venous distention
- positive hepatojugular reflux
- weak or irregular pulses
- pulsus alternans (in LV failure)
- holosystolic murmur at lower left sternal border if RV failure (from relative tricuspid insufficiency) or at apex if LV failure (from relative mitral insufficiency)
- point of maximum intensity displaced leftward of and below normal point

Pulmonary

- crackles, usually bibasilar
- cough
- frothy sputum (if pulmonary edema is present)
- air hunger
- wheezing
- hyperventilation

Gastrointestinal
• liver tenderness
• liver enlargement
• ascites

Integumentary
• dependent edema, usually pitting
• cyanosis
• diaphoresis
• pallor

Renal
• oliguria

DIAGNOSTIC STUDIES
• arterial blood gas (ABG) analysis—may reveal respiratory alkalosis (early stage) or hypoxemia and respiratory acidosis (late stage).
• serum digitalis level—may reveal subtherapeutic range.
• 12-lead EKG—reveals sinus tachycardia, frequent premature ventricular contractions, atrial fibrillation, or other dysrhythmias; it may reveal P-mitrale if atrial distention is present, or P-pulmonale if cor pulmonale is present.
• pulmonary artery pressures—reveal elevated pulmonary artery diastolic pressure and pulmonary capillary wedge pressure (PCWP) in LV failure and elevated right atrial pressure in RV failure.
• chest X-ray—reveals pulmonary infiltrates or cardiac enlargement.
• complete blood count—may reveal dilutional changes.
• liver enzyme levels—may be elevated with liver congestion.
• serum albumin values—may be decreased because of impaired protein synthesis from liver congestion.
• gated blood pool imaging—may reveal reduced ejection fraction.
• echocardiography—may reveal chamber enlargement, ventricular dyskinesia, or valvular abnormalities.

POTENTIAL COMPLICATIONS
• refractory heart failure
• cardiac arrest
• pulmonary edema
• fluid and electrolyte imbalance

Collaborative problem: *Potential hypoxemia related to pulmonary congestion, decreased systemic perfusion, or both*

NURSING PRIORITY: Maintain optimal gas exchange.

Interventions	Rationales
1. Monitor pulmonary status as needed, typically every 15 minutes until stable and then every 2 hours. Observe for:	1. Baseline and ongoing monitoring of pulmonary status provides data to guide priority setting and interventions.
• dyspnea, orthopnea, shallow respirations, accessory muscle use, cough, or adventitious breath sounds	• Left ventricular end-diastolic pressure (LVEDP) is the pressure that most directly determines the strength of LV contraction and the resulting adequacy of stroke volume. As the heart fails, decreased ventricular compliance raises this pressure beyond the level that produces optimal stretch of myocardial fibers and, according to the Frank-Starling mechanism, optimal contractility. The elevated LVEDP is reflected backward into the pulmonary capillary bed and produces pulmonary congestion. Elevated pulmonary capillary hydrostatic pressure causes fluid to shift across capillary walls into the interstitium and eventually into the alveoli. Interstitial edema produces dyspnea, shallow respirations, and accessory muscle use, whereas alveolar edema produces orthopnea, cough, and adventitious breath sounds.
• tachypnea, cyanosis, restlessness, irritability, confusion, somnolence, or slow or irregular respirations.	• Fluid-filled alveoli cannot oxygenate the capillary blood flowing past them, thereby producing a pulmonary shunt and hypoxemia. Tachypnea is an early compensatory mechanism for hypoxemia, whereas cyanosis is a late reflection of it. Decreased cardiac output (forward failure) produces cerebral ischemia, resulting in an altered level of consciousness. Ischemia of medullary and pontine respiratory centers causes altered breathing patterns.

(continued)

Interventions

2. Monitor ABG values as ordered, typically every 4 hours until stable or as needed. Obtain chest X-rays, as ordered.

Rationales

2. ABG values provide objective evidence of hypoxemia and accompanying respiratory and metabolic acidosis, whereas chest X-rays provide objective evidence of pulmonary fluid infiltration.

3. Place the patient in semi-Fowler's or high Fowler's position.

3. Elevating the head of the bed improves diaphragmatic excursion, thus facilitating ventilation.

4. Administer supplemental oxygen, as ordered, typically by nasal cannula at 6 liters/minute (or, if the patient has chronic obstructive pulmonary disease [COPD], at 2 liters/minute).

4. Supplemental oxygen helps to saturate hemoglobin maximally, thus raising arterial oxygen content and improving oxygen transport. The cannula is used to avoid the feeling of suffocation that air-hungry patients experience with a mask. The oxygen flow rate must be low for a COPD patient to avoid removing the hypoxic drive to breathe and inducing a respiratory arrest.

5. Suction as needed.

5. The heart failure patient may produce sputum so rapidly that he cannot clear it spontaneously. Prompt suctioning not only improves gas exchange but also lessens the anxiety experienced by the patient with a compromised airway.

6. Administer narcotics, sedatives, and tranquilizers, as ordered, only if the respiratory rate is >12/minute. Titrate doses to achieve desired effects without causing respiratory depression.

6. These drugs decrease pain, anxiety, catecholamine stimulation, and tachypnea, thus lessening the work of breathing. In a patient with preexisting respiratory center depression, however, they cause further depression and may precipitate a respiratory arrest. Titrating doses minimizes the risk of side effects.

7. Alert the doctor immediately if the patient develops severe dyspnea, pink frothy sputum, marked neck-vein distention, or describes a sense of impending doom. See the "Hypervolemia" collaborative problem later in this care plan for interventions.

7. These findings indicate pulmonary edema, a life-threatening development. Immediate medical intervention is crucial. The "Hypervolemia" collaborative problem covers appropriate interventions in detail.

8. Additional individualized interventions: ____________

8. Rationales: ____________

Target outcome criteria

Within 3 days, the patient will:

- show no signs or symptoms of hypoxemia
- have ABG levels within normal limits for patient
- display a level of consciousness similar to or better than before admission
- show no restlessness, irritability, confusion, or somnolence.

Collaborative problem: *Inadequate cardiac output related to heart rate abnormalities and/or diminished contractility*

NURSING PRIORITY: Maintain adequate cardiac output (CO).

Interventions

1. Observe for signs and symptoms of decreased CO, such as:

Rationales

1. CO falls in heart failure because of several interrelated mechanisms. Decreased contractility makes the heart unable to clear volume efficiently. The resulting distention causes ventricular fibers to exceed the optimal range of stretch on the Frank-Starling curve, so the ejection fraction falls and systemic perfusion suffers. Forward failure of the LV affects all body systems.

Interventions	Rationales
• arterial hypotension, tachycardia, narrowed pulse pressure, weak peripheral pulses	• Systemic vascular resistance (SVR) increases initially in an attempt to maintain mean arterial pressure (MAP). Pulse pressure narrows because the decreased CO lowers systolic pressure, whereas the increased SVR elevates diastolic pressure. Tachycardia, although a compensatory response for decreased CO, may actually impair it further by limiting ventricular filling time.
• restlessness, irritability, confusion, somnolence	• Changes in level of consciousness or mentation reflect cerebral hypoxemia or ischemia.
• weakness and fatigue	• Weakness and fatigue result from diminished skeletal muscle perfusion, excessive work of breathing, and sleep disturbances.
• cool, mottled, or cyanotic skin	• Skin changes reflect shunting away from skeletal muscle beds as the body attempts to preserve perfusion to core organs.
• decreased urine output	• Decreased urine output reflects diminished renal perfusion resulting from decreased circulating blood volume and intense sympathetic vasoconstriction of afferent arterioles.
• pulsus alternans (alternating volume of arterial pulse).	• Pulsus alternans, a classic finding in heart failure, may reflect varying degrees of contractility resulting from beat-to-beat variation in end-diastolic volume, according to the Frank-Starling curve.
2. Monitor the EKG continuously. Document and report significant findings (see "Monitoring Standards" appendix, page 314, for details).	2. Because CO depends on the heart rate and stroke volume, dysrhythmias can affect CO significantly. Continuous monitoring allows for prompt treatment of dysrhythmias, before CO drops so dramatically that cardiac arrest occurs.
3. Assist with insertion of a pulmonary artery (PA) catheter, as ordered.	3. The multiple therapies used in HF can have differing and sometimes opposing effects on the determinants of CO. Basing interpretation of these effects on clinical signs alone can be confusing. Insertion of a PA catheter allows objective measurement of CO and monitoring of PCWP. The latter is particularly important because PCWP monitoring provides the most direct bedside indication of the functional state of the LV myocardium. In mitral valve or pulmonary disease, however, PCWP alterations do not necessarily reflect LV performance.
4. Monitor cardiac index (CI) and PCWP every hour, as ordered. Calculate CI by dividing CO by body-surface area (determined from a DuBois body-surface area nomogram). Note both isolated values and the trend of values.	4. Objective measurements provide a means of evaluating the adequacy of CI and level of PCWP. CI adjusts CO according to the patient's size, so it provides a more precise indication of the appropriateness of CO for a given patient than does CO alone. Whereas isolated values provide immediate data, the trend of values indicates whether failure is resolving or worsening over time.
5. Classify the patient according to the Forrester subsets:	5. The Forrester classification is useful to distinguish disease patterns and anticipate therapy. Forrester classified hemodynamic subsets of acute myocardial infarction patients according to levels of PCWP and CI, which are closely correlated to clinical signs of failure.
• Subset I: PCWP <18 mm Hg and CI >2.2 liters/minute/m^2 (no failure)	• A PCWP of 18 mm Hg is the level above which signs of pulmonary congestion appear and a CI of 2.2 liters/minute/m^2 is the level below which signs of peripheral hypoperfusion appear. Increased PCWP and depressed CI are the "final common pathways" for almost all signs of HF. In Subset I, a relatively normal PCWP and CI indicate no failure is present.

(continued)

Interventions	Rationales
• Subset II: PCWP >18 mm Hg and CI >2.2 liters/minute/m^2 (pulmonary congestion)	• In Subset II, PCWP is elevated, but CI is relatively normal. Clinically, the patient shows signs of pulmonary congestion.
• Subset III: PCWP <18 mm Hg and CI <2.2 liters/minute/m^2 (peripheral hypoperfusion)	• In Subset III, PCWP is relatively normal, but CI is depressed. Clinically, the patient shows signs of peripheral hypoperfusion.
• Subset IV: PCWP >18 mm Hg and CI <2.2 liters/minute/m^2 (pulmonary congestion and peripheral hypoperfusion).	• In Subset IV, PCWP is elevated and CI is depressed. Clinically, the patient presents with both pulmonary congestion and peripheral hypoperfusion.
6. Anticipate medical therapy consistent with Forrester subsets. Administer therapy as ordered.	6. Anticipation of therapy allows systematic planning rather than implementing interventions in a hectic, crisis-ridden atmosphere. Goals and therapeutic measures follow logically from the characteristics of each subset.
• For patients with no signs of failure (Subset I), observe for possible development of failure.	• Patients in Subset I have acceptable PCWP and CI. However, because critically ill patients are notorious for rapid decompensation, continuing observation always is warranted.
• For patients with only pulmonary congestion (Subset II), see the "Hypervolemia" collaborative problem in this care plan.	• That collaborative problem deals with pulmonary congestion in detail.
• For patients with hypoperfusion but no pulmonary congestion (Subset III):	• Measures for patients in Subset III are designed to increase CO and therefore increase peripheral perfusion.
□ if heart rate (HR) is elevated, administer volume. Document effectiveness and observe for side effects, especially fluid overload.	□ Tachycardia is a primary compensatory response to hypovolemia. Administering volume increases preload and thus increases CO. The resulting increase in circulating blood volume restores peripheral perfusion and relieves the tachycardia because SV × HR = CO; as stroke volume (SV) increases, HR returns toward normal.
□ if HR is depressed, assist with pacemaker insertion. Document effectiveness and observe for pacemaker malfunction.	□ Because HR is a primary determinant of CO, bradycardia with hypoperfusion strongly suggests the need to restore a normal HR. Pacemaker insertion provides an immediate way to increase HR while the underlying problem, such as heart block, is identified and, if possible, resolved.
• For patients with both pulmonary congestion and hypoperfusion (Subset IV), see the "Hypervolemia" collaborative problem below.	• That collaborative problem addresses the care of patients in Subsets II and IV.
7. Additional individualized interventions: ____________	7. Rationales: ____________

Target outcome criteria

Within 3 days, the patient will have:

- vital signs within normal limits for patient
- no significant dysrhythmias
- CI >2.2 liters/minute/m^2 and PCWP <18 mm Hg
- strong, bilaterally equal peripheral pulses.

Collaborative problem: *Hypervolemia related to sodium and water retention from compensatory release of antidiuretic hormone and aldosterone*

NURSING PRIORITY: Reduce excess fluid volume.

Interventions	**Rationales**
1. Monitor for signs and symptoms of fluid volume excess:	1. Conscientious monitoring allows early detection of problems and facilitates prompt corrective intervention.
• neck-vein distention, dependent edema, liver congestion, or ascites	• As the RV fails, inefficient RV systolic emptying causes back pressure to build up in neck veins and then in systemic veins. Increased hydrostatic pressure in systemic capillaries causes fluid transudation into interstitial spaces. The resulting edema is most noticeable in dependent areas, because they are most affected by gravity. Ascites results from fluid accumulation in the peritoneal cavity.
• crackles, rhonchi, wheezes, cough, or S_3 and S_4 heart sounds	• LV failure causes increased hydrostatic pressure in pulmonary capillaries. Crackles may result from pulmonary interstitial fluid compressing alveoli or from fluid accumulating in alveoli. Rhonchi and wheezes indicate fluid accumulation in large airways. S_3 and S_4 heart sounds reflect decreased ventricular compliance or volume overload of the ventricles.
• elevated PCWP.	• The level of PCWP correlates with the degree of pulmonary congestion. Usually, 18 to 20 mm Hg correlates with the onset of congestion, 20 to 25 mm Hg with moderate congestion, 25 to 30 mm Hg with severe congestion, and >30 mm Hg with pulmonary edema.
2. Monitor hourly intake and output and 24-hour fluid balance. Weigh the patient daily.	2. Intake and output monitoring provides an objective method of tracking incremental gains or losses of fluid, whereas 24-hour summaries indicate net fluid balance. Daily weights are a cruder measure of fluid status; a weight change of 2.2 lb (1 kg) corresponds with a 1-liter change in fluid balance.
3. Administer I.V. solutions, as ordered. Avoid saline solutions.	3. The selection of an appropriate type and amount of I.V. fluid depends upon the patient's current condition and the cause of failure. Saline solutions are usually avoided because the salt content causes obligatory water retention.
4. If the patient is placed on fluid restrictions:	4. Fluid restrictions help limit excessive preload.
• explain the rationale to the patient and family	• Enlisting the patient's and family's support of fluid restrictions increases the likelihood of compliance. Thirst is a powerful need and restricting its satisfaction may cause the patient to feel deprived or punished. Explaining the rationale may help reframe the situation so that the patient can view it more positively.
• establish a fluid intake schedule, teach the patient how to record oral fluid intake, and use microdrip tubing or an infusion pump to control I.V. intake.	• A concrete schedule, consistent measurements, and use of microdrip tubing or infusion devices help ensure maintenance of fluid restrictions.
5. For patients with pulmonary congestion (Subset II), administer pharmacologic therapy, as ordered.	5. Subset II patients have an elevated PCWP and good CI. Therapy is designed to decrease circulating blood volume, thereby relieving pulmonary congestion.

(continued)

Interventions	Rationales
• If blood pressure is normal, administer diuretics, typically furosemide (Lasix) or bumetanide (Bumex). Document effectiveness. Monitor for side effects, especially excessive diuresis or electrolyte imbalances (particularly hypokalemia).	• Diuretics reduce preload rapidly and effectively, moving the patient to a more favorable point on the ventricular compliance curve. Because they block renal reabsorption of fluid and increase renal tubular flow, potassium excretion increases. Excessive diuresis and hypokalemia are exaggerations of their therapeutic effects.
• If blood pressure is elevated, administer vasodilators, typically:	• When blood pressure is high enough to cause pulmonary congestion interfering with oxygenation, rapid lowering of blood pressure becomes too urgent to wait for the slow action of diuretics. By expanding the vascular bed, vasodilators allow the vessels to accommodate the same amount of fluid in a larger cross-sectional area, thus lowering pressure. The increased vessel capacitance also lowers preload, which improves LV performance.
□ venodilators, such as nitroglycerin or morphine. Observe for and report side effects, especially hypotension and, with morphine, respiratory depression.	□ Nitroglycerin produces significant venodilation and relatively little arteriolar dilation. Used primarily for its venodilating properties, it decreases preload and pulmonary congestion. It also redistributes myocardial blood flow, causing greater dilation of large vessels than of small ones, thus increasing flow to ischemic areas. As myocardial perfusion improves, more efficient contraction increases CO. Morphine, the drug of choice in pulmonary edema, also induces vasodilation. The resulting reductions in preload, afterload, and myocardial work all improve CO. It also induces euphoria, particularly helpful in lessening the severe anxiety present with pulmonary edema.
□ arteriolar dilators, such as sodium nitroprusside (Nipride). Monitor for and report side effects, especially hypotension, signs of hypoxemia, and thiocyanate and cyanide toxicity.	□ Although sodium nitroprusside dilates both arteriolar and venous beds, it is used primarily for its arteriolar effects. Because it reduces afterload, systolic emptying is improved, and myocardial work decreases. As a result, it produces a greater increase in CO than nitroglycerin. Hypotension results from excessive dosage. Hypoxemia may result from reversal of pulmonary vasoconstriction, a compensatory mechanism in areas of pulmonary hypoxemia that shunts blood to better-aerated alveoli. Thiocyanate and cyanide toxicity may develop from accumulation of toxic metabolites with long-term use, high dosage, or impaired liver or renal perfusion.
6. For patients with pulmonary congestion and peripheral hypoperfusion (Subset IV), administer pharmacologic therapy, as ordered.	6. Subset IV patients have an elevated PCWP and depressed CI, so the treatment goals are to lower PCWP and improve CI.
• If blood pressure is depressed, administer positive inotropes, typically:	• The constellation of elevated PCWP, depressed CI, and depressed blood pressure strongly suggests that depressed myocardial contractility is the culprit. Positive inotropic agents increase myocardial contractility, thus improving CI and lowering PCWP as fluid is moved more efficiently through the heart.
□ digitalis preparations. Observe for and report signs of toxicity, including gastrointestinal distress, bradycardia, atrioventricular block, premature beats, and atrial tachycardia with block.	□ Digitalis improves contractility, but it also slows HR and cardiac conduction. It also may provoke various dysrhythmias by increasing automaticity.
□ dopamine hydrochloride (Intropin). Observe for and report hypotension, tachydysrhythmias, ectopic beats, vasoconstriction with high doses, and I.V. fluid infiltration.	□ Dopamine has complex pharmacologic actions that are dose-related. In failure, mid-range doses of dopamine (2 to 10 mcg/kg/minute) increase renal perfusion, via dopaminergic effects, and increase HR and contractility, via $beta_1$-adrenergic stimulating effects.

Interventions

□ dobutamine hydrochloride (Dobutrex). Monitor for and report side effects, especially tachycardia and dysrhythmias.

Rationales

□ Dobutamine, primarily a direct $beta_1$ stimulator, is a potent inotropic agent with relatively less chronotropic effect than dopamine. As such, it significantly improves contractility with less tendency to cause dysrhythmias than dopamine.

□ combined inotrope and vasodilator therapy, such as dopamine and sodium nitroprusside or amrinone (Inocor). With dopamine and sodium nitroprusside, monitor for and report adverse reactions, especially chest pain or increased ventricular dysrhythmias. With amrinone, observe for and report adverse reactions, including dysrhythmias, hypotension, and GI distress.

□ Combination therapy involves two drugs whose synergistic effects result in greater and safer improvement of CO than with either agent used alone. The combination of dopamine and sodium nitroprusside, for example, causes greater preload reduction, better augmentation of contractility, and better afterload reduction than either agent alone. However, both agents may decrease myocardial oxygen supply. Amrinone is a drug with both inotrope and vasodilator properties that lessens pulmonary congestion and improves cardiac output. It is used commonly for short-term management of HF patients refractory to other therapies.

• If blood pressure is normal, administer vasodilators. See intervention 5 above for details.

• Patients with congestion, hypoperfusion, and normal blood pressure may benefit from afterload reduction achieved with administration of vasodilators. Vasodilators have been previously discussed, under intervention 5.

7. Additional individualized interventions: ______________

7. Rationales: ______________

Target outcome criteria

Within 2 days, the patient will have:

- blood pressure within normal limits for the patient
- absent neck-vein distention and pedal edema
- PCWP within normal limits for the patient
- lungs clear to auscultation
- heart rate within normal limits for the patient, ideally 60 to 100 beats/minute
- fluid intake and output in approximate balance
- normal chest X-ray.

Nursing diagnosis: *Activity intolerance related to hypoxemia, weakness, or diminished cardiovascular reserve*

NURSING PRIORITY: Promote rest.

Interventions

1. Assess for signs and symptoms of activity intolerance, such as HR increase >25%, blood pressure increase >25%, any HR or blood pressure decrease, chest pain, dysrhythmias, exertional dyspnea, decreased level of consciousness, or complaints of weakness or fatigue.

Rationales

1. Dysfunctional myocardium may be unable to adjust SV and oxygen uptake appropriately with exertion. The unmet oxygen demand may precipitate tachycardia and myocardial or cerebral ischemia. Anaerobic metabolism resulting from impaired perfusion of skeletal muscle results in weakness or fatigue.

2. During periods of physiologic instability, place the patient on complete bed rest or chair rest. Assist with activity, as needed. Implement measures in the "Impaired Physical Mobility" care plan, page 33, as appropriate.

2. Bed or chair rest decreases myocardial work load. Also, bed rest induces a peripheral fluid shift of approximately 500 ml, thus lowering preload, and decreases antidiuretic hormone production, resulting in diuresis. Assisting with activity conserves cardiovascular and energy reserves. The "Impaired Physical Mobility" care plan contains measures to combat the hazards of immobility.

(continued)

Interventions	Rationales
3. Pace nursing care to promote rest. If possible, allow at least 90 minutes at a time of uninterrupted sleep.	3. The numerous medical and nursing measures necessary to treat HF may provide little uninterrupted rest, resulting in an exhausted patient. The average length of a sleep cycle is 90 minutes. Providing at least this much uninterrupted rest at a time allows the patient to progress through both rapid eye movement (REM) sleep, which helps restore psychological equilibrium, and non-REM sleep, which helps restore physiologic well-being.
4. When the patient stabilizes, increase activity gradually, as ordered.	4. Gradual activity increase allows time for neurovascular compensatory mechanisms to accommodate increased demands.
• Maintain supplemental oxygen.	• Supplemental oxygen provides optimal arterial oxygen content to meet increased tissue oxygen demands with exercise.
• Monitor the patient's response to increased activity. Slow or discontinue activity progression if any signs of activity intolerance appear.	• Close monitoring provides for appropriate matching of exercise demands and energy resources.
5. Additional individualized interventions: ______	5. Rationales: ______

Target outcome criteria
By transfer, the patient will engage in self-care activities without displaying signs or symptoms of activity intolerance.

Nursing diagnosis: *Knowledge deficit related to disease process and complex therapeutic regimen*

NURSING PRIORITY: Prevent recurrent episodes of heart failure, when possible.

Interventions	Rationales
1. Implement the following measures only as the patient's condition allows. See the "Knowledge Deficit" care plan, page 45, for details.	1. Patients in the critical care unit, in many cases, are too ill for sustained teaching. The "Knowledge Deficit" care plan contains information on assessing readiness to learn and information on teaching methodologies.
2. Briefly explain the pathophysiology of heart failure.	2. Although extensive teaching probably should be deferred until after transfer from the unit, a brief explanation provides the context within which the patient can better understand the rationales for therapy.
3. Emphasize the patient's role in controlling the disease and the importance of medical follow-up.	3. Heart failure commonly becomes chronic or recurrent. Active participation by the patient in implementing and monitoring treatment and conscientious medical care can be instrumental in limiting the disease's progression.

Interventions	Rationales
4. In collaboration with the dietitian, instruct the patient and family about the prescribed diet, typically low in sodium, fat, cholesterol, and (if the patient is overweight) calories. Refer the patient to a smoking-cessation program, if appropriate. Stress the value of family support in making the necessary life-style modifications.	4. Many of the therapies for chronic or recurrent HF involve life-style modifications, such as low-sodium diet preparation, that may affect other family members. Others may involve changing habits the patient finds pleasurable, such as smoking. In either case, family support can smooth the transition to a healthier life-style.
5. Instruct the patient and family about discharge medications, typically diuretics, digitalis, or antihypertensive agents.	5. Treatment of HF usually involves a complex regimen of ongoing medications. Information about the medications with which the patient is discharged better equips the patient and family to manage the medication regimen.
6. Emphasize signs and symptoms requiring immediate medical attention after discharge, such as shortness of breath, rapid weight gain, increasing fatigue, or increasing edema. Instruct the patient and family to contact the clinician if these indicators occur or worsen.	6. An alert, informed patient and family are the patient's first line of defense against recurrence or aggravation of HF. Knowing what to observe for and appropriate measures to take increases the likelihood that the clinician will be alerted promptly if these indicators develop or exacerbate.
7. Additional individualized interventions: ____________	7. Rationales: ____________

Target outcome criteria

By transfer, the patient will:
- display beginning interest in ways to implement prescribed life-style modifications
- display a personal conviction of the necessity for his future well-being.

Transfer planning

NURSING TRANSFER CRITERIA

Upon transfer, documentation shows evidence of:
- blood pressure within 30 mm Hg of normal value for at least 12 hours without I.V. vasoactive drug support
- no significant dysrhythmias for at least 12 hours without I.V. antiarrhythmic agents
- absence of arterial and pulmonary artery line
- stable respiratory status for at least 12 hours without mechanical ventilation.

PATIENT-FAMILY TEACHING CHECKLIST

Document evidence that patient and family demonstrate understanding of:

__ cause and implications of HF
__ purpose of medications
__ activity restrictions
__ rationales for other therapeutic interventions
__ need for life-style modifications.

DOCUMENTATION CHECKLIST

Using outcome criteria as a guide, document:

__ clinical status on admission
__ significant changes in status
__ pertinent laboratory and diagnostic test findings
__ hemodynamic measurements
__ oxygen therapy
__ fluid therapy or restrictions
__ response to inotropes, vasodilators, or other pharmacologic agents
__ dietary modifications
__ activity restrictions
__ patient-family teaching
__ transfer planning.

ASSOCIATED CARE PLANS

Acute Myocardial Infarction
Impaired Physical Mobility
Knowledge Deficit
Shock

REFERENCES

Forrester, J., et al. "Medical Therapy of Acute MI by Application of Hemodynamic Subsets," *New England Journal of Medicine* 295:1356-62, December 1976.

Holloway, N., and Kern, L. "Cardiovascular Disorders," in *Nursing the Critically Ill Adult,* 3rd ed. Edited by Holloway, N. Menlo Park, Calif.: Addison-Wesley Publishing Co., 1988.

Acute Myocardial Infarction

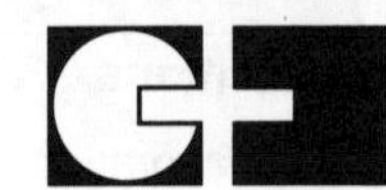

DRG information

DRG 121 Circulatory Disorders With Acute Myocardial Infarction (AMI) and Cardiovascular Complications, Discharged Alive.
Mean LOS = 11.1 days
Principal diagnoses include:
- heart aneurysm
- cardiac arrest
- atrioventricular or bundle branch blocks
- benign or malignant hypertensive heart disease with congestive heart failure (CHF)
- pulmonary embolism or infarction
- heart failure
- acute renal failure
- atrial or ventricular fibrillation or flutter
- shock without mention of trauma
- supraventricular or unspecified paroxysmal tachycardia.

Additional DRG information: The assignment of DRG 121 is dependent on the presence of AMI plus one or more of the listed cardiovascular complications.

DRG 122 Circulatory Disorders With AMI, Without Cardiovascular Complications, Discharged Alive.
Mean LOS = 9.4 days
Principal diagnoses include AMI, any site, with other circulatory disorders, for example, coronary arteriosclerotic heart disease.
Additional DRG information: Patients with any of the cardiovascular complications listed for DRG 121 are excluded from DRG 122.

DRG 123 Circulatory Disorders With AMI, Expired.
Mean LOS = 2.9 days
Principal diagnoses include selected principal diagnoses listed under DRG 121 or 122. The distinction in this DRG is that the patient expires as a result of the AMI.

Introduction

DEFINITION AND TIME FOCUS

Acute myocardial infarction (AMI) is the necrosis of myocardial tissue, usually resulting from coronary artery occlusion or spasm. It may present as subendocardial infarction, involving the inner myocardial layer, or transmural infarction, involving the full thickness of the myocardium. Mortality depends on the extent and location of the infarct, the patient's preexisting health status, and the speed and effectiveness of therapy.

This clinical plan focuses on the patient admitted for diagnosis and management during an attack of severe crushing chest pain, the classic presentation in AMI.

ETIOLOGY AND PRECIPITATING FACTORS

- coronary artery disease, coronary artery spasm, hypotension, hypoxemia, severe bradycardia or tachycardia (especially with poor cardiac reserve), or other factors decreasing myocardial oxygen supply
- exercise, emotional stress, exposure to extreme heat or cold, eating, tachycardia, or other factors increasing myocardial oxygen demand

Focused assessment guidelines

NURSING HISTORY (Functional health pattern findings)

Health perception–health management pattern

- may experience sudden onset of severe chest pain—heavy, tight, crushing, or constricting quality; usually retrosternal; usually radiating to left arm, but may radiate to right arm, back, epigastrium, jaw, or neck; lasting longer than 30 minutes; unrelieved by rest or nitroglycerin. In some instances, AMI is painless.
- may be under treatment for angina, atherosclerosis, hyperlipidemia, hypertension, CHF, dysrhythmias, stroke, peripheral vascular disease, or diabetes mellitus
- may have history of previous MI, cardiac surgery, or oral contraceptive use
- may have positive coronary artery disease risk factors, such as obesity or cigarette smoking
- may fall into other high-risk categories—a man over age 40 or postmenopausal woman.

Nutritional-metabolic pattern

- may report indigestion, nausea, or vomiting
- commonly reports a diet high in calories, fat, and salt

Elimination pattern

- may report feeling of fullness or bowel movement coinciding with onset of chest pain

Activity-exercise pattern

- may experience shortness of breath
- commonly reports sporadic exercise or sedentary lifestyle

Sleep-rest pattern

- may report sleep disturbances

Cognitive-perceptual pattern

- may report history of recurrent chest pain

Self-perception–self-concept pattern

- may express great concern about ability to return to work as soon as possible

Role-relationship pattern
- may describe self as someone on whom others depend
- may report family history of death from MI (especially before age 50)

Coping–stress tolerance pattern
- usually anxious, tense, Type A personality
- may report fear of death or of the unknown

Value-belief pattern
- may have delayed seeking medical attention or express disbelief over current experience (denial)

PHYSICAL FINDINGS
Cardiovascular
- hypotension or hypertension
- tachycardia or, uncommonly, bradycardia
- other dysrhythmias
- S_3 or S_4 heart sounds
- slowed capillary refill time (if shock present)

Pulmonary
- crackles (if heart failure present)

Gastrointestinal
- vomiting
- abdominal distention

Neurologic
- restlessness
- irritability
- confusion

Integumentary
- diaphoresis
- cool, clammy skin
- variable skin color (may be normal, pale, ashen, or cyanotic)

Musculoskeletal
- pained or anxious facial expression
- tense posture

DIAGNOSTIC STUDIES
Note: Initial laboratory data may reflect no significant abnormalities; however:
- cardiac isoenzymes—show characteristic trends, particularly elevated creatine-phosphokinase-2 (CPK_2) and "flipped" lactic dehydrogenase (LDH) pattern (LDH_1 greater than LDH_2).
- arterial blood gas (ABG) levels—may reveal hypoxemia and acid-base abnormalities.
- electrolyte panel— used to rule out disturbances affecting cardiac conduction and contractility (such as hypokalemia or hyperkalemia and hypocalcemia or hypercalcemia).
- white blood cell count and sedimentation rate—usually rise on second day because of inflammatory response.
- blood urea nitrogen levels and creatinine clearance—may rise, indicating diminished renal perfusion.
- serum cholesterol and triglyceride levels—may be elevated, indicating increased risk of atherosclerosis.
- serum drug levels—may indicate subtherapeutic or toxic levels of antiarrhythmic agents, such as digitalis.
- 12-lead EKG—shows characteristic changes: with transmural infarction, ST elevation and upright T waves in hyperacute phase, progressing to deeply inverted T waves and pathologic Q waves in leads overlooking the infarcted area; with subendocardial infarction, ST depression.
- chest X-ray—may show cardiac enlargement produced by CHF.
- myocardial imaging (radionuclide) studies—demonstrate areas of poor or absent perfusion, wall motion abnormalities, and reduced ejection fraction.
- echocardiography—may illustrate structural or functional cardiac abnormalities.

POTENTIAL COMPLICATIONS
- dysrhythmias
- sudden death
- cardiogenic shock
- CHF
- pulmonary edema
- papillary muscle dysfunction or rupture
- ventricular rupture
- pericarditis
- pulmonary embolism
- ventricular aneurysm
- cardiac tamponade

Collaborative problem: *Potential cardiogenic shock related to dysrhythmias, impaired contractility, or thrombosis*

NURSING PRIORITY: Optimize cardiac output and cellular perfusion.

Interventions	Rationales
1. Institute and document continuous EKG monitoring on admission, with alarms on at all times. Preferably, monitor lead MCL_1 or MCL_6. See the "Potential for injury" nursing diagnosis later in this plan for details about specific dysrhythmias.	1. Dysrhythmias are the primary cause of death in the first 24 hours after infarction. MCL_1 and MCL_6 best differentiate supraventricular aberration from ventricular ectopy.
2. Record and analyze rhythm strips routinely every 4 hours and as needed for significant variations. Mount strips in chart.	2. Systematic analysis may provide warning of impending problems with impulse initiation or conduction.
3. Obtain serial 12-lead EKGs on admission, daily for 3 days, and as needed for chest pain.	3. The EKG obtained on admission provides a baseline for infarct localization. Serial EKGs monitor evolutionary changes.
4. Evaluate and document hourly or as needed: level of consciousness, pulse, blood pressure, heart sounds, breath sounds, urine output, skin color and temperature, and capillary refill time.	4. Level of consciousness is a sensitive indicator of cerebral ischemia. Pulse rate, rhythm, and volume may indicate fluid deficit or overload or ectopic beats. A systolic blood pressure reading more than 20 mm Hg below the patient's normal value or a systolic blood pressure of 80 mm Hg or less indicates shock. Abnormal heart sounds indicate the presence of various problems: S_3 or S_4, congestive heart failure; murmurs, incompetent or stenotic valves; and a pericardial friction rub, pericarditis. Abnormal breath sounds (particularly crackles that do not clear with coughing) suggest CHF. A urine output <60 ml/hour suggests decreased renal perfusion. Pale, cyanotic, mottled, or cool skin indicates decreased peripheral perfusion, as does a capillary refill time >3 seconds.
5. Establish and maintain a patent I.V. line on admission. Document accumulative intake and output hourly.	5. This "I.V. lifeline" is necessary for emergency venous access for fluid and drug administration. The usual order is for dextrose 5% in water to keep the vein open (KVO). If the patient does not need fluid, a heparin lock may be ordered instead. Intake and output records provide clues to developing fluid imbalances.
6. Administer heparin, warfarin sodium (Coumadin), or both, as ordered.	6. Heparin commonly is ordered prophylactically to minimize the risk of thromboembolism from dysrhythmias or immobility. It also may be used to limit extension of a thrombus that produced an AMI. Long-term anticoagulation is achieved with Coumadin.
7. Prepare the patient for aggressive treatment measures, as ordered, which may include:	7. Infarctions that are impending, in progress, or complicated may require immediate aggressive interventions.
• emergency coronary arteriography	• Coronary arteriography normally is not performed during AMI, because of the risk of furthering the infarct. It is a necessary precursor to angioplasty or emergency bypass surgery, however, to locate the site of occlusion precisely.
• streptokinase infusion	• Intracoronary or I.V. streptokinase may be administered to lyse fresh clots, thus relieving the occlusion and reestablishing perfusion to the damaged area.

Interventions	Rationales
• tissue plasminogen activator (tPA)	• tPA lyses clots at their sites, reestablishing perfusion with less risk of bleeding than streptokinase.
• percutaneous transluminal coronary angioplasty (PTCA)	• PTCA may increase coronary artery blood flow by compressing occluding lesions and dilating the vessel lumen. The resulting increase in luminal cross-sectional area improves blood flow to ischemic tissue.
• coronary artery bypass surgery.	• Emergency surgery may be necessary to bypass life-threatening lesions.
8. Additional individualized interventions: ____________	8. Rationales: ____________

Target outcome criteria

Within 24 hours of admission, the patient will:
- display vital signs within normal limits for this patient
- show normal skin color
- have a capillary refill time <3 seconds.

Within 3 days of admission, the patient will experience no life-threatening dysrhythmias.

Collaborative problem: *Hypoxemia related to ventilation-perfusion imbalance*

NURSING PRIORITIES: (a) Optimize myocardial oxygen demand-supply ratio and (b) minimize the risk of further infarction.

Interventions	Rationales
1. Observe for signs and symptoms of hypoxemia, such as tachycardia, restlessness, irritability, or tachypnea. Monitor ABG values, as ordered.	1. Hypoxemia commonly results from impaired coronary artery perfusion, decreased systemic perfusion, and respiratory depressant effects of analgesics and sedatives. ABG values provide objective evidence of the degree of hypoxemia. Prompt treatment minimizes ischemic damage.
2. Administer and document oxygen therapy on admission, according to medical protocol and nursing judgment, typically 3 to 5 liters/minute by nasal cannula for the first 24 to 48 hours.	2. Supplemental oxygen will elevate arterial oxygen content and may relieve myocardial ischemia.
3. If blood pressure is stable within normal limits, place the patient in semi-Fowler's position.	3. The semi-upright position facilitates diaphragmatic movement.
4. During the period of acute instability, place the patient on bed rest or chair rest. Once stabilized, progress activity as tolerated. See the "Activity intolerance" nursing diagnosis, page 147, in the "Acute Heart Failure" care plan.	4. Rest reduces myocardial oxygen demands. Controlling oxygen demands helps limit the risk of infarct extension. Gradual resumption of activity as physical condition allows helps promote a sense of well-being. The "Activity intolerance" nursing diagnosis contains detailed information on assessing activity tolerance and promoting safe resumption of physical activity.
5. Provide adequate rest periods. For example, set priorities for care and group procedures. Refer to the "Sensory-Perceptual Alteration" care plan, page 60, for further suggestions.	5. Sleep deprivation, endemic to critical care units, can lead to increased irritability, confusion, increased sensitivity to pain, and other problems. The "Sensory-Perceptual Alteration" care plan provides detailed interventions and rationales related to sleep deprivation.
6. Additional individualized interventions: ____________	6. Rationales: ____________

Target outcome criteria
Within 24 hours of admission, the patient will:
- show no dyspnea
- manifest arterial PO_2 >80 mm Hg
- display normal sinus rhythm or controlled dysrhythmias
- have normal skin color
- be resting comfortably.

Collaborative problem: *Chest pain related to myocardial ischemia*

NURSING PRIORITY: Relieve chest pain.

Interventions	Rationales
1. On admission, teach the patient to report any chest pain immediately along with tightness, heaviness, or burning.	1. Symptoms other than obvious pain may indicate ischemia. Awareness of more subtle symptoms suggesting ischemia facilitates early intervention.
2. Monitor continuously for chest pain: verbalizations or complaints, sternal rubbing, tense posture, emotional withdrawal, facial grimacing, shortness of breath, diaphoresis, or restlessness.	2. The patient may not report pain, but astute observation may detect associated signs and symptoms and facilitate early intervention. Shortness of breath and diaphoresis may result from sympathetic stimulation, whereas restlessness may reflect cerebral ischemia.
3. Document pain episodes: analyze pain characteristics, record a monitor rhythm strip, and obtain a 12-lead EKG.	3. Careful analysis of characteristics aids differential diagnosis of pain. The rhythm strip can document new dysrhythmias, whereas the 12-lead EKG can document infarct extension.
4. Medicate and document promptly at onset of pain, according to medical protocol or orders. Evaluate and document blood pressure, pulse, and respirations before and after pain medication. Assess pain relief 30 minutes after medicating.	4. Pain medication is more effective when given before severe pain. Pain may stimulate the sympathetic nervous system and increase myocardial work load. Vital sign measurements before medication provide objective indicators of the degree of physiologic stress imposed by pain, whereas those afterward indicate relief of such stress.
5. During the initial period of cardiovascular instability, titrate morphine I.V., typically in 2- to 5-mg doses (if ordered), according to the level of pain and vital signs. Withhold morphine and contact the doctor if (a) the respiratory rate <12 breaths/minute, or (b) the systolic blood pressure is <90 mm Hg (for a previously normotensive patient) or >20 mm Hg below the baseline value, for a previously hypertensive patient.	5. Administering narcotics I.V relieves pain more rapidly and reliably than by the I.M. route, because I.M. medications are absorbed erratically from poorly perfused muscles. I.M. injections also elevate CPK levels, obscuring their diagnostic value. Morphine is the drug of choice for pain associated with AMI, because it is a potent analgesic, causes peripheral vasodilation (thus lessening venous return and myocardial work load), and causes euphoria. The vital sign parameters listed indicate respiratory depression and excessive vasodilation, both possible side effects of morphine.
6. Remain with the patient until pain is relieved.	6. The presence of a competent, confident caregiver may reassure the patient, relieving anxiety and, therefore, lessening sympathetic stimulation.
7. Position the patient comfortably. Use noninvasive pain-relief measures and medications, as appropriate. See the "Acute Pain" care plan, page 10, for details.	7. Comfortable positioning and noninvasive pain-relief measures such as rhythmic breathing, distraction, and relaxation may reduce the perception of incoming pain stimuli and promote endorphin release. The "Acute Pain" care plan discusses numerous alternate pain-relief strategies.
8. Additional individualized interventions: ________	8. Rationales: ________

Target outcome criteria
Within 1 to 2 hours of admission, the patient will:
- verbalize relief of pain
- display no associated signs and symptoms of pain
- assume a relaxed posture
- have a relaxed facial expression.

Nursing diagnosis: *Potential ineffective coping related to fear of death, anxiety, denial, or depression*

NURSING PRIORITY: Promote healthy coping.

Interventions	Rationales
1. Implement measures in the "Ineffective Coping" care plan, page 26, as appropriate.	1. AMI is a major threat to psychological equilibrium and may provoke a wide variety of protective responses. The "Ineffective Coping" care plan contains comprehensive information on evaluating and promoting healthy rather than dysfunctional responses.
2. Administer tranquilizers, as ordered, typically diazepam (Valium).	2. Minor tranquilizers may be used to keep anxiety at a tolerable level and avoid the deleterious physiologic effects of anxiety-triggered catecholamine release.
3. Additional individualized interventions: ____________	3. Rationales: ____________

Target outcome criteria
Within 24 hours, the patient will:
- display feelings appropriate to initial stage of coping
- display beginning signs of effective coping.

Nursing diagnosis: *Constipation related to diet, bed rest, immobility, or medications*

NURSING PRIORITY: Prevent or minimize constipation.

Interventions	Rationales
1. Encourage intake of the prescribed diet—which is usually low in calories, salt, and fat—at mealtimes. Limit intake of caffeine. Document intake, likes, and dislikes.	1. Dietary prescriptions vary with the patient's needs. Caffeine is avoided because it is a cardiac stimulant.
2. Supply a bedside commode when the patient's condition allows.	2. A bedside commode requires less energy to use than a bedpan so constipation can be relieved with less myocardial oxygen demand.
3. Administer stool softeners and laxatives judiciously, as ordered, and document. Use alternatives and supplements to stool softeners and laxatives, such as increased dietary fiber and prune juice. Encourage increased fluid intake, if appropriate to medical status.	3. Straining to defecate produces Valsalva's maneuver, which can cause bradycardia and decrease cardiac output. Rebound tachycardia and myocardial ischemia may follow. Dependence on laxatives, however, causes diminished urge for spontaneous defecation.
4. Provide privacy, a room deodorizer, and television or radio noise while the patient is defecating.	4. Without such measures, the patient may inhibit defecation because of embarrassment over expulsive sounds and odors.

(continued)

Interventions

5. Additional individualized interventions: ____________

____

Rationales

5. Rationales: ____________

____

> **Target outcome criteria**
> Within 3 days, the patient will:
> • resume a regular bowel elimination pattern
> • experience no straining during defecation
> • have a soft stool.

Nursing diagnosis: *Potential for injury: complications related to myocardial ischemia, injury, necrosis, inflammation, or dysrhythmias*

NURSING PRIORITY: Prevent or minimize complications.

Interventions

1. Monitor constantly for general complications of MI, including:

Rationales

1. Numerous complications can impair the recovery of the MI patient. Many occur with any type of infarct and are associated less with its location than with the extent of myocardial damage and degree of the underlying coronary artery disease. Others more commonly have a pathophysiologic correlation with a specific type of infarct. This section presents general complications first, followed by specific ones related to the infarct type in which they most commonly occur.

DYSRHYTHMIAS

• Observe constantly for ventricular dysrhythmias: ventricular premature beats (VPBs), accelerated ventricular rhythm, ventricular tachycardia, and ventricular fibrillation.

• Ventricular dysrhythmias are the most common complication of MI. In the first few hours postinfarct, they probably result from an ischemia-induced reentry mechanism, whereas later dysrhythmias probably result from increased automaticity.

• Observe constantly for supraventricular dysrhythmias: premature atrial or junctional beats; atrial tachycardia, flutter, or fibrillation; or supraventricular tachycardia.

• Supraventricular dysrhythmias may result from ischemia, heart failure, catecholamine stimulation, and other factors. Though less serious than ventricular dysrhythmias, they may contribute to an unstable physiologic status or to thromboembolism. Tachycardias increase myocardial oxygen demand, reduce left ventricular (LV) filling time, and reduce coronary artery perfusion time. The loss of atrial "kick" (normally coordinated atrial contraction) also may reduce cardiac output (CO).

• Administer and document antiarrhythmic agents, as ordered. Monitor effectiveness and side effects. Typical agents are:

□ Class IA agents, such as procainamide (Pronestyl), quinidine, and disopyramide (Norpace)

□ Class IB agents, such as lidocaine, ordered prophylactically or as needed for warning VPBs (more than 6/minute, sequential, multifocal, or close to the preceding T wave), ventricular tachycardia, or ventricular fibrillation

• Dysrhythmias may impair CO or progress to cardiac arrest. Antiarrhythmic agents are classified according to their electrophysiologic properties.

□ Used for both atrial and ventricular dysrhythmias, particularly reentrant ones, Class IA drugs decrease automaticity, conduction, and repolarization.

□ Class IB agents, used to prevent and treat ventricular dysrhythmias, inhibit ventricular automaticity. Lidocaine also increases the threshold for fibrillation. Prophylactic lidocaine may be ordered because of AMI's high incidence of ventricular fibrillation, which commonly occurs without premonitory signs.

Interventions	Rationales
□ Class II agents, such as propranolol (Inderal)	□ Class II agents, beta-adrenergic blockers, are used to control supraventricular dysrhythmias. Their complex mechanisms include suppressing sinus node automaticity and decreasing atrioventricular (AV) conduction.
□ Class III agents, such as bretylium tosylate (Bretylol)	□ Bretylium suppresses reentrant ventricular dysrhythmias and elevates the threshold for ventricular fibrillation.
□ Class IV agents, such as verapamil (Calan).	□ Class IV drugs, calcium channel blockers, inhibit sinoatrial (SA) and AV automaticity and prolong AV conduction. They are particularly useful in treating supraventricular tachycardias.
• Implement and document emergency measures as needed, based on medical protocol and nursing judgment.	• Protocols usually allow for emergency treatment of warning and lethal dysrhythmias (ventricular premature beats, tachycardia, fibrillation, asystole; symptomatic sinus bradycardia; Mobitz II second-degree and third-degree AV blocks).
ACUTE HEART FAILURE	
• Implement measures contained in the "Acute Heart Failure" care plan, page 140, and the "Shock" care plan, page 173, as appropriate.	• Varying degrees of failure are common during the first week after the infarction. Numerous factors place the MI patient at risk for myocardial failure, which may appear as CHF or cardiogenic shock. They include myocardial ischemia, hypoxemia, acidosis, hypotension, and paradoxical movement of the injured myocardial wall.
INFARCT EXTENSION	
• Monitor for new, increased, or persistent chest pain. Obtain a 12-lead EKG reading and administer pain medication, as ordered. Notify the doctor about the pain and about any new indicators of infarction on the 12-lead EKG reading.	• Infarct extension may result from progressive ischemia of the myocardium secondary to swelling of damaged cells and inflammatory responses that compress surrounding tissue. Other factors that may be implicated include hypoxemia and microemboli.
PERICARDITIS	
• Observe for pericardial chest pain, typically, stabbing localized pain that worsens on deep inspiration and with movement. Also observe for fever, tachycardia, and pericardial friction rub.	• Pericardial sac inflammation is a relatively benign complication. Focal pericarditis usually develops within 5 days, whereas generalized pericarditis (Dressler's syndrome) typically develops within 14 days.
• If signs or symptoms are present, notify the doctor. Administer anti-inflammatory agents, as ordered, typically aspirin, corticosteroids, or nonsteroidal anti-inflammatory agents.	• Administering anti-inflammatory agents reduces the inflammatory process, relieving the signs and symptoms and reducing the risk of pericardial effusion.
• Monitor for indicators of a pericardial effusion: weak peripheral pulses, pulsus paradoxus >10 mm Hg, or a decreased level of consciousness. If present, notify the doctor promptly.	• A pericardial effusion represents transudation of fluid across the walls of inflamed cells. The degree may vary from mild to major. Left untreated, an effusion may produce a cardiac tamponade large enough to induce cardiac arrest.
• Monitor for indicators of a cardiac tamponade: Beck's triad (elevated central venous pressure [CVP], arterial hypotension, and distant heart sounds), neck-vein distention, tachycardia, decreased pulse pressure, paradoxical pulse, profound hypotension, and a pericardial friction rub. Summon immediate medical assistance and prepare for emergency pericardial aspiration.	• A cardiac tamponade is a medical emergency. Because it impinges on ventricular expansion, it severely limits ventricular filling and therefore CO. Immediate removal of the pericardial fluid is necessary to permit ventricular filling and prevent cardiac arrest.

(continued)

Interventions	Rationales
VENTRICULAR ANEURYSM	
• Observe for signs and symptoms of a possible ventricular aneurysm: those of congestive heart failure, thromboembolism, or persistent ectopy. Alert the doctor and prepare the patient for surgery, as ordered.	• Ventricular aneurysm is thought to occur in about 10% of MI patients. Aneurysmal dilation most commonly occurs in the anterolateral area, although it may also occur in the posterior or septal walls or the apical area. The systolic outward bulging of the area weakened by the infarction lessens stroke volume. In addition, clots may occur in the dilated area and embolize to other organs. Aneurysmectomy removes the bulging, weakened area and prevents potentially fatal myocardial rupture.
RUPTURE	
• Monitor for signs and symptoms of papillary muscle rupture: sudden shock, a loud holosystolic murmur radiating from the apex to the left axilla, and signs of severe left ventricular failure. Obtain immediate medical assistance. Assist with treatment of cardiogenic shock or prepare the patient for surgery, as ordered.	• Papillary muscle rupture results from necrosis of the muscles that anchor the chordae tendineae of the mitral valve. It occurs most commonly with inferior infarction involving the posterior papillary muscle, although the anterior papillary muscle may be damaged with an anteroseptal infarct. The resulting acute mitral insufficiency may be so pronounced as to severely limit CO. Definitive treatment is mitral valve replacement.
• Observe for signs and symptoms of potential septal rupture: severe chest pain, severe heart failure, a loud holosystolic murmur at apex and lower left sternal border, or sudden cardiac death. Initiate cardiopulmonary resuscitation (CPR), if necessary, and obtain immediate medical assistance. Implement measures to treat cardiogenic shock or prepare the patient for surgery, as ordered.	• Septal rupture, a rare but life-threatening emergency, results from necrosis of the interventricular septum. It may occur in inferior or anteroseptal infarcts and is most likely if significant disease is present in both the right and left anterior descending coronary arteries. CPR and measures to combat cardiogenic shock may keep the patient alive until the ventricular septal defect can be repaired surgically.
• Be alert for signs and symptoms of a possible impending myocardial rupture, especially in a patient with a transmural infarction who is on anticoagulant therapy: persistent chest pain without EKG changes, persistent hypertension postinfarct, M-shaped QRS complexes, or pericardial blood or fluid detected by an echocardiogram. Notify the doctor immediately. Assist with emergency pericardiocentesis and treatment of cardiogenic shock, as ordered.	• Rupture of the free ventricular wall, a devastating complication, occurs most commonly in the anterior or lateral walls. It may occur anywhere from 3 days to 3 weeks after the infarction, during the healing stage when leukocytic removal of myocardial debris thins the myocardial wall. Hypertension, anticoagulation, and full-thickness infarction increase the risk of rupture. The resulting massive cardiac tamponade leads to death. The invariable mortality from rupture emphasizes the urgency of action when any signs and symptoms of impending rupture are detected.
2. Monitor constantly for specific complications of particular types of MI.	2. Specific complications commonly correlate with particular types of infarcts, because they stem from a common pathophysiologic cause.
ANTERIOR, ANTEROSEPTAL, OR ANTEROLATERAL INFARCT	
• Monitor for signs or symptoms of potential bundle branch block (BBB). Constantly monitor QRS complex width and the pattern of deflections in V_1 and V_6 (or MCL_1 and MCL_6). On serial EKGs, note axis deviation.	• Because the left anterior descending coronary artery nourishes the ventricular septum, where the bundle branches are located, an anterior infarct may produce septal ischemia or necrosis with resulting BBB. BBB widens the QRS complex beyond the normal limit because it disrupts the usual sequence or speed of depolarization. Because V_1 (MCL_1) is oriented to the right ventricle and V_6 (MCL_6) to the left, the patterns of deflections in these leads best indicate the timing and sequence of bundle branch conduction.
• Document and alert the doctor to the presence of any of the following:	• Untreated, BBB increases risk of mortality from AMI.

Interventions	Rationales
□ Right BBB (RBBB): QRS >0.12 seconds, RSR′ pattern in V_1	□ RBBB produces delayed right ventricular (RV) stimulation, prolonging the QRS duration. It also alters the usual sequence of deflections, in which septal depolarization is followed by simultaneous depolarization of both ventricles. Instead, RBBB produces a small positive wave of septal depolarization, a large negative wave of LV depolarization, and a large positive wave of RV depolarization.
□ Left BBB (LBBB): QRS >0.12 seconds, absent Q wave, and large monophasic R wave in V_6	□ LBBB disrupts the depolarization pattern to a greater extent than RBBB. It causes loss of the normal septal Q waves in leads oriented to the LV and allows the RV to depolarize before the LV.
□ Left anterior hemiblock (LAH) or left posterior hemiblock (LPH)	□ Hemiblocks are blocks of one fascicle of the left bundle branch. Left anterior hemiblock is more common than left posterior hemiblock because the anterior fascicle is thinner and has a more vulnerable blood supply. LAH is considered relatively benign, whereas LPH is more serious because it implies extensive infarction.
• Observe closely for development of Mobitz II second-degree AV block or complete heart block, particularly if RBBB with LAH or LPH is present. Prepare for prophylactic pacemaker insertion, as ordered.	• Progression to a more advanced degree of block is possible at any time. RBBB with hemiblock represents blockage of two of the three fascicles responsible for ventricular conduction, leaving the patient dependent on the sole remaining fascicle. Mobitz II block is an ominous sign because it represents intermittent blockage of all three fascicles. It implies extensive myocardial necrosis and commonly heralds complete heart block. Prophylactic pacemaker insertion prevents ventricular asystole if complete heart block should occur.
INFERIOR INFARCT	
• Monitor for sinus bradycardia and AV block, particularly first-degree AV block and Mobitz I second-degree AV block.	• Although these rhythms may occur with any type of infarct from excess vagal stimulation, they are most common in inferior infarction. An inferior infarct typically is produced by occlusion of the right coronary artery (RCA), the artery that nourishes the SA node in about 90% of the population and the AV node in about 55%. Ischemia of the SA node produces sinus arrhythmias, whereas AV nodal ischemia above the bundle of His produces progressive slowing of impulse conduction through the AV node. Such ischemia usually is transient and responds promptly to administration of atropine.
□ Correlate rhythm with clinical status, noting the presence of hypotension, altered level of consciousness, chest pain, or increased VPBs.	□ The clinical signs listed indicate the dysrhythmia is decreasing CO.
□ If the patient is symptomatic, administer atropine, as ordered and per unit protocol. Notify the doctor and document the episode.	□ Atropine blocks vagal stimulation, thereby increasing SA node impulse formation and AV node conduction.
• Observe for indicators of RV infarction, such as:	• RV infarction rarely occurs alone but more commonly is associated with inferior or posterior LV infarction, because these areas all are perfused by the RCA. RV infarction is estimated to occur in about 30% of inferior MIs.
□ neck-vein distention, positive hepatojugular reflux, Kussmaul's sign (increased neck-vein distention on inspiration), or elevated CVP or right atrial pressure (RAP) with normal or mildly elevated pulmonary capillary wedge pressure (PCWP).	□ These signs reflect the increased venous pressure that results from impaired RV compliance and inability to pump blood effectively.

(continued)

Interventions	Rationales
□ widely split S_2; S_3 or S_4 heart sounds audible at the third to fourth intercostal space at the left sternal border (right ventricular S_3 or S_4); or murmur of tricuspid insufficiency	□ The wide split of S_2 reflects delayed pulmonic valve closure, the result of prolonged RV ejection caused by the increased RV volume and pressure. The S_3 or S_4 indicates decreased RV compliance, whereas the murmur of tricuspid insufficiency reflects a functional valvular insufficiency secondary to RV dilatation.
□ bradycardia, AV blocks, and hypotension.	□ Bradycardia probably reflects SA nodal ischemia, blocks indicate AV nodal ischemia, and hypotension results from impaired RV stroke volume.
• If the patient is volume depleted on admission, be especially alert for the above signs after I.V. hydration is achieved.	• Because MI patients may be volume depleted on admission from nausea, vomiting, and diaphoresis, signs of RV infarction may appear only after rehydration.
• When recording 12-lead EKGs on patients with suspected inferior or posterior infarction, routinely record right ventricular leads, such as V_4R.	• The routine 12-lead EKG is not helpful in detecting RV infarction per se, although it will reveal signs of concomitant inferior or posterior infarction. Right ventricular leads typically reveal Q waves, ST elevation, and T-wave inversion with acute RV infarction.
• If indicators of RV infarction are present, alert the doctor. Obtain a chest X-ray and other noninvasive diagnostic studies, as ordered.	• A chest X-ray and other diagnostic studies provide objective evidence of RV infarction. With RV infarction alone, the chest X-ray typically is clear. An echocardiogram helps differentiate RV infarction from cardiac tamponade, whereas radionuclide studies visualize areas of infarction or decreased RV ejection fraction. Diagnostic studies also aid in differentiation of hypotension resulting primarily from RV dysfunction from that resulting from LV dysfunction—an important distinction because therapy for each is quite different.
• If an RV infarction is confirmed, collaborate with the doctor to modify therapy. Typically:	• Although the treatment of RV infarction differs from that for LV infarction, the goal is the same: to improve LV filling pressure and thereby optimize CO.
□ Avoid diuretics. Administer fluid boluses, as ordered, typically to maintain RAP at 20 to 25 mm Hg and PCWP at 15 to 18 mm Hg.	□ Because strong RV contraction is absent with RV infarction, blood flow from the right to the left side of the heart becomes passive and dependent on preload. Diuretics are avoided because they lower preload. Fluid is administered, rather than limited as in LV infarction, to improve preload-dependent RV systolic ejection, thereby increasing LV filling pressure and CO.
□ Administer inotropes and vasodilators judiciously, as ordered.	□ Inotropes may increase RV contractility. Vasodilators may be used to decrease pulmonary vascular resistance; the resulting RV afterload reduction may improve LV filling, whereas the simultaneous LV afterload reduction may improve LV systolic emptying.
• Monitor hemodynamic parameters and clinical indicators of the effectiveness of therapy closely.	• The association of RV infarction with LV infarction can be confusing to interpret and a challenge to manage. The treatment of RV infarction described above must be tempered with consideration of therapy for LV infarction. Continual surveillance is necessary to make sure that therapies are titrated and modified as necessary to achieve optimal cardiac output.
3. Additional individualized interventions: ______________	3. Rationales: ______________

Target outcome criteria
Within 24 hours of admission, the patient will:
• display normal sinus rhythm or a controlled dysrhythmia with a ventricular rate of 60 to 100 beats/minute
• manifest strong, bilaterally equal peripheral pulses.

Within 3 days of admission, the patient will:
• have hemodynamic values within expected limits
• manifest strong, bilaterally equal peripheral pulses
• have clear breath sounds
• have clear heart sounds with decreasing or no S_3 or S_4, rub, or new murmurs
• experience no further episodes of chest pain
• show decreasing or no neck-vein distention.

Nursing diagnosis: *Knowledge deficit related to diagnostic procedures, therapeutic interventions, and long-range implications for life-style changes*

NURSING PRIORITY: Educate the patient and family about health status, as appropriate.

Interventions	Rationales
1. Implement measures in the "Knowledge Deficit" care plan, page 45, as appropriate.	1. The "Knowledge Deficit" care plan contains detailed information helpful in assessing and meeting learning needs for all patients. This plan focuses on information specific to AMI.
2. Defer participation in a formal rehabilitation and education program until the period of physiologic instability has passed. In the meantime:	2. Attempting to implement a major teaching program during this period is inappropriate, because physiologic recovery is a higher priority. Nevertheless, capitalizing on serendipitous teaching opportunities provides a way to assess learning needs and meet immediate concerns.
• Establish rapport. Use eye contact, reflective listening, and nonverbal communication. Emphasize and display consistency as much as possible.	• Excessive anxiety interferes with learning. Establishing rapport through consistent, caring contact helps promote trust and relaxation, which are conducive to retention of new information.
• Assess immediate learning needs, encourage questions, and provide brief explanations, correcting any misconceptions; repeat as necessary.	• The sobering experience of AMI usually raises major questions for the patient and family related to health and life-style considerations. Responding to expressed needs displays sensitivity to the patient and family. Brief, repeated explanations may be necessary because high anxiety levels or medication effects may cause the patient to unconsciously "screen out" information.
• As appropriate, provide brief information about pathophysiology of AMI, risk factor reduction, medications, dietary recommendations, activity restrictions, rehabilitation programs, community agencies, and support groups. Consult the "Acute Myocardial Infarction" care plan in *Medical-Surgical Care Plans*, which explains post-CCU care.	• Judicious selection of initial teaching content helps prevent information overload. The "Acute Myocardial Infarction" care plan in *Medical-Surgical Care Plans* contains comprehensive information on long-range learning needs and rehabilitation programs, usually addressed after the patient has progressed from the phase of intensive care.
• Note and document long-range learning needs. Upon transfer, communicate them to the new unit's staff.	• Documentation and communication of long-range learning needs allows continuity of care and personalization of ongoing educational efforts.
3. Additional individualized interventions: ____________	3. Rationales: ____________

Target outcome criteria
Within 48 hours of admission, the patient and family will:
• provide feedback indicating an adequate knowledge base for immediate needs (for example, by asking appropriate questions and by respecting dietary restrictions)
• express beginning identification of long-range learning needs.

Transfer planning

NURSING TRANSFER CRITERIA

Upon transfer, documentation shows evidence of:
• stable blood pressure within normal limits without I.V. inotrope or vasodilator support
• stable cardiac rhythm with dysrhythmias (if any) controlled by oral, sublingual, or transdermal medications or by permanent pacemaker
• spontaneous ventilation.

PATIENT-FAMILY TEACHING CHECKLIST

Document evidence that patient and family demonstrate understanding of:
__ the extent of infarction
__ activity restrictions
__ recommended dietary modifications
__ smoking-cessation program as needed
__ common changes in feelings postinfarct
__ community resources for life-style modification support and cardiac rehabilitation.

DOCUMENTATION CHECKLIST

Using outcome criteria as a guide, document:
__ clinical status on admission
__ significant changes in status
__ pertinent diagnostic test findings
__ chest pain episodes
__ pain-relief measures
__ rhythm strip analyses
__ use of emergency protocols
__ hemodynamic and other trend data
__ I.V. line patency
__ oxygen therapy
__ other therapies
__ nutrition intake
__ patient-family teaching
__ transfer planning.

ASSOCIATED CARE PLANS

Acute Heart Failure
Acute Pain
Grieving and Dying
Impaired Physical Mobility
Ineffective Coping
Knowledge Deficit
Shock

REFERENCES

Guzzetta, C., and Dossey, B. *Cardiovascular Nursing.* St. Louis: C.V. Mosby Co., 1984.
Hoaglund, P. "Right Ventricular Infarction," *Critical Care Quarterly* 7:19-25, March 1985.
Holloway, N., ed. *Nursing the Critically Ill Adult,* 3rd ed. Menlo Park, Calif.: Addison-Wesley Publishing Co., 1988.
Lewis, P. "Evaluation of the Patient Sustaining a Right Ventricular Infarction and Nursing Implications," *Critical Care Nurse* 3(1):50-54, January/February 1983.
Rossignol, M., et al. "Assessment and Treatment of Right Ventricular Infarction," *Focus on Critical Care* 12(6):20-25, 1985.
Vaughan, P., and Rice, V. "Complications of Myocardial Infarction," *Critical Care Nurse* 2(3):44-51, May/June 1982.

Cardiac Surgery

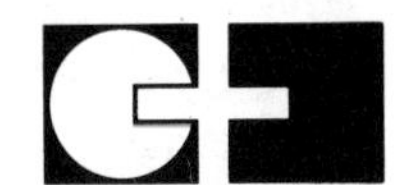

DRG information

Cardiac surgery may be classified under several DRGs, depending on the principal operating room procedure and whether cardiac catheterization was performed.

DRG 104 Cardiac Valve Procedure With Pump and With Cardiac Catheterization.
Mean LOS = 17.4 days
Principal operating room procedures include:
- open-heart mitral, aortic, pulmonic, or tricuspid valvuloplasty without replacement
- replacement of mitral, aortic, pulmonic, or tricuspid valve with tissue graft or prosthetic device
- implantation or replacement of automatic cardioverter/defibrillator, total system.

DRG 105 Cardiac Valve Procedure With Pump and Without Cardiac Catheterization.
Mean LOS = 13.2 days

DRG 106 Coronary Bypass With Cardiac Catheterization.
Mean LOS = 14.2 days
Principal operating room procedures include aortocoronary bypass of 1, 2, 3, 4, or >4 coronary arteries.

DRG 107 Coronary Bypass Without Cardiac Catheterization.
Mean LOS = 11.1 days

DRG 108 Other Cardiothoracic or Vascular Procedures With Pump.
Mean LOS = 11.0 days
Principal operating room procedures include:
- percutaneous transluminal coronary angioplasty (PTCA) to remove artery obstruction, with pump
- biopsy of pericardium
- cardiotomy
- excision of aneurysm or other heart lesion
- open chest cardiac massage
- operations on structures adjacent to heart valves
- pericardiotomy
- pericardiectomy
- repair of atrial or ventricular septa with tissue graft or prosthetic device
- repair, total, of certain congenital cardiac anomalies
- closed cardiac valvotomy.

Additional DRG information: Hundreds of additional vascular operating room procedures also are classified under DRG 108. The above list details only coronary procedures. Other cardiac surgical procedures not addressed in the following care plan (such as permanent pacemaker insertion) have still other DRG numbers.

Introduction

DEFINITION AND TIME FOCUS

Cardiac surgery is performed for numerous reasons, indicated below. During surgery, the heart's activity is arrested and the lungs collapsed; to preserve organ viability, cardiopulmonary bypass (CPB) maintains systemic perfusion and gas exchange during this time. CPB results in some predictable changes in physiologic function and in hemodynamics during the early postoperative period. Nursing care during this period is based on astute patient assessment for these anticipated changes, maintaining organ function, preventing complications, and providing emotional support to the patient and family.

This clinical plan focuses on the coronary artery bypass graft (CABG) or valve replacement patient during the first 2 to 3 postoperative days, the period of recovery in the critical care unit (CCU). It assumes that preoperative teaching has been provided by a cardiovascular nurse specialist or other members of a heart surgery teaching program and that a formal postoperative teaching and rehabilitation program is provided after transfer from the CCU. (For preoperative and postoperative teaching plans, the reader is referred to the excellent presentation in Sadler, 1984.)

ETIOLOGY AND PRECIPITATING FACTORS

- severe coronary artery disease of one or more vessels, particularly the left anterior descending coronary artery
- acute myocardial infarction, especially if complicated by cardiogenic shock, infarct extension, uncontrollable failure, papillary muscle rupture, or septal rupture
- unstable or crescendo angina pectoris
- previous bypass grafting with recurrent angina or angiographic evidence of graft closure
- ventricular aneurysm
- valvular stenosis or insufficiency with hemodynamic compromise

Focused assessment guidelines

NURSING HISTORY (Functional health pattern findings)

Health perception–health management pattern

- may have history of acute or chronic coronary artery disease or valvular dysfunction
- may have preexisting condition that has become refractory to less invasive therapies, such as medications

Note: Remaining health pattern findings are those of the underlying disease; refer to care plans in "Acute Myocardial Infarction," page 150, and "Acute Heart Failure," page 140, for examples.

PHYSICAL FINDINGS

Because the preoperative physical findings are those of the underlying disorder, they are not repeated here; instead, this section presents typical postoperative findings.

General appearance

- weight increase of 1 to 8 kg above preoperative weight

Cardiovascular

- blood pressure variable
- dysrhythmias
- heart sounds variable; if valve replacement done, may have early flow murmur or audible clicking
- chest tube drainage variable
- peripheral pulses usually equal bilaterally
- slow capillary refill

Pulmonary

- variable rate and depth, depending on ventilator settings
- breath sounds usually diminished in left base
- crackles or rhonchi

Neurologic

- level of consciousness variable (patient usually can be awakened)
- confusion
- disorientation

Integumentary

- cool skin
- dry skin
- pallor
- generalized edema
- serosanguinous oozing from incisions

Gastrointestinal

- absent bowel sounds

Renal

- polyuria

DIAGNOSTIC STUDIES

All the following tests are performed preoperatively for baseline data. This section details common early postoperative findings.

- hemoglobin and hematocrit levels—decreased because of hemodilution; hematocrit value is commonly about 25%.
- coagulation panel—reveals prolonged prothrombin time (PT) and partial thromboplastin time (PTT), reflecting intraoperative heparinization; and decreased platelet level, reflecting platelet destruction by CPB equipment, especially roller and filtration unit.
- serum glucose level—elevated because of stress-induced glycogenolysis and decreased insulin production.
- serum electrolyte values—vary, depending on preexisting status, operative replacement, fluid shifts, and other factors.
- cardiac isoenzymes—may be elevated if myocardial infarction is present.
- 12-lead EKG—findings vary, depending on preexisting disorders (such as myocardial infarction), acid-base status, electrolyte status, or medications.
- chest X-ray—used to evaluate cardiac size, mediastinal position, and pulmonary status; postoperatively, it is used to confirm placement of endotracheal and chest tubes.
- preoperative cardiac catheterization and coronary arteriography—reveal critical coronary artery occlusion, poor left ventricular function, or hemodynamically significant valve stenosis or insufficiency as manifested by elevated left ventricular end-diastolic pressure, cardiac index <2.5 liter/minute/m^2, ejection fraction <0.5, tight valve areas, increased valvular gradients, or occlusive lesions.

POTENTIAL COMPLICATIONS

- cardiogenic shock
- hypovolemic shock
- myocardial infarction
- heart failure
- endocarditis
- graft occlusion
- thromboembolism
- atelectasis

Collaborative problem: *Potential low cardiac output syndrome related to hypothermia, excessive vasoconstriction, myocardial depression, dysrhythmias, or cardiac tamponade*

NURSING PRIORITY: Maintain optimal cardiac output.

Interventions	Rationales
1. Monitor blood pressure continuously with an arterial catheter. Maintain mean arterial pressure (MAP) within desired limits; determine limits in consultation with the surgeon. Generally, report any values abnormal for the patient or systolic blood pressure <80 or >180 mm Hg, diastolic blood pressure >100 mm Hg, or MAP <60 or >100 mm Hg.	1. Low cardiac output syndrome, a common postoperative problem, may result from preexisting abnormalities or the stress of surgery. Arterial monitoring provides the most direct and accurate blood pressure measurements. Because perfusion is directly related to blood pressure, maintenance of optimal MAP ensures adequate organ perfusion. Hypothermia, used during surgery to lower metabolic demand and protect organs from ischemic damage, induces vasoconstriction, which increases systemic vascular resistance and the risk of hypertension. Also, the stress-triggered release of catecholamines, antidiuretic hormone (ADH), and aldosterone may produce hypertension. Persistent hypertension can cause leaking or rupture of suture lines. Hypotension may be triggered by numerous factors, discussed later in this plan.
2. Measure cardiac output (CO), as ordered, typically every hour until normal and then every 2 hours. Calculate cardiac index (CI) by dividing CO by body-surface area (BSA); obtain BSA value from a BSA chart or nomogram. Calculate systemic vascular resistance (SVR) by subtracting right atrial pressure (RAP) from MAP and dividing the result by CO. Follow the trend of CI and SVR values, comparing them to normal ranges and previous values.	2. CO may drop in the postoperative period because of decreased preload from a fluid volume deficit (discussed in a later problem), increased afterload from elevated SVR, or impaired contractility (discussed below). Any of these factors may precipitate failure of the already stressed heart. CO measurements and CI calculations provide objective data on the adequacy of output, whereas calculation of SVR values provides objective evidence of the degree of resistance to ventricular ejection. Increased afterload and hypertension both increase myocardial work load. SVR values typically are elevated in the early postoperative period. SVR and blood pressure values should return to normal gradually as rewarming occurs.
3. Monitor pulmonary artery diastolic pressure (PADP) continuously until stable. Monitor RAP, pulmonary artery systolic pressure (PASP), and pulmonary capillary wedge pressure (PCWP), as ordered, typically every hour until stable. Compare to preoperative values and to desired limits; determine limits in consultation with the surgeon.	3. Because PADP indirectly reflects the functional state of the left ventricle, it is a useful indicator of left ventricular performance. RAP reflects central venous pressure; PASP, the force of right ventricular ejection; and PCWP, the functional state of the left ventricle. Values provide objective data for assessing the patient's fluid volume, cardiovascular function, and pulmonary status.
4. Provide constant EKG monitoring. Observe for indicators of possible myocardial damage (ST-segment deviation, T-wave inversion, pathologic Q waves) and for dysrhythmias, typically atrial fibrillation and heart block in valve replacement patients, and ventricular dysrhythmias in all patients. If present, assess for underlying causes, treat (according to standing orders) with medications or temporary pacing, and document.	4. Constant monitoring provides early warning of possible myocardial damage or dysrhythmias. Underlying causes may include pain, anxiety, hypokalemia, hypoxemia, and volume depletion. Often dysrhythmias respond to standard protocols, such as lidocaine administration for premature ventricular beats. In many cases, pacing wires are inserted during surgery and brought out through the chest wall. If necessary, they can be connected to a pacemaker to provide a stable cardiac rhythm until cardiac irritability or underlying causes resolve.

(continued)

Interventions	Rationales
5. Monitor level of consciousness; apical pulse rate; skin color, warmth, and temperature; peripheral pulse rates; and urine output every 15 minutes to 1 hour until normal and stable. Report any abnormalities to the surgeon promptly.	5. These parameters indicate the adequacy of central and peripheral perfusion. Abnormalities may signal the development of numerous complications and need medical evaluation.
6. Monitor core body temperature continuously via rectal probe or every hour with a rectal thermometer until normal and then every 4 hours.	6. Body temperature usually is low on patient's arrival in the CCU from hypothermia and heat loss from the open chest during surgery. The temperature then typically rises somewhat above normal (because of the inflammatory response after surgery) and gradually returns to normal in approximately 3 days.
7. If the temperature is low, cover the patient with warmed blankets until the temperature returns to normal. As temperature rises, monitor for signs of fluid volume deficit. If the temperature rises above 101° F. (38.3° C.), assess for underlying causes; administer antipyretics, such as acetaminophen (Tylenol), as ordered; and use a hypothermia blanket, as ordered, for high fever.	7. Gradual rewarming is desirable in order to allow time for the heart to adjust to the expanded vascular bed as vasoconstriction lessens. As temperature rises, vasodilation may occur precipitously and unmask a previously hidden fluid volume deficit. Temperatures above 101° F. suggest a cause other than the normal inflammatory response, such as dehydration or sepsis. Fever increases cardiac work load, so such measures as administering acetaminophen or hypothermia precautions may be used. Aspirin is usually avoided because it decreases platelet aggregation and may contribute to postoperative bleeding.
8. Administer vasodilators, such as sodium nitroprusside (Nipride), as ordered. Refer to the "Acute Heart Failure" care plan, page 140, for details regarding administration. Correlate vasodilator administration with body temperature and rewarming.	8. Vasodilator administration is used to achieve controlled dilation of the vascular bed and to control hypertension. Because afterload reduction lessens resistance to ventricular ejection, it also lessens myocardial work load. The "Acute Heart Failure" care plan covers nursing care for vasodilator administration. Vasodilator administration, fever, and rewarming all cause vasodilation; correlation is necessary to avoid unintended excessive expansion of the vascular bed.
9. Administer positive inotropic agents, as ordered, typically dopamine (Intropin) or dobutamine (Dobutrex). Refer to the "Acute Heart Failure" care plan, page 140, for details on administration.	9. Mild, transient depression of contractility is common because of hypothermia and myocardial edema. Dopamine improves contractility through its beta$_1$-adrenergic effects but may cause tachycardia and dysrhythmias. Dobutamine also increases contractility and is less likely to cause tachycardia and dysrhythmias. In uncomplicated situations, an inotrope may be used for the first 12 to 24 hours; in cases with preoperative myocardial depression or intraoperative infarction, it may be used for a longer period. The "Acute Heart Failure" care plan presents nursing care on administration of inotropic agents.
10. Monitor for indicators of cardiac tamponade, even when mediastinal chest tubes are draining. Observe for rapid hypotension, marked central venous pressure (CVP) elevation, neck-vein distention, muffled heart sounds, paradoxical pulse, or decreased QRS voltage on EKG; also observe for suddenly decreased chest tube drainage.	10. Cardiac tamponade may result from pericardial accumulation of blood or fluid, which may occur despite draining mediastinal chest tubes if the fluid accumulates in an area not drained by the tubes. Tamponade can rapidly interfere with ventricular filling and cardiac output.
11. Additional individualized interventions: ________	11. Rationales: ________

Target outcome criteria

Within 24 hours after surgery, the patient will:
- have MAP 70 to 100 mm Hg
- have regular supraventricular rhythm with ventricular rate 60 to 100 beats/minute (ideally, normal sinus rhythm)
- have peripheral pulses bilaterally equal and full
- have warm, dry arms and legs
- have a temperature of 98.6° to 101° F. (37° to 38.3° C.)
- display no signs of cardiac tamponade
- have RAP, PADP, PASP, and PCWP within desired limits.

Collaborative problem: *Interstitial edema related to hemodilution, excessive fluid replacement, and stress adaptation syndrome*

NURSING PRIORITY: Restore normal fluid volume.

Interventions	Rationales
1. Expect signs and symptoms of interstitial fluid overload; monitor degree of overload and speed of resolution, for example:	1. During CPB, hemodilution is achieved with crystalloid I.V. solution. Because hemodilution decreases blood viscosity and peripheral vascular resistance, it minimizes microcirculatory sludging, thus protecting organs from ischemic damage during the period of decreased perfusion during surgery.
• Monitor generalized edema and tissue turgor.	• Hemodilution lowers plasma oncotic pressure, which allows fluid to shift from the vascular to interstitial spaces, producing generalized edema.
• Monitor daily weights. Compare to preoperative and previous day's values.	• Weight gain from hemodilution may be as much as 8 kg. Daily weight comparisons provide objective evidence of the degree of fluid retention and the speed with which fluid is mobilized and excreted after surgery.
• Monitor for neck-vein distention or S_3 heart sounds, and if present, notify the doctor.	• Although most of the fluid overload is sequestered in the interstitial space, some increase in central blood volume may occur. These findings may reflect such an increase or may result from cardiac dysfunction, as described in a later problem. In either case, they require medical evaluation.
2. Administer I.V. solutions, as ordered. Unless the patient is hypovolemic, limit fluid intake from all sources to 100 ml/hour or less.	2. Early hypovolemia is common, and administration of I.V. fluid may be needed initially to compensate for interstitial fluid shifts, to increase plasma volume, and to optimize preload. Hemodilution during bypass causes fluid to be sequestered in the interstitial space; however, this fluid shifts back into the vascular space on about the second through fifth postoperative day. In addition, because of the large number of I.V. lines, it is easy to overload the patient with fluid unless total fluid intake is monitored.
3. Monitor intake and output measurements, usually hourly on the first postoperative day and then every 8 hours. Monitor specific gravity every 2 hours for the first 24 hours. Report urine output <0.5 ml/kg/hour and abnormal specific gravity values.	3. The stress reaction triggered by surgery causes the release of ADH, the secretion of aldosterone, and sympathetic stimulation of the kidneys, all of which result in fluid retention. Monitoring intake and output records provides objective data with which to judge the patient's tendency toward fluid retention and on which to base further therapeutic decisions. Urine output may be as much as 1 liter/hour for the first 4 hours. Oliguria with high specific gravity may indicate hypovolemia, whereas oliguria with low specific gravity may indicate renal damage.
4. Administer diuretics, such as furosemide (Lasix) I.V., if ordered.	4. Aggressive diuresis may be used to eliminate the fluid that has shifted into the interstitial space.

(continued)

Interventions

5. Monitor for signs and symptoms of electrolyte imbalance, particularly hypokalemia. See the "Fluid and Electrolyte Imbalances" appendix, page 317, for details. If hypokalemia is present:
- observe for dysrhythmias
- add potassium to I.V. fluids, as ordered
- monitor serum levels closely, typically every 4 hours in the first 24 hours
- monitor for development of hyperkalemia.

Rationales

5. Hypokalemia is very common postoperatively. It may result from preoperative diuretic administration, hemodilution, or postoperative diuresis. Supplemental I.V. potassium administration usually is necessary. Close monitoring of potassium level is essential to guide replacement and to avoid hyperkalemia from the combination of exogenous potassium administration and endogenous potassium release from hemolyzed blood cells.

6. Additional individualized interventions: ______________

6. Rationales: ______________

Target outcome criteria

Within 4 hours after surgery, the patient will display a urine output >0.5 ml/kg/hour.

Within 24 hours after surgery, the patient will have a 24-hour fluid output greater than intake.

Within 3 days after surgery, the patient will:
- display a return to preoperative weight
- have normal serum electrolyte levels.

Collaborative problem: *Hypovolemia related to bleeding or diuresis*

NURSING PRIORITY: Maintain normal fluid volume.

Interventions

1. Monitor PT, PTT, and platelet counts, as ordered. Consult surgeon about reportable values, particularly prolonged PT, prolonged PTT, or low platelet level.

Rationales

1. Blood loss has multiple etiologies during and after the surgery. During the surgery, a certain amount of blood loss is inevitable, and heparin is used to prevent clotting in the extracorporeal circuit. This anticoagulation is reversed with protamine sulfate at the end of the procedure, but inadequate reversal may result in bleeding. Heparin rebound also may occur from the release of heparin previously sequestered in the tissues. Finally, the cardiopulmonary bypass equipment, especially the roller pump and filtration unit, damages platelets. All of these factors may alter normal coagulation, so values below normal are expected postoperatively. Reportable values vary among surgeons.

2. Monitor hemoglobin (Hgb) and hematocrit (HCT) levels. Consult surgeon about reportable values, particularly declining Hgb or HCT levels.

2. Hgb and HCT levels are expected to be low postoperatively, as a result of hemodilution. As postoperative diuresis occurs, the values should return toward normal. Failure to do so implies continued bleeding. Usually, the patient will be transfused when the hematocrit reaches 25% to 30%.

3. Measure and document chest tube drainage. Report to the surgeon drainage that is >200 ml/hour, constant, or increasing.

3. Postoperative sources of bleeding include oozing of incisions or suture disruption. Chest drainage exceeding the indicated parameters is considered an indication for surgical reexploration.

4. Observe for other signs and symptoms of bleeding, such as excessive oozing from incisions, petechiae, and ecchymoses. If HCT and Hgb levels or coagulation values are abnormal, test urine, feces, and vomitus for occult blood.

4. Although laboratory tests provide valuable objective data of bleeding tendencies, they are no substitute for astute clinical assessment. Signs or symptoms of frank or occult bleeding may be the first tip-offs to a state of abnormal coagulation.

Interventions	Rationales
5. Monitor vital signs for tachycardia or hypotension.	5. Vital sign changes commonly are nonspecific and may be relatively late indicators of bleeding; however, tachycardia is a compensatory response for hypovolemia, whereas hypotension reflects loss of a significant portion of blood volume.
6. Administer protamine sulfate, platelet concentrate, fresh frozen plasma, or whole blood, as ordered.	6. Protamine sulfate treats anticoagulation from inadequate heparin reversal. Platelet concentrate restores missing platelets, whereas fresh frozen plasma replaces both platelets and clotting factors. Whole blood provides platelets, clotting factors, red blood cells, hemoglobin, white blood cells, and volume.
7. Monitor for urine output >1 liter/hour for the first 4 hours, or increasing output thereafter. Monitor serum glucose levels, as ordered. Correlate glucose values with urine output.	7. Mannitol, usually administered during surgery to maintain cardiac output, produces osmotic diuresis. In addition, diuretics may be administered postoperatively to eliminate retained fluid, as explained previously. Hyperglycemia results from stress-induced glycogenolysis and decreased insulin production. Hyperglycemia produces osmotic diuresis. Correlating glucose levels with urine output may identify hyperglycemia as the culprit in excessive diuresis.
8. Additional individualized interventions: ______	8. Rationales: ______

Target outcome criteria

Within 3 hours after surgery, the patient will manifest chest tube drainage <200 ml/hour and declining.

Within 24 hours after surgery, the patient will:
- display minimal drainage from incisions
- have vital signs within normal limits
- show Hgb, HCT, PT, PTT, and platelet levels returning to normal
- experience no signs or symptoms of excessive bleeding.

Collaborative problem: *Potential hypoxemia related to alveolar collapse, increased pulmonary shunt, increased secretions, and capillary leak*

NURSING PRIORITY: Maintain oxygenation and ventilation.

Interventions	Rationales
1. Monitor pulmonary status and conscientiously provide standard postoperative care to prevent pulmonary complications. See "Postoperative Considerations" appendix, page 323, for details.	1. Many factors place the cardiac surgical patient at risk for impaired gas exchange. Lung collapse during CPB results in atelectasis. Absent alveolar expansion during CPB lessens surfactant production, making lungs more difficult to expand postoperatively. Hemodilution promotes interstitial fluid accumulation. CPB also activates complement and kinin systems, creating a capillary leak syndrome. Microcirculatory clotting increases pulmonary shunt. Anesthesia irritates the airways, increasing production of secretions, and depressed ciliary action impairs secretion removal. Postoperatively, lingering anesthetic effects and narcotics cause respiratory depression, whereas pain and splinting lessen lung expansion. These factors all make close observation of pulmonary status and aggressive pulmonary hygiene important postoperatively. The "Postoperative Considerations" appendix details the nursing measures used to achieve these goals.

(continued)

Interventions	Rationales
2. Provide care according to the "Mechanical Ventilation" care plan, page 108.	2. The cardiac surgical patient is usually mechanically ventilated for several hours postoperatively to re-expand collapsed alveoli and lessen cardiopulmonary work load. The "Mechanical Ventilation" care plan details appropriate nursing care.
3. Additional individualized interventions: ____________	3. Rationales: ____________

Target outcome criteria
Within 24 hours after surgery, the patient will:
• have a spontaneous respiratory rate of 12 to 24 breaths/minute
• maintain arterial blood gas levels within normal limits.

Nursing diagnosis: *Potential sensory-perceptual alteration: postcardiotomy delirium related to sensory overload/deprivation from CCU environment, anesthesia, or prolonged CPB*

NURSING PRIORITY: Optimize sensory-perceptual processing.

Interventions	Rationales
1. Implement measures contained in the "Sensory-Perceptual Alteration" care plan, page 60, as appropriate.	1. The "Sensory-Perceptual Alteration" care plan describes measures that are applicable to any CCU patient to reduce or eliminate sensory-perceptual dysfunction.
2. Assess for indicators of postcardiotomy delirium (PCD) every 4 hours while the patient is awake, for the first 5 postoperative days, or more frequently if the patient is disoriented. Use a standardized assessment tool, such as the accompanying checklist (see *Delirium Assessment Checklist* on page 171). If indicators of delirium are present, reassure the patient and family that they usually are transient, continue implementing the measures in the "Sensory-Perceptual Alteration" care plan, and arrange for early transfer to a telemetry unit, if the patient's condition allows.	2. Postcardiotomy delirium is a syndrome that involves disorientation, perceptual illusions, hallucinations, or paranoid ideation. In mild form, it may affect up to 70% of cardiac surgery patients. PCD may result from many factors present in the critical care setting, including anxiety, sensory deprivation and overload, and sleep disruption; personality factors also play a role. In addition, causative factors from cardiac surgery may include prolonged cardiopulmonary bypass, decreased cardiac output, hypotension, and vasoactive medications. The syndrome typically develops on the second to fifth postoperative day, abates within 2 to 3 days, and resolves after transfer from the unit. Measures in the "Sensory-Perceptual Alteration" care plan are helpful, as is early transfer to a less hectic environment.
3. Additional individualized interventions: ____________	3. Rationales: ____________

Target outcome criteria
By the end of the first postoperative week, the patient will return to his normal level of mentation.

DELIRIUM ASSESSMENT CHECKLIST

Disorientation to time*
- What time of day is it? What day of the week is it? 1 pt ___

Disorientation to time last 24 hours*
- Have you lost track of time since yesterday? 1 pt ___

Disorientation to place*
- What is the name of this place? 2 pt ___

Disorientation to place last 24 hours*
- At any time since yesterday, have you not recognized where you were? 2 pt ___

Disorientation to identity*
- What is your name? 3 pt ___

Failure to recognize family (observed or reported by family) 3 pt ___

Perceptual illusions
- Are you seeing or hearing strange things now? 3 pt ___

Perceptual illusions last 24 hours
(Sometimes people who have had heart surgery see or hear things and wonder if they are real.)
- Have you seen things like shadows in the room which seemed strange or unusual? 2 pt ___
- Have you heard things which seemed strange? 2 pt ___
- Have you felt any sensations which seemed unusual? 2 pt ___
- Have you had any unusually vivid dreams? 2 pt ___
- Have objects around you been changing shape or size or seemed to be floating? 2 pt ___

Hallucinations
- Have objects, voices, sounds, or colors appeared out of nowhere? 5 pt ___

Paranoid reaction
- Have you had the feeling that people are making you suffer on purpose? 1 pt ___

*½ point if correct response after prompting.

KEY: pt = point; 0 = no delirium; 1 to 5 points = 1+ delirium; 6 to 13 points = 2+ delirium; 14 to 20 points = 3+ delirium; 21 or more points = 4+ delirium.

From Sadler, P.D.: "Nursing assessment of postcardiotomy delirium." *Heart & Lung* 8:745-50, 1979.

Nursing diagnosis: *Knowledge deficit related to postoperative care*

NURSING PRIORITY: Educate the patient and family about the early postoperative period, as needed.

Interventions	Rationales
1. Refer to the "Knowledge Deficit" care plan, page 45.	1. The "Knowledge Deficit" care plan contains general information on assessing and meeting learning needs.
2. Ascertain whether preoperative teaching was provided. If the patient and family did receive preoperative teaching, reinforce explanations, as necessary. If emergency surgery was performed, provide explanations as the opportunity arises.	2. The elective cardiac surgery patient and his family usually receive extensive preoperative teaching. However, anxiety may limit retention of information, and for the patient, pain and medications affecting consciousness further limit recall. The emergency cardiac surgery patient and his family may have received only minimal preoperative preparation, so teaching should be done as learning opportunities occur.
3. Encourage questions.	3. Questions provide an opportunity for dealing with initial concerns, clarifying misconceptions, and filling in gaps in knowledge.
4. Begin discharge planning. Evaluate needs for discharge teaching. Explain to the family that detailed discharge education will be done after CCU transfer. Document and communicate needs to staff on surgical floor when the patient is transferred from the unit.	4. Discharge planning is most effective when awareness of its importance pervades all phases of hospitalization. Detailed discharge education is most appropriate after the patient has achieved physiologic stability. Early identification of needs sets the stage for later teaching, whereas documentation and communication enhance continuity of care.
5. Additional individualized interventions: ___	5. Rationales: ___

Target outcome criteria
Throughout the unit stay, the patient (after extubation) and family will verbalize questions and concerns.

Transfer planning

NURSING TRANSFER CRITERIA

Upon transfer, documentation shows evidence of:
- blood pressure within normal limits for 12 hours without I.V. pharmacologic agents
- normal sinus rhythm or acceptable variant for 12 hours without I.V. antiarrhythmic drugs
- CI, SVR, and other hemodynamic values within desired limits
- removal of pulmonary artery catheter, arterial line, and chest tubes
- spontaneous ventilation within normal limits for at least 12 hours
- arterial blood gas, Hgb, HCT, and electrolyte levels and coagulation panel within normal limits.

PATIENT-FAMILY TEACHING CHECKLIST

Document evidence that patient and family demonstrate understanding of:
__ surgical procedure
__ anticipated postoperative course
__ rationale for interventions
__ common emotional reactions
__ discharge planning.

DOCUMENTATION CHECKLIST

Using outcome criteria as a guide, document:
__ clinical status on admission
__ significant changes in status
__ pertinent diagnostic test findings
__ CI, SVR, and other hemodynamic parameters
__ diuretic, inotropic, or vasodilator administration
__ routine postoperative care
__ emotional response
__ fluid and electrolyte status
__ pulmonary care
__ complications, if any, and related interventions
__ patient-family teaching
__ transfer planning.

ASSOCIATED CARE PLANS

Acute Heart Failure
Acute Pain
Grieving and Dying
Impaired Physical Mobility
Ineffective Coping
Knowledge Deficit
Mechanical Ventilation
Sensory-Perceptual Alteration
Shock

REFERENCES

Guzzetta, C., and Dossey, B. *Cardiovascular Nursing: Bodymind Tapestry.* St. Louis: C.V. Mosby Co., 1984.

Sadler, D. *Nursing for Cardiovascular Health.* Norwalk, Conn.: Appleton-Century-Crofts, 1984.

Shinn, J. "Cardiopulmonary Bypass," in *Nursing the Critically Ill Adult,* 3rd ed. Edited by Holloway, N. Menlo Park, Calif.: Addison-Wesley Publishing Co., 1988.

Young, L. "Coronary Artery Bypass Surgery: Commonplace Yet Complicated," *Critical Care Nurse* 1(6):24-25, 1981.

Shock

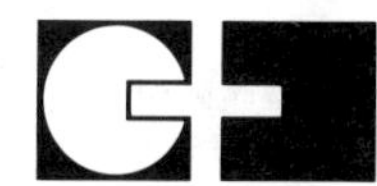

DRG information

DRG 127 Heart Failure and Shock.
Mean LOS = 6.2 days
Principal diagnoses include:
- benign, malignant, or unspecified hypertensive heart disease with congestive heart failure
- heart failure
- congestive heart failure
- shock without trauma.

Introduction

DEFINITION AND TIME FOCUS

Shock is a complex, life-threatening process of hemodynamic and metabolic derangements that cause impaired tissue perfusion. Shock is usually classified into hypovolemic, cardiogenic, and vasogenic types, according to its cause: in hypovolemic shock, decreased blood volume; in cardiogenic shock, impaired cardiac pumping; and in vasogenic shock, excessive expansion of the vascular bed.

No matter what the initiating mechanism, however, all types of shock share a final common pathway: microcirculatory dysfunction and altered cellular metabolism. Shock's systemic effects are mediated by sympathetic stimulation, which causes constriction of precapillary sphincters and venules. The resulting low capillary pressure promotes an interstitial-to-intravascular fluid shift that temporarily compensates for diminished circulating blood volume and maintains capillary flow. As shock progresses, however, this powerful compensatory mechanism fails. Decompensation results in capillary hypoxemia and acidosis, which promote sphincter relaxation, allowing capillary pressure to rise. Increased capillary permeability permits fluid to leak into the tissues, and the resulting decreased circulating blood volume increases hypoxemia and acidosis, creating a vicious circle that ultimately causes irreparable damage.

On a cellular level, shock disrupts vital processes. Delicate sodium-potassium transport mechanisms are paralyzed, allowing sodium to accumulate inside the cell and produce swelling. Mitochondrial depression impairs energy production; oxygen deprivation causes cells to switch from aerobic to anaerobic metabolism. Anaerobic metabolism, an inefficient energy-generating process, also depletes glucose stores and produces lactic acid, creating metabolic acidosis. As cells die, lysosomal destruction causes release of proteases and other enzymes. These enzymes wreak havoc on surrounding cells' integrity and trigger release of vasoactive substances, including myocardial depressant factor, that cause myocardial depression and severe vasodilation, further accelerating the vicious circle.

This clinical plan focuses on the patient admitted to the critical care unit with any of the three major types of shock.

ETIOLOGY AND PRECIPITATING FACTORS

- fluid volume loss, as in hemorrhage, severe dehydration, excessive diuresis, burns, surgical or accidental trauma, diabetes mellitus, or diabetes insipidus
- cardiac pump failure, as in acute myocardial infarction, congestive heart failure, massive pulmonary embolism, acute cardiac tamponade, papillary muscle rupture, valvular insufficiency, or ventricular septal defect
- vasomotor tone loss, as in spinal cord injury, or release of vasodilating substances, as in anaphylaxis or sepsis

Focused assessment guidelines

NURSING HISTORY (Functional health pattern findings)

Health perception–health management pattern

- may have a history of diabetes mellitus, pancreatitis, hypertension, myocardial infarction (MI), congestive heart failure (CHF), or other factor affecting fluid balance or cardiovascular function
- may have undergone a recent invasive procedure, especially abdominal or genitourinary surgery
- may report recent trauma (particularly to the chest, abdomen, or spinal cord) or burns
- may report exposure to various allergens, including food, drugs, or venom from insect bite or sting
- may have recently received blood transfusion or undergone a diagnostic procedure using contrast media
- may have compromised immune system

Nutritional-metabolic pattern

- may describe intense thirst

Elimination pattern

- may describe increased urination or severe diarrhea (early) or oliguria (late)

Activity-exercise pattern

- typically complains of weakness and fatigue

Cognitive-perceptual pattern

- commonly shows reduced alertness or restlessness or anxiety

PHYSICAL FINDINGS

Cardiovascular

- orthostatic hypotension in early hypovolemic shock
- supine hypotension in late hypovolemic and other types of shock
- tachycardia
- dysrhythmias
- decreased or thready peripheral pulses
- capillary filling time >3 seconds
- neck-vein distention (in cardiogenic shock)

Pulmonary

- tachypnea
- dyspnea (in cardiogenic shock)
- crackles (in cardiogenic shock)

Neurologic

- altered level of consciousness (LOC), ranging from confusion, irritability, or restlessness (early) to coma (late)

Integumentary

- altered skin temperature, ranging from increased warmth in early septic shock to coolness in early hypovolemic shock and to coldness in late septic and hypovolemic shock
- pallor
- mottling
- cyanosis

Gastrointestinal

- pale or cyanotic oral mucous membranes

Renal

- polyuria in early septic shock
- oliguria or anuria in late septic shock and in other types of shock

DIAGNOSTIC STUDIES

- complete blood count (CBC)—may vary, depending on the shock type and stage. Typically, hemoglobin level decreases in hemorrhagic hypovolemic shock, hematocrit increases in early hemorrhagic shock and decreases later; red blood cell count decreases in hemorrhagic shock; white blood cell count increases in septic shock.
- blood glucose level—elevated, reflecting stress-induced sympathetic stimulation.
- blood urea nitrogen (BUN) and creatinine levels—elevated, reflecting decreased renal perfusion.
- serum electrolyte levels—may vary, depending on the underlying problem and shock stage. Commonly, hypernatremia reflects increased sodium retention by the kidneys in response to volume losses; hypokalemia reflects urinary potassium losses in exchange for sodium; and hyperkalemia reflects acidosis, decreased glomerular filtration, and cell necrosis.
- arterial blood gas (ABG) levels—reveal increased pH level and decreased $PaCO_2$ in early shock, reflecting respiratory alkalosis caused by hyperventilation, or decreased pH level, increased $PaCO_2$, and decreased bicarbonate level in late shock, reflecting respiratory acidosis caused by hypoventilation and metabolic acidosis caused by anaerobic metabolism.
- cardiac enzymes—reveal elevated total creatine phosphokinase (CPK) level, CPK cardiac fraction (CPK_2), and lactic dehydrogenase isoenzyme (LDH_1) when patient has cardiac damage.
- blood cultures—may be positive in septic shock.
- clotting profile—may reveal coagulopathy, shown by decreased platelet level, decreased fibrinogen level, and increased fibrin split products in septic shock.
- serum osmolality—may increase, reflecting fluid loss.
- urine osmolality or specific gravity—increase, reflecting water retention.
- 12-lead EKG—may reveal dysrhythmias or changes reflecting myocardial ischemia, MI, or electrolyte imbalances.
- chest X-ray—may reveal enlarged cardiac shadow in CHF, pneumothorax, or hemothorax.

POTENTIAL COMPLICATIONS

- renal failure
- adult respiratory distress syndrome
- disseminated intravascular coagulation
- heart failure
- liver failure
- acute MI
- irreversible brain damage

Collaborative problem: *Potential hypovolemic shock related to blood loss, diuresis, dehydration, or third-space fluid shift*

NURSING PRIORITY: Restore fluid volume.

Interventions	Rationales
1. Observe for signs and symptoms of fluid loss:	1. Signs and symptoms correlate with the approximate percentage of volume loss.
• minimal volume loss: Slight tachycardia; normal supine blood pressure; positive postural vital signs (systolic blood pressure decrease >10 mm Hg or pulse increase >20 beats/minute); capillary refill time >3 seconds; urine output >30 ml/hour; cool, pale skin of arms and legs; and anxious mental status	• Powerful compensatory mechanisms produce these signs, which correlate with blood volume loss between 10% and 15%. Medullary vasomotor center stimulation via the baroreceptor reflex causes tachycardia and vasoconstriction. Also, release of antidiuretic hormone (ADH) and aldosterone cause renal retention of sodium and water. All of these mechanisms help to maintain blood volume and normal supine blood pressure. However, postural vital signs are positive because homeostatic mechanisms cannot compensate for the added stress of a position change. Prolonged capillary refill time and slight oliguria reflect decreased circulating volume. Cool, pale skin with normal mental status reflects shunting of blood away from the periphery to preserve function of core organs (brain and heart).
• moderate volume loss: Rapid, thready pulse; supine hypotension; cool truncal skin; urine output 10 to 30 ml/hour; severe thirst; and restlessness, confusion, or irritability	• These signs correlate with a volume loss of approximately 25%. As circulating blood volume drops to this level, compensatory mechanisms are no longer sufficient and decompensation occurs. Oliguria reflects decreased renal perfusion, whereas mental changes indicate decreased cerebral perfusion.
• severe volume loss: Marked tachycardia and hypotension; weak or absent peripheral pulses; cold, mottled, or cyanotic skin; urine output <10 ml/hour; and unconsciousness.	• These signs reflect a volume loss of at least 40% and severely decreased vital organ perfusion.
2. If the patient has active external bleeding (for example, from an arm laceration), apply direct, continuous pressure and elevate the area, if possible.	2. Direct pressure to bleeding sites provides mechanical control of hemorrhage and aids in promoting clot formation by obstructing flow.
3. Elevate the patient's legs above heart level, unless he has active bleeding from the head and neck or suspected increased intracranial pressure or cardiogenic shock.	3. Elevation promotes venous drainage from the legs and increases circulating blood volume as much as 800 ml. This measure will exacerbate the conditions indicated, however.
4. Obtain initial and serial diagnostic tests, including CBC, blood type and cross matching, serum electrolyte levels, ABG levels, urinalysis, 12-lead EKG, and chest X-ray.	4. Serial data provide objective evidence of the disorder's severity and the effectiveness of interventions.
5. Insert and maintain the following, as ordered:	5. These invasive measures will combat shock.
• two or more large-bore I.V. lines	• Large-bore I.V. lines allow rapid infusion of large fluid volumes.
• urinary catheter	• The catheter facilitates monitoring of urine output, the most easily assessed indicator of renal perfusion.
• central venous pressure (CVP) catheter.	• CVP measurements can be used to guide fluid volume replacement and may be ordered for patients with lesser degrees of shock. For patients with severe shock or undetermined shock type, a pulmonary artery (PA) catheter is preferred because it allows measurement of pulmonary capillary wedge pressure (PCWP), which reflects left ventricular filling pressures more accurately than CVP does.

(continued)

FLUID CHALLENGE ALGORITHM

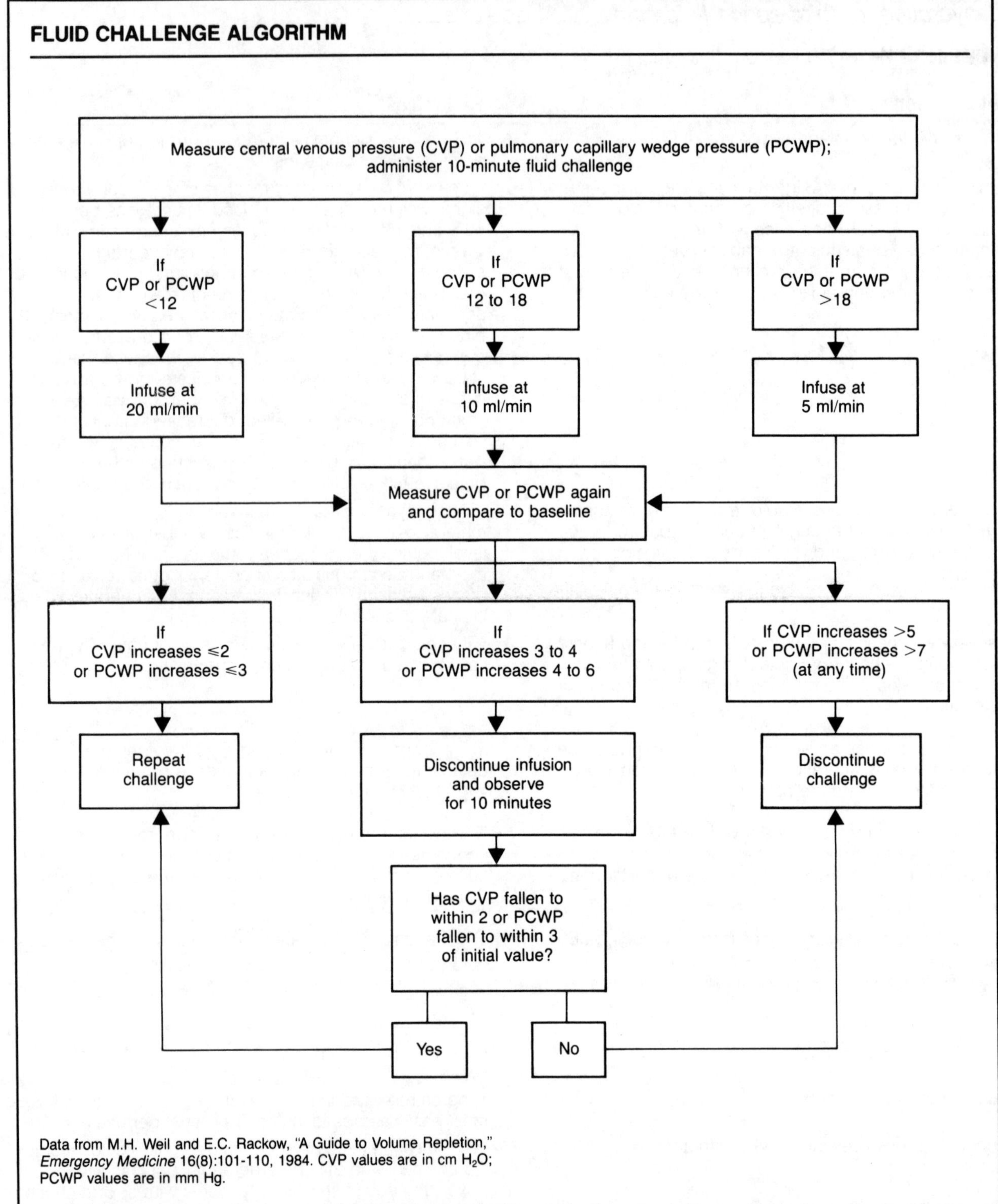

Data from M.H. Weil and E.C. Rackow, "A Guide to Volume Repletion," *Emergency Medicine* 16(8):101-110, 1984. CVP values are in cm H_2O; PCWP values are in mm Hg.

Interventions

6. Monitor urine output and CVP every 15 minutes to 1 hour. Determine the frequency of measurement according to the depth of shock and rapidity of its progression.

Rationales

6. These measurements help determine the degree of shock and evaluate the effectiveness of interventions.

7. Administer a fluid challenge, if ordered. See *Fluid Challenge Algorithm* for details.

7. A fluid challenge involves administration of a bolus of fluid over a limited period. It allows assessment of hemodynamic response to rapid volume administration, which proves helpful in determining whether shock is hypovolemic or cardiogenic.

8. Administer crystalloid or colloid I.V. solutions, as ordered. Refer to *Guide to Parenteral Fluids,* pages 178 to 183, for details.

8. Various I.V. solutions may be used; their advantages and drawbacks remain controversial. The table identifies common solutions, including their indications and special considerations. Colloids—solutions containing protein— help expand intravascular volume via their osmotic pull; however, proteins may leak into the interstitial space, causing such complications as pulmonary edema. Crystalloid solutions—solutions containing salt, sugar, or both—do not cause protein leakage but require relatively large volumes because they leave the vascular space quickly.

9. Monitor arterial blood pressure and mean arterial pressure (MAP) by arterial line or sphygmomanometer.

9. Arterial pressure measurements provide objective data that help gauge the adequacy of cardiac output and the amount of peripheral vascular resistance. MAP reflects the average pressure at which organs are perfused.

• Assist with insertion of an arterial line, if ordered. Monitor blood pressure continuously and measure MAP electronically.

• Direct blood pressure measurement is preferred because it provides more accurate data than sphygmomanometric measurement.

• If an arterial line is not in place, measure cuff blood pressure every 5 to 15 minutes until stable, then every hour. Calculate MAP by adding one third of pulse pressure to diastolic pressure, or by using this formula:

$$\frac{SP + (DP \times 2)}{3}$$

where SP equals systolic pressure and DP equals diastolic pressure.

• Sphygmomanometric blood pressure measurement and arithmetic MAP calculation, though less desirable than intra-arterial measurement, provide valuable data. MAP is closer to diastolic blood pressure than to systolic blood pressure because diastole is about twice as long as systole in the cardiac cycle.

• Maintain MAP within the desired range—usually at least 70 mm Hg. Consult with the doctor about the appropriate range for the patient.

• Maintaining MAP within the desired range provides for adequate organ perfusion. In most cases, MAP must be maintained above 70 mm Hg in a previously normotensive patient. A higher MAP is appropriate for the patient with chronic hypertension. An MAP that's too low promotes ischemia; an MAP that's too high contributes to such complications as cerebral and pulmonary edema.

10. During all fluid administration, monitor the trend of hemodynamic measurements and urine output. Observe for signs of fluid overload, such as crackles, neck-vein distention, or a third heart sound (S_3).

10. Because the shock patient is hemodynamically unstable and has compromised compensatory mechanisms, volume administration may cause rapid progression from fluid depletion to fluid overload. If not detected promptly, fluid overload may precipitate pulmonary edema, CHF, or cerebral edema.

(continued on page 184)

GUIDE TO PARENTERAL FLUIDS[1]

Type	Description	Composition	Uses and indications
BLOOD AND BLOOD PRODUCTS			
Whole blood	500-ml unit of complete blood	Red blood cells, leukocytes, plasma, platelets, and clotting factors[2]	• To replace blood volume and maintain hemoglobin (Hgb) at 12 to 14 g/dl
Red blood cells (packed, concentrated)	—	—	• To increase the hematocrit to a minimum level of 30% • To correct red blood cell deficiency and improve the oxygen-carrying capacity of the blood • Used in anemia and for modest blood loss (when hematocrit is below 25% or 30%)
fresh	300-ml unit of whole blood minus 80% of plasma (hematocrit 70%)	Red blood cells, 20% plasma, and some leukocytes and platelets	
frozen (also called leukocyte-poor)	200- to 250-ml unit with 85% to 90% of red blood cell mass contained in one unit of whole blood	Red blood cells, no plasma, and almost no leukocytes or platelets	
Human plasma (fresh, frozen, or dried)	200-ml unit of uncoagulated, unconcentrated plasma (separated from one unit of whole blood)	Plasma, all plasma proteins, including albumin, and clotting factors (no red cells, white cells, or platelets)	• To restore plasma volume in hypovolemic shock without increasing the hematocrit • To restore clotting factors (except platelets)
Platelets	Platelet sediment from platelet-rich plasma, resuspended in 30 to 50 ml of plasma	Platelets, lymphocytes, and some plasma	• To control bleeding caused by thrombocytopenia • To maintain normal blood coagulability
Plasma protein fraction (e.g., Plasmanate and Plasma-Plex)	250- and 500-ml units of a 5% solution of human plasma proteins in normal saline	Albumin, 44 g/liter; alpha and beta globulins, 6 g/liter; sodium, 130 to 160 mEq/liter; potassium, 2 mEq/liter; osmolality, 290 mOsm/liter; pH, 6.7 to 7.3	• To expand plasma volume in hypovolemic shock (while crossmatching is being completed) • To increase the serum colloid osmotic pressure

[1] From Rice, V. "Shock Management, Part I. Fluid Volume Replacement," *Critical Care Nurse* 4(6):71-73, November/December 1984, with permission.

[2] The concentration and state of preservation of clotting factors in whole blood depends on the duration of storage and other variables.

Advantages	Disadvantages	Special considerations
• Provides intravascular volume • Increases the oxygen-carrying capacity of the blood	• Possibility of limited supply • Potential associated risks of hepatitis and allergic reactions • Delayed administration because of necessary typing and crossmatching • Possibility of type and crossmatch errors	• Whole blood should be stored at 0 to 10° C., but warmed at least 20 to 30 minutes before administration. (Never infuse cold blood.) • Use *fresh* whole blood whenever possible to avoid adverse metabolic changes related to stored blood.
• Concentrated form helps to prevent excess fluid administration in patients with cardiogenic shock (increases the oxygen-carrying capacity with less volume loading) • Associated with fewer risks of metabolic complications when compared to stored whole blood (decreased amount of transfused antibodies and electrolytes) • Provides economical use of blood as a resource; frees other blood components, such as platelets and clotting factors, to be concentrated and stored	• Slow infusion rate because of increased viscosity • Decreased content of plasma proteins and coagulation factors when compared to whole blood • Inadequate (alone) for volume replacement and correction of hypovolemia • Altered blood clotting with administration of more than 20 units; for every four units of red blood cells over 20, one unit of fresh frozen plasma should be administered to replenish clotting factors • High cost of frozen (thawed) red blood cells	• Administer via Y-connector tubing with normal saline to increase infusion flow rate. • Washed red blood cells (resuspended in saline) can be given in shock to decrease red cell adhesiveness. (Washing decreases the cell's fibrinogen coating.)
• Effective for rapid volume replacement • Contains clotting factors	• Expensive • Deficient of red blood cells	• Human plasma carries the risk of viral hepatitis and allergic reactions. • Administer from frozen plasma promptly after thawing to prevent deterioration of clotting Factors V and VIII.
—	• Deficient of other coagulation factors	—
• Can be used interchangeably with 5% human serum albumin • Osmotically equivalent to plasma • Associated with low risk of hepatitis	• Expensive • Deficient of clotting factors • Associated with larger number of side effects, such as hypotension and hypersensitivity, than those reported with 5% albumin (from the presence of globulins) • Hypotension induced by rapid intravenous administration (>10 ml/minute)	• Plasma protein fraction is prepared from pooled plasma heated to 60° C. for 10 hours. This procedure reduces the risk of transmission of hepatitis viruses. • Rapid administration of large dosages can alter blood coagulation. • This solution should be used cautiously in patients with congestive heart failure (because of added fluid and rapid plasma volume expansion) and in patients with renal failure (because of added proteins).

(continued)

GUIDE TO PARENTERAL FLUIDS *(continued)*

Type	Description	Composition	Uses and indications
BLOOD AND BLOOD PRODUCTS *(continued)*			
Albumin	Aqueous fraction of pooled plasma prepared from whole blood in buffered normal saline	—	• To increase the plasma colloid osmotic pressure • To rapidly expand the plasma volume
5%	250- and 500-ml units	Albumin, 50 g/liter; sodium, 130 to 160 mEq/liter; potassium, 1 mEq/liter; osmolality, 300 mOsm/liter; colloid osmotic pressure, 20 mm Hg; pH, 6.4 to 7.4	
25% (salt-poor)[4]	25-, 50-, and 100-ml units	Albumin, 240 g/liter; globulins, 10 g/liter; sodium, 130 to 160 mEq/liter; osmolality, 1,500 mOsm/liter; pH, 5.4 to 7.4	
PHARMACEUTICAL PLASMA EXPANDERS			
Dextran	Biosynthesized, water-soluble, large polysaccharide polymer of glucose	—	• To rapidly expand plasma volume
Low molecular weight dextran (LMWD) (Dextran 40, Gentran 40, and Rheomacrodex)	500-ml unit of solution contining 10% dextran in either normal saline or 5% dextrose in water	Glucose polysaccharides with average molecular weight of 40,000	
High molecular weight dextran (HMWD) (Dextran 70, Gentran 70-75, and Macrodex)	500-ml unit of solution which contains 6% dextran in either normal saline or dextrose 5% in water	Glucose polysaccharides with average molecular weight of 70,000	
Hetastarch (Hespan)	500-ml unit of 6% solution containing a synthetic polymer of hydroxyethyl starch in normal saline	• Globular and branched-chain hydroxyethyl starch prepared from amylopectin • Average molecular weight, 69,000 to 70,000; sodium, 154 mEq/liter; chloride, 154 mEq/liter; osmolality, 310 mOsm/liter; colloid osmotic pressure, 30 to 35 mm Hg	• To expand plasma volume

[3] Ross, A.D., and Angaran, D.M. "Colloids vs. Crystalloids—A Continuing Controversy," *Drug Intelligence and Clinical Pharmacy* 18(3):202-212, 1984.

[4] The term salt-poor designates the 25% albumin concentration and is a carryover from the days when acetyltryptophan replaced a 1.9% salt solution to increase the thermal stability of the product. The term salt-poor is erroneous because both concentrations of albumin contain sodium carbonate or sodium bicarbonate to adjust the pH and sodium caprylate and sodium acetyltryptophan as stabilizers.

[5] Collins, J.A., et al. "Massive Transfusion in Surgery and Trauma," *Progress in Clinical and Biological Research* 108:5-29, 1982.

[6] Rackow, E.C., et al. "Fluid Resuscitation in Circulatory Shock: A Comparison of the Cardiorespiratory Effects of Albumin, Hetastarch, and Saline Solutions in Patients with Hypovolemic and Septic Shock," *Critical Care Medicine* 11(11):839-850, 1983.

[7] Sjogren, E.R. "Hespan (Hetastarch)," *Critical Care Nurse* 3(4):38-40, 1983.

Advantages	Disadvantages	Special considerations
• Rare allergic reactions (<0.011% in all albumin solutions combined)[3] • Rare transmission of hepatitis virus because of heating process (transmission only occurs secondary to accidents in its preparation)	• Potential leakage from capillaries in shock states associated with increased capillary permeability • Possible precipitation of congestive heart failure following rapid infusion in patients with circulatory overload and compromised cardiovascular function	• Albumin does not contain preservatives, so each opened bottle should be used at once. • The administration rate of 5% albumin should not exceed 2 to 4 ml/minute. • The administration rate of 25% albumin should not exceed 1 ml/minute. • Use of 25% albumin is reserved for patients with pulmonary or peripheral edema and hypoproteinemia. Administer with a diuretic to ensure diuresis.
• LMWD and HMWD: associated with low incidence of anaphylactic reactions (<0.01%)[5] • LMWD and HMWD: less expensive than protein solutions • LMWD: associated with fewer allergic reactions than HMWD • LMWD: facilitates blood flow by decreasing red blood cell adhesiveness • HMWD: leaks from the capillaries less readily than LMWD; can effectively increase plasma volume for up to 24 hours	• LMWD: 70% excreted unchanged in the urine, so the urine osmolality and specific gravity are altered[3] • LMWD: potential osmotic nephrosis and renal tubular shutdown • LMWD: possible bleeding from raw surfaces caused by decreased platelet adhesiveness; side effects include decreased hemoglobin, hematocrit, fibrinogen, and clotting Factors V, VIII, and IX • HMWD: 50% excreted unchanged in the urine, so the urine osmolality and specific gravity are altered[3] • HMWD: higher incidence of allergic reactions when compared to LMWD • HMWD: increases blood viscosity and platelet adhesiveness	• Avoid the use of dextrans in patients with active hemorrhage, hemorrhagic shock, coagulation disorders, and thrombocytopenia. • Bleeding time can be prolonged when the correct dose of Dextran 70 (1.2 g/kg/day) or Dextran 40 (2 g/kg/day) are exceeded.[3] • Administer dextran in dextrose solutions to patients with sodium restriction. • Dextran administration can interfere with typing and crossmatching of blood when the older (outdated) enzyme method is used.
• Same volume expansion characteristics of albumin but with longer duration of action (up to 36 hours)[3] • Associated with low risk of allergic and anaphylactic reactions (0.085%)[6] • Cost of hetastarch is about half that of plasma protein fraction and albumin • Nonantigenic • No danger of hepatitis transmission	• Potential dilution of plasma proteins and decreased plasma colloid osmotic pressure • Potential dilution of clotting factors with resultant coagulation changes • Potential circulatory overload in patients with severe congestive heart failure and compromised renal function • Increased serum amylase level (>200 Somogyi units/dl), peaking within 1 hour of I.V. administration of hetastarch and persisting for 3 to 4 days (from the action of amylase in hetastarch degradation)	• Do not use if the solution is cloudy or deep brown or if it contains crystals. • Monitor clotting studies and platelet counts, observing for prolonged prothrombin and partial thromboplastin times and thrombocytopenia. • The safety and compatibility of additives with hetastarch have not been established; the manufacturer recommends infusing hetastarch through a separate line, when possible, or piggybacking the second drug. • The maximum infusion rate in acute hemorrhagic shock is 20 ml/kg/hour.[7] • Monitor serum albumin; if it falls below 2 g/dl, consider substituting albumin for hetastarch.

(continued)

GUIDE TO PARENTERAL FLUIDS *(continued)*

Type	Description	Composition	Uses and indications
PHARMACEUTICAL PLASMA EXPANDERS *(continued)*			
Mannitol (Osmitrol)	Solution of mannitol in water or normal saline	Mannitol (inert form of sugar mannose)	• To raise intravascular volume • To reduce interstitial and intracellular edema • To promote osmotic diuresis
CRYSTALLOID SOLUTIONS—ISOTONIC			
Normal saline	0.9% sodium chloride in water	Sodium, 154 mEq/liter; chloride, 154 mEq/liter; osmolality, 308 mEq/liter	• To raise plasma volume when red blood cell mass is adequate • To replace body fluid
Lactated Ringer's solution (Hartmann's solution)	0.9% sodium chloride in water with added electrolytes and buffers	Sodium, 130 mEq/liter; potassium, 4 mEq/liter; calcium, 2.7 mEq/liter; chloride, 109 mEq/liter; lactate, 27 mEq/liter; pH, 6.5	• To replace body fluid • To buffer acidosis
Ringer's solution	0.9% sodium chloride in water with added potassium and calcium	Sodium, 147 mEq/liter; potassium, 4 mEq/liter; calcium, 5 mEq/liter; chloride, 156 mEq/liter	• To replace body fluid • To provide additional potassium and calcium
CRYSTALLOID SOLUTIONS—HYPOTONIC			
½ normal saline	0.45% sodium chloride in water	Sodium, 77 mEq/liter; chloride, 77 mEq/liter	• To raise total fluid volume
dextrose 5% in water (D_5W)	dextrose 5%	—	• To raise total fluid volume • To provide calories for energy (200 calories/1,000 ml)

Advantages	Disadvantages	Special considerations
• Reduces intracellular swelling • Increases urine output	• Potential circulatory overload in patients with congestive heart failure, pulmonary congestion, and renal dysfunction	—
• Considered by some to be the single most important salt for maintaining and replacing intracellular fluid • Increases plasma values without altering normal sodium concentration or serum osmolality	• Potential fluid retention and circulatory overload because of sodium content	—
• Lactate is converted to bicarbonate in the liver, which buffers acidosis • Lactate replaces bicarbonate, preventing precipitation of calcium bicarbonate and calcium carbonate • Lactate is more stable than bicarbonate and more compatible with ions present in the solution	• Increased lactic acidosis in shock caused by lactate • Fluid retention and circulatory overload caused by sodium content	• Lactate conversion requires aerobic metabolism, so it should be used cautiously in shock and other hypoperfusion states.
• Does not contain lactate, so can be given to patients with hypoperfusion	• Potential hyperchloremic metabolic acidosis caused by chloride concentration • Potential fluid retention and circulatory overload caused by sodium content	—
—	• Potential interstitial and intracellular edema caused by rapid movement of this fluid from the vascular space • Dilution of plasma proteins and electrolytes	—
• Distributed evenly in every body compartment (acts like free water) • Reverses dehydration • Prevents hyperosmolar state • Maintains adequate renal tubular flow (facilitates water excretion)	• Dilution of plasma proteins and electrolytes caused by rapid metabolism of glucose and resultant free water	—

Interventions

11. Additional individualized interventions: ___________

Rationales

11. Rationales: ___________

Target outcome criteria
Within 48 hours, the patient will:
- maintain arterial pressure within normal limits
- maintain strong peripheral pulses
- maintain capillary refill time <3 seconds
- maintain CVP within normal limits
- show no signs of fluid overload
- have warm, dry skin
- return to previous LOC—ideally, alert and oriented.

Collaborative problem: *Potential cardiogenic shock related to decreased myocardial contractility, dysrhythmias, or excessive vasoconstriction*

NURSING PRIORITY: Optimize cardiac output (CO).

Interventions

1. Observe for signs and symptoms of poor arterial perfusion, such as hypotension, tachycardia, dysrhythmias, oliguria, weak peripheral pulses, or decreased LOC.

Rationales

1. The decreased CO that typifies all shock types except early septic shock results from various factors. In cardiogenic shock (described below), cardiac dysfunction is the primary problem. In other shock types, cardiac dysfunction occurs secondary to ischemia, acidosis, electrolyte imbalances, or release of myocardial depressant factor, triggered by splanchnic bed ischemia.

Decreased CO may cause signs of poor arterial perfusion, sometimes referred to as forward failure, or signs of venous congestion, sometimes referred to as backward failure. Signs and symptoms listed indicate forward failure.

Interventions

2. Observe for signs and symptoms of venous congestion, such as S_3 heart sounds, crackles, neck-vein distention, or liver congestion.

Rationales

2. Signs and symptoms listed indicate backward failure, most commonly seen when decreased CO stems from cardiogenic factors.

Interventions

3. Monitor EKG continuously. Promptly report to the doctor any new or worsening signs of ischemia or infarction, such as T-wave inversion, ST-segment displacement, or abnormal Q waves; or significant dysrhythmias, such as premature ventricular beats or severe sinus bradycardia.

Rationales

3. Decreased CO threatens coronary artery perfusion and myocardial oxygenation.

Interventions

4. Assist with insertion of a thermodilution catheter, if ordered. Measure CO, as ordered, typically every hour until stable and then every 2 to 4 hours. Calculate cardiac index (CI) by dividing CO by the patient's body-surface area, a value obtained from a DuBois body-surface area chart. Monitor pressure trends. Notify the doctor of any abnormal values.

Rationales

4. CO measurement provides an objective indication of the amount of CO, whereas CI value individualizes the amount to a particular patient. The trend of pressures indicates whether cardiac function is improving or deteriorating. Abnormal values require medical evaluation.

Interventions

5. Monitor right arterial pressure (RAP), pulmonary artery pressure (PAP), and PCWP, as ordered, typically every hour and as needed. Correlate values with each other and with the patient's signs and symptoms.

Rationales

5. Hypovolemic shock and cardiogenic shock cause many similar signs and symptoms but produce different characteristic patterns of hemodynamic values. Cardiac pressures are elevated in cardiogenic shock, reflecting pulmonary congestion, but decreased in hypovolemic shock, reflecting low circulating blood volume. Correlation of values with the clinical picture enhances accurate assessment and intervention.

Interventions	Rationales
6. Calculate systemic vascular resistance (SVR) by dividing CO into MAP minus RAP. Monitor trend in readings.	6. SVR refers to resistance of systemic vessels. Although it cannot be measured directly, it can be calculated by the formula given. Normally, SVR changes in the opposite direction of CO (that is, as CO falls, SVR rises). SVR trends provide objective assessment of the degree of compensation for decreased CO and can be used to evaluate efficacy of therapy. SVR values also indicate the amount of afterload (resistance to left ventricular ejection).
7. Construct a ventricular function curve, if used in your unit, by plotting CO against PCWP.	7. These curves help determine the PCWP (representing left ventricular filling pressure) that produces the best CO.
8. Administer I.V. solutions, as ordered—in cardiogenic shock, typically 5% dextrose in water at a minimal rate.	8. Because hypovolemia is not the basic problem in cardiogenic shock, aggressive fluid replacement usually is not necessary. Fluid administration may be ordered to elevate filling pressures to a range that produces optimal CO.
9. Administer I.V. medications to improve CO, as ordered. Refer to the "Acute Heart Failure" care plan, page 140, for details. Typically administered drugs include the following:	9. Various pharmacologic agents can improve CO. The "Acute Heart Failure" care plan gives specific information about their use.
• positive inotropic agents, such as digoxin, dopamine, dobutamine, or amrinone	• Positive inotropic agents increase $beta_1$-adrenergic stimulation of the myocardium to improve its contractility.
• vasodilators, such as sodium nitroprusside and nitroglycerin.	• Vasodilators reduce afterload, thus improving myocardial efficiency and reducing myocardial work load.
10. Assist with insertion of an intra-aortic balloon pump (IABP), if used, and provide appropriate nursing care.	10. Intra-aortic balloon counterpulsation can compensate temporarily for impaired myocardial contractility by increasing CO and improving coronary artery perfusion pressure. Placed in the descending aorta, the balloon pulsates counter to cardiac contraction, inflating during diastole and deflating during systole. Diastolic inflation increases intra-aortic volume and pressure, thus augmenting coronary artery flow and improving myocardial oxygen supply. Systolic deflation creates a space into which blood ejected from the heart can flow, thus reducing afterload, myocardial work load, and myocardial oxygen demand.
• Maintain optimal timing of balloon inflation and deflation.	• Balloon timing proves critical. Optimal timing includes inflation just after aortic valve closure and deflation just before systole.
• Prevent or minimize complications:	• IABP is a complex therapy with numerous potential patient and technical complications.
□ Monitor peripheral pulses and tissue perfusion every hour.	□ Arterial occlusion may result from decreased circulation in the catheterized leg or from balloon displacement.
□ Elevate the head of the bed no more than 20 degrees. Do not flex the catheterized leg. Turn the patient side-to-side every 1 to 2 hours.	□ Proper positioning minimizes the risk of catheter displacement or damage.
□ Administer prophylactic heparinization, if ordered. Maintain balloon quivering during periods when it is not inflating fully.	□ The doctor must carefully weigh the risk of thrombus formation around the catheter against the risk of bleeding from anticoagulation. Blood stasis around the balloon during periods of prolonged deflation may cause thromboembolism.

(continued)

Interventions	Rationales
□ Maintain strict aseptic technique at the balloon insertion site. Administer prophylactic antibiotics, as ordered.	□ The balloon and its line provide direct access to the vascular system and heart. Infection is a grave complication. Aseptic technique and antibiotic prophylaxis decrease the infection risk.
□ Maintain proper balloon function, for example, through periodic purging and refilling. Consult the manufacturer and special training programs for details.	□ Numerous technical complications may occur. Technical expertise to prevent or deal with these requires special training and supervised clinical experience.
11. Additional individualized interventions: ____________	11. Rationales: ____________

Target outcome criteria

Within 72 hours, the patient will:

- display blood pressure and pulse within normal limits
- have PCWP <24 mm Hg
- show CI >2.2 liters/minute/m^2
- manifest capillary refill time <3 seconds.

Collaborative problem: *Potential vasogenic shock related to vasomotor tone loss or release of vasodilating substances*

NURSING PRIORITIES: (a) Expand circulating blood volume and (b) restore vasomotor tone, if possible.

Interventions	Rationales
1. Observe for general signs and symptoms of vasogenic shock, such as hypotension and decreased SVR.	1. In vasogenic shock, vascular bed expansion creates relative hypovolemia. The clinical picture varies, however, depending on the cause. General signs and symptoms result from widespread vasodilation in neurogenic shock and early anaphylactic and septic shock. Arteriolar vasodilation lowers systemic vascular resistance, causing hypotension, whereas venodilation reduces venous return to the heart, usually reducing CO.
2. Observe for additional evidence of specific types of vasogenic shock:	2. Additional signs and symptoms vary with the cause. Treatment differs depending on the underlying problem.
• neurogenic shock: history of spinal cord injury, head injury, or drug overdose; decreased filling pressures; normal or increased CO	• In neurogenic shock, normal sympathetic vasoconstriction stimulation ceases from interrupted spinal cord pathways or vasomotor center depression.
• anaphylactic shock: history of allergen exposure, itching, hives, angioneurotic edema, stridor, or wheezing	• Anaphylactic shock is characterized by release of chemical mediators that produce increased capillary permeability and vasodilation.
• septic shock: history of exposure to infectious agents, reduced disease resistance, or reduced ability to detect or report signs and symptoms of infection, plus signs of early-stage or late-stage septic shock.	• Septic shock results from overwhelming infection, typically from aerobic, gram-negative organisms such as *Escherichia coli*, the *Klebsiella-Enterobacter-Serratia* family, and *Pseudomonas aeruginosa*. As these bacteria die, they release endotoxin, causing such complex effects as immunologic system stimulation and complement cascade activation. Powerful inflammatory chemical mediators are then released from damaged cells, causing massive vasodilation and increased capillary permeability.

Interventions	Rationales
□ Early stage (hyperdynamic, or warm, shock): warm, dry, or flushed skin; tachycardia; decreased filling pressures; decreased SVR; increased CO; confusion; restlessness; hyperventilation; and fever.	□ Warm, dry, flushed skin reflects vasodilation. Sepsis produces profound sympathetic nervous system stimulation, resulting in increased heart rate and contractility. Although filling pressures decrease from vasodilation, increased heart rate and contractility combine with reduced afterload to increase CO. However, despite increased CO, blood pressure remains low from the disparity between vascular bed capacity and the volume available to fill it. Low blood pressure impairs cerebral perfusion, producing intellectual deterioration. Endotoxin release causes hyperventilation via respiratory center stimulation. Fever reflects pyrogen release and endotoxic stimulation of the hypothalamus.
□ Late stage (hypodynamic, or cold, shock): increased SVR and decreased CO; cold, clammy skin; oliguria; pulmonary congestion; generalized edema; and decreased temperature.	□ As septic shock progresses, vasodilation changes to vasoconstriction. Increased capillary permeability causes massive fluid loss into interstitial spaces, creating functional hypovolemia. This massive fluid loss, plus release of myocardial depressant factor from the ischemic splanchnic bed, causes a dramatic CO decrease. Also catecholamine release and prostaglandin release from damaged tissues causes severe vasoconstriction. The clinical picture then resembles that of classic hypovolemic shock, with such signs and symptoms as cold, clammy skin and oliguria. Pulmonary congestion reflects capillary leakage and direct damage to the pulmonary vascular endothelium by endotoxin, whereas generalized edema reflects interstitial fluid accumulation. Decreased temperature, an ominous sign, probably reflects impaired hypothalamic perfusion.
3. Administer I.V. fluids, as ordered, typically isotonic saline solution.	3. I.V. fluid replacement usually must be aggressive; large volumes are necessary to replace intravascular losses. Solutions containing lactate may be avoided in patients with septic shock because of their impaired lactate metabolism.
4. Administer pharmacologic agents, as ordered, typically epinephrine and antihistamines in patients with anaphylactic shock; antibiotics, antipyretics, or naloxone in patients with septic shock; or norepinephrine (Levophed) or phenylephrine (Neo-Synephrine) in patients with decreased SVR.	4. Pharmacologic therapy aims to combat the cause or harmful effects of vasogenic shock. Antihistamines block histamine, a major chemical mediator; antibiotics fight infectious organisms; antipyretics reduce fever. Naloxone may reverse endotoxin-triggered beta-endorphin release, which contributes to hypotension. Norepinephrine and phenylephrine are used for their alpha-adrenergic properties—blood vessel constriction and normalization of SVR.
5. Additional individualized interventions: ______________	5. Rationales: ______________

Target outcome criteria

Within 72 hours, the patient will:
- display blood pressure within normal limits
- have strong arterial pulses
- have SVR between 800 and 1600 and CI >2.2 liters/minute/m^2
- have clear lung sounds.

Collaborative problem: *Hypoxemia related to ventilation-perfusion imbalance and diffusion defect*

NURSING PRIORITY: Maintain ventilation and oxygenation.

Interventions	Rationales
1. Provide standard nursing care related to impaired gas exchange: maintain airway patency; monitor respiratory status; suction as necessary; provide supplemental oxygen, as ordered; assist with intubation and mechanical ventilation, if indicated.	1. Numerous factors may cause ventilation-perfusion imbalance in shock, including atelectasis, microemboli, pulmonary congestion, and impaired capillary perfusion. The general measures listed apply to the care of any critically ill patient. Additional interventions below focus on measures specific to patients with shock.
2. Monitor ABG levels, as ordered—typically, at least every 4 hours.	2. ABG levels show the type and degree of acid-base imbalance. Values vary depending on the shock type and stage. In septic shock, endotoxin initially stimulates the respiratory center, resulting in hyperventilation and respiratory alkalosis. Next, metabolic alkalosis may develop, probably from impaired anaerobic metabolism. Early hypovolemic or cardiogenic shock commonly is characterized by respiratory alkalosis induced by hyperventilation, a compensatory response to hypoxemia. Late shock of all types is characterized by combined metabolic acidosis (from lactic acid production during anaerobic metabolism) and respiratory acidosis (from impaired oxygen diffusion resulting from pulmonary congestion and decreased capillary perfusion).
3. Administer sodium bicarbonate I.V., as ordered.	3. Sodium bicarbonate administration may be necessary to restore acid-base balance in severe acidosis.
4. Additional individualized interventions: ____________	4. Rationales: ____________

Target outcome criteria
Within 48 hours, the patient will:
- maintain patent airway
- have clearing breath sounds bilaterally
- show ABG levels within expected limits.

Nursing diagnosis: *Potential for injury: complications related to ischemia*

NURSING PRIORITY: Prevent or minimize complications.

Interventions	Rationales
1. Prevent paralytic ileus and stress ulcers. Withhold food and fluids; insert a nasogastric tube connected to suction, as ordered; administer cimetidine (Tagamet), ranitidine (Zantac), or antacids, as ordered. Monitor bowel sounds.	1. Paralytic ileus may result from mesenteric ischemia. The resulting gastric distention provokes vomiting, which can lead to chemical pneumonitis if aspiration occurs. Withholding food and fluids prevents introduction of food and fluids that the stomach cannot handle. Nasogastric drainage decompresses the stomach. The medications listed decrease hydrochloric acid secretion and reduce the risk of stress ulcers.

Interventions	Rationales
2. Observe for signs and symptoms of adult respiratory distress syndrome (ARDS), such as tachypnea, progressive dyspnea, increased inspiratory pressure (if the patient's on a ventilator), ABG levels revealing hypoxemia and an increased A-a gradient, bilateral diffuse exudates on chest X-ray, or lung compliance <50 ml/cm H_2O. If you detect these problems, document them and alert the doctor. Implement measures described in the "Adult Respiratory Distress Syndrome" care plan, page 101, as appropriate.	2. Shock ranks as a major risk factor for developing ARDS, because of such factors as decreased perfusion, hypoxemia, increased capillary permeability, and high oxygen levels used in treatment. Septic shock patients have a particularly high risk, because endotoxin directly damages the pulmonary vascular endothelium. The care plan for ARDS comprehensively describes this ominous complication and related care.
3. Observe for signs and symptoms of acute myocardial infarction (AMI), such as severe chest pain, shortness of breath, hypotension, diaphoresis, pained facial expression, elevated cardiac isoenzymes, or EKG showing ST-segment displacement, T-wave inversion, or pathologic Q waves. See the "Acute Myocardial Infarction" care plan, page 150, for more details.	3. Decreased perfusion, catecholamine stimulation, hypoxemia, and increased afterload all may precipitate AMI. The AMI care plan gives details on this complication.
4. Observe for signs and symptoms of heart failure, such as tachycardia, dysrhythmias, S_3 or S_4 heart sounds, neck-vein distention, crackles, dependent edema, or elevated PCWP. See the "Acute Heart Failure" care plan, page 140.	4. Cardiac failure may result from decreased coronary artery perfusion, hypoxemia, acidosis, and numerous other factors present in shock. The "Acute Heart Failure" care plan presents comprehensive information for this development.
5. Observe for signs and symptoms of disseminated intravascular coagulation (DIC), such as blood oozing from multiple sites, repeated bleeding episodes, acral cyanosis, petechiae, ecchymoses, hematomas, prolonged prothrombin time, prolonged partial thromboplastin time, decreased fibrinogen level, decreased platelet count, or elevated fibrin split products level. See the "Disseminated Intravascular Coagulation" care plan, page 253, for details.	5. Shock is a major risk factor for DIC because of such factors as capillary sludging; acidosis; and sepsis, trauma, or other underlying causes. The septic shock patient has a particularly high risk for DIC because sepsis triggers the complement cascade, which in turn provokes accelerated coagulation and fibrinolysis, the key pathophysiologic mechanisms in DIC. The "Disseminated Intravascular Coagulation" care plan describes this devastating development in depth.
6. Observe for signs and symptoms of acute renal failure, such as oliguria or anuria, weight gain, neck-vein distention, crackles, dependent edema, or elevated BUN and serum creatinine levels. As appropriate, implement measures described in the "Acute Renal Failure" care plan, page 227.	6. Constriction of renal blood vessels occurs as an early compensatory mechanism in shock. Although this constriction limits glomerular filtration, thus conserving fluid volume, it does so at a price: impaired perfusion of renal cells, which may result in acute renal failure. The "Acute Renal Failure" care plan describes this complication in detail.
7. Observe for signs and symptoms of liver failure, such as drowsiness, intellectual deterioration, personality changes, septicemia, fever, hyperkinetic circulation, jaundice, hepatomegaly, ascites, easy bruising, increased prothrombin time, elevated serum glutamic-oxaloacetic transaminase level, or increased bilirubin level. See the "Liver Failure" care plan, page 199.	7. Although shock may damage liver parenchymal cells, prompt correction of shock may allow these cells to regenerate. Early detection of signs and symptoms of liver failure may prevent severe damage to this critical organ. The "Liver Failure" care plan presents the pathophysiology of this disorder and related care.
8. Additional individualized interventions: ____________	8. Rationales: ____________

Target outcome criteria

By the time of transfer from the unit, the patient will show no signs of the complications described above.

Nursing diagnosis: *Fear related to threat to life*

NURSING PRIORITY: Provide emotional support to the patient and family.

Interventions	Rationales
1. Implement measures described in the "Ineffective Coping" care plan, page 26, and the "Grieving and Dying" care plan, page 15, as appropriate.	1. Families (and alert patients) are aware that shock poses a life threat, and they react to the possibility of death in various ways. Measures to help them cope with their realistic fear and other emotional responses are described in these two care plans.
2. Additional individualized interventions: ____________	2. Rationales: ____________

Target outcome criteria
By the time of transfer, the patient will:
- meet outcome criteria identified in the "Ineffective Coping" care plan
- meet outcome criteria identified in the "Grieving and Dying" care plan.

Transfer planning

NURSING TRANSFER CRITERIA

Upon transfer, documentation shows evidence of:
- blood pressure within normal limits without I.V. inotrope or vasodilator support
- pulse and respirations within normal limits
- ABG levels within expected limits for recovery stage
- urine output within normal limits
- no evidence of major complications.

PATIENT-FAMILY TEACHING CHECKLIST

Document evidence that patient and family demonstrate understanding of:
__ cause and significance of shock
__ expectations for recovery
__ purpose of monitoring devices
__ rationales for therapeutic interventions.

DOCUMENTATION CHECKLIST

Using outcome criteria as a guide, document:
__ clinical status on admission
__ significant changes in status
__ pertinent diagnostic test findings
__ care for invasive monitoring lines
__ fluid administration
__ inotropes, vasodilators, or other pharmacologic agents
__ intra-aortic balloon pump, if used
__ measures to support ventilation and oxygenation
__ emotional support
__ patient-family teaching
__ transfer planning.

ASSOCIATED CARE PLANS

Acute Heart Failure
Acute Myocardial Infarction
Adult Respiratory Distress Syndrome
Disseminated Intravascular Coagulation
Grieving and Dying
Impaired Physical Mobility
Ineffective Coping
Liver Failure
Major Burns
Mechanical Ventilation
Multiple Trauma
Pulmonary Embolism

REFERENCES

Perry, A., and Potter, P. *Shock: Comprehensive Nursing Management.* St. Louis: C.V. Mosby Co., 1983.
Proctor, R.H. *Clinical Aspects of Endotoxin Shock.* New York: Elsevier Science Publishers, 1986.
Rice, V. "The Clinical Continuum of Septic Shock," *Critical Care Nurse* 4(5):86-109, 1984.
Rice, V. "Shock Management. Part I: Fluid Volume Replacement," *Critical Care Nurse* 4(6):69-82, 1984.
Rice, V. "Shock Management. Part II: Pharmacologic Intervention," *Critical Care Nurse* 5(1):52-57, 1985.
Rock, P., et al. "Efficacy and Safety of Naloxone in Septic Shock," *Critical Care Medicine* 28-33, 1985.
Root, R.K., and Merle, A.S. *Septic Shock.* New York: Churchill Livingstone, 1985.
Weil, M.H., and Rackow, E.C. "A Guide to Volume Repletion," *Emergency Medicine* 16:101-10, 1984.

Gastrointestinal Hemorrhage

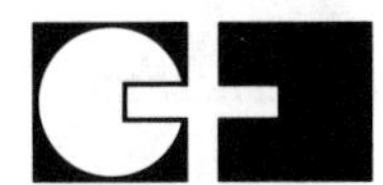

DRG information

DRG 174 Gastrointestinal Hemorrhage. With Complication or Comorbidity (CC).
Mean LOS = 7.1 days
Principal diagnoses include:
- GI hemorrhage—site or etiology unspecified
- hemorrhage of anus or rectum
- acute ulcer (gastric, peptic, duodenal, jejunal, or a combination of sites) with hemorrhage
- esophageal varices with hemorrhage.

DRG 175 Gastrointestinal Hemorrhage. Without CC.
Mean LOS = 5.3 days
Principal diagnoses include selected principal diagnoses listed under DRG 174. The distinction is that patients grouped under DRG 175 have no CC.

Introduction

DEFINITION AND TIME FOCUS

In the critical care setting, acute gastrointestinal (GI) bleeding is most commonly associated with upper GI pathology; although bleeding can occur anywhere in the GI tract, patients with lower GI bleeding are less likely to be admitted to the critical care unit because lower GI bleeding is usually less severe. Bleeding may occur as a direct manifestation of an underlying condition, such as ulcers, invasive tumors, or esophageal varices. (Gastritis or gastric ulcer is estimated to account for up to 80% of all GI bleeding episodes.) Bleeding may also develop as an untoward effect of therapeutically administered medications, such as anti-inflammatory drugs or anticoagulants. Trauma, burns, sepsis, and other conditions may cause stress ulcers, which usually manifest as sudden, severe, and painless bleeding. Regardless of the cause, acute GI bleeding may be life-threatening unless diagnosis and treatment are prompt. Delay in diagnosis is associated with higher mortality and increased complications. This care plan focuses on the critical care patient experiencing an acute episode of upper GI bleeding.

ETIOLOGY AND PRECIPITATING FACTORS

- gastric irritation or altered gastric pH, as with medication use (for example, salicylates, steroids, or other anti-inflammatory drugs), alcohol or caffeine abuse, toxic or allergic reactions, ingestion of corrosive substances, peptic or gastric ulcer, gastritis, and stress reactions
- altered gastric function or circulation, as with tumors, portal hypertension or esophageal varices, or Mallory-Weiss laceration of gastric mucosa
- altered blood coagulation, as with the use of anticoagulants or blood dyscrasias, cancer, shock, sepsis, uremia, and disseminated intravascular coagulation (DIC)

Focused assessment guidelines

NURSING HISTORY (Functional health pattern findings)

Health perception–health management pattern

- commonly gives a history of gastric ulcer or gastritis
- may have history of heavy alcohol intake or cigarette smoking (associated with gastritis and esophageal varices)
- may give a history of long-term steroid, salicylate, or other anti-inflammatory therapy

Nutritional-metabolic pattern

- commonly complains of nausea
- may complain of a "fullness" in the abdomen
- may complain of thirst
- may complain of "heartburn"

Elimination pattern

- may describe dark or tarry stools
- may give history of "coffee-ground" emesis

Activity-exercise pattern

- commonly describes weakness and easy fatigability

Cognitive-perceptual pattern

- if bleeding is related to ulcer disease, may complain of gnawing, aching, or burning abdominal pain, which may be relieved by eating
- if bleeding is related to stress ulcer, may be painless

Coping–stress tolerance pattern

- likely to express extreme fear in reaction to sight of own blood

PHYSICAL FINDINGS

General appearance

- frightened or anxious facial expression

Cardiovascular

- tachycardia
- orthostatic hypotension
- weak, thready peripheral pulse

Gastrointestinal

- melena
- hematemesis (associated with upper GI bleeding)
- "coffee-ground" vomitus (indicates slower upper GI bleeding)

• hematochezia (bright, bloody stools—usually indicates lower GI bleeding but may occur with rapid upper GI hemorrhage)

Pulmonary
• hyperventilation

Neurologic
• restlessness
• decreased alertness (with shock)

Integumentary
• pallor
• diaphoresis

DIAGNOSTIC STUDIES

• blood urea nitrogen (BUN) levels—elevated because of accumulated blood breakdown by-products and overload of renal clearance system. Elevated BUN level, when creatinine level remains normal, indicates blood loss >1 liter.
• complete blood count (CBC)—obtained for baseline; may reflect minimal abnormalities for up to 36 hours if bleeding is slow. Eventually, reduced hemoglobin, hematocrit, and red blood cell count reflect overall blood loss; reticulocyte count may be elevated in response to bleeding.
• blood typing and cross matching—obtained in anticipation of blood replacement; in acute bleeding, type-specific, non–cross-matched blood may be administered as an emergency measure.
• prothrombin time, partial thromboplastin time—obtained for baseline and for evaluation of altered coagulation status as cause of bleeding. Further clotting studies may also be obtained if coagulation defects are suspected.
• gastric aspiration—provides information regarding amount and time of bleeding; results are used to guide further intervention. For example, a small aspiration of material resembling coffee grounds may indicate "old" bleeding that only warrants close observation of the patient; aspiration of fresh bright red blood is evidence of active hemorrhage and demands prompt intervention.
• endoscopic examination—provides fiber-optic visualization of bleeding site and associated pathology; may permit direct coagulation of bleeding sites via endoscope or tissue biopsy.
• abdominal angiography—allows visualization of abdominal vasculature; used to locate bleeding sites and may be used for localized treatment by infusion of vasopressin or injection of clot formation material (embolization).
• computed tomography (CT) scan—may be used to detect tumors or polyps
• barium studies—may be used to identify gastric erosions or tumors as bleeding source if angiography is not available; used as a last resort in patients with active bleeding as barium obscures the field for subsequent endoscopic or angiographic assessment.

POTENTIAL COMPLICATIONS

• shock
• renal failure
• disseminated intravascular coagulopathy
• hepatic encephalopathy
• myocardial ischemia or infarction

Collaborative problem: *Potential hypovolemic shock related to blood loss*

NURSING PRIORITIES: (a) Assess amount of blood loss, (b) restore blood and fluid volume, and (c) help identify the source or cause and provide treatment.

Interventions	Rationales
1. See the "Shock" care plan, page 173.	1. The "Shock" care plan provides detailed interventions for assessment and treatment of the patient in actual or impending shock.
2. Assess the amount of blood loss using the following procedures:	2. Prevention of shock depends on accurate status assessment.
• Maintain accurate intake and output records, including precise measurement and guaiac testing of all vomitus and stools.	• Direct measurement of bloody output is essential to guide replacement therapy. Guaiac testing provides objective assessment for the presence of blood. Careful monitoring of urine output is vital because a drop in hourly urine output (<60 ml/hour) may signal the development of shock.

Interventions	Rationales
• Evaluate orthostatic vital signs every 4 hours, unless the patient is syncopal, frankly hypotensive, or severely tachycardic when supine. Note and report promptly to the doctor a systolic blood pressure decrease of >10 mm Hg or a pulse increase of >20 beats/minute.	• Compensatory neurovascular mechanisms may be able to maintain normal supine blood pressure when blood loss is <500 ml. Moving from a supine to a sitting position adds an orthostatic stress that may unmask hidden hypotension. A pulse increase of 20 to 30 beats/minute correlates with a blood loss of 500 ml, whereas a pulse increase of >30 beats/minute and systolic blood pressure drop of >10 mm Hg may indicate a blood loss of 1,000 ml or more. Although many critically ill patients are too unstable to tolerate orthostatic assessment, it may provide useful data in the stable patient. However, when clear evidence of hypotension already exists, the test may accelerate shock progression.
• Evaluate vital signs, hemodynamic pressures, and EKG findings according to "Monitoring Standards" appendix, page 314, or unit protocol.	• These parameters provide additional data useful in judging the degree of shock present.
• Obtain appropriate laboratory studies, as ordered, including CBC, BUN, and creatinine for baseline and ongoing monitoring.	• Hemoglobin and hematocrit values reflect blood volume status but may show no changes initially. BUN and creatinine levels are of greater diagnostic value. An elevated BUN level in the presence of normal creatinine level indicates a likely blood loss of >1,000 ml.
• Assess the patient frequently for clinical signs of hypovolemia. Note constellations of signs and symptoms, such as those of mild shock (for example, anxiety, perspiration, or weakness); moderate shock (for example, hyperactive bowel sounds, tachycardia, fever, or thirst); or severe shock (for example, pallor, cool and clammy skin, decreased level of consciousness, decreased urine output, and thready pulse).	• Clinical parameters help define stages of blood loss. Signs and symptoms of mild shock (<500 ml blood loss) are nonspecific. Signs of moderate shock (500 to 1,000 ml blood loss) reflect progressive activation of sympathetic nervous system compensatory mechanisms and other homeostatic mechanisms. Signs of severe shock (>1,000 ml blood loss) reflect ischemia of core organ systems.
• Insert and maintain a gastric tube, as ordered, and check drainage for blood.	• Gastric intubation permits removal and accurate measurement of accumulated blood from the stomach. It is also therapeutic because blood in the stomach may stimulate vomiting and excess gastric acid secretion, both of which may precipitate or accelerate bleeding. Finally, blood that passes into the intestines is broken down into ammonia, which may have toxic metabolic effects.
3. Replace blood loss by:	3. Prompt replacement therapy is essential to prevent hypovolemia and hypoxemia related to reduced hemoglobin level.
• establishing and maintaining I.V. access with a large-bore cannula	• A large-bore cannula is necessary for rapid infusion of blood and fluids.
• administering and monitoring the response to transfusion of packed red blood cells, fresh frozen plasma, or other blood components as well as volume expanders, such as plasma protein fraction (Plasmanate), or albumin, as ordered.	• Replacement of blood components and restoration of circulating volume is essential to minimize cell death from hypoxemia. If congestive heart failure is present, packed cells may be administered with minimal additional fluid to avert fluid overload. The hematocrit should increase with each unit of packed cells administered. Persistent bleeding is present if hematocrit does not improve. For other patients, volume expanders may be indicated. Albumin, for example, provides an osmotically induced fluid expansion equal to five times its volume. Blood that has been stored for a period of time may be deficient in some clotting factors, so the administration of fresh frozen plasma or other components may be needed.

(continued)

Interventions	Rationales
4. Initiate measures to stop bleeding, as ordered, such as:	4. As many as 90% of upper GI hemorrhages cease spontaneously, but severe bleeding constitutes a medical or surgical emergency, and prompt corrective treatment is warranted.
• maintaining activity restrictions, which usually includes strict bed rest	• Activity may increase intra-abdominal pressure and accelerate bleeding.
• performing gastric lavage, usually with room temperature normal saline solution, with or without addition of norepinephrine (Levophed) to the solution. If norepinephrine is used, the usual dilution is 2 ampules to 1,000 ml normal saline solution in a continuous irrigation. Question orders for iced lavage.	• Gastric lavage removes accumulated blood and clots and clears the stomach for endoscopic examination. Norepinephrine may be added for its local vasoconstrictive effects. Systemic effects are minimized when norepinephrine is administered in this way because the drug is metabolized in the liver immediately after gastric absorption. Iced lavage, which was traditionally ordered based on the theory that gastric cooling decreased blood flow, has become controversial as a therapeutic measure. Recent studies have actually demonstrated prolonged clotting times in response to iced irrigation.
• administering vasopressin (Pitressin) I.V., unless the patient has a history of coronary artery disease or other vascular problems. The dose range is 0.02 to 0.06 mcg/minute I.V. or through an arterial catheter placed near the bleeding site.	• Vasopressin causes vasoconstriction and contraction of smooth muscle in the GI tract. It also increases reabsorption of water in the renal tubules. However, in a patient with cardiovascular disease, its use may precipitate myocardial ischemia, infarction, or hypertension.
• instilling topical thrombin, via gastric tube. Dilute the drug in normal saline solution at the recommended dilution. Check for fresh bleeding 30 minutes after administration by aspirating stomach contents.	• Thrombin reacts with fibrinogen to produce a fibrin clot. Because of its powerful and immediate clotting effects, thrombin is never injected into blood vessels, where it could result in extensive rapid clotting and death. Usually, 5,000 units of thrombin dissolved in 5 ml of diluent is capable of clotting as much as 1,000 ml of blood in less than 1 minute. Because direct contact with bleeding vessels is necessary for the effective action of thrombin, gastric tube administration may be ineffective, depending on the bleeding site.
• assisting with insertion, monitoring, and maintaining the placement of Sengstaken-Blakemore tube or other compression tubes. Elevate the head of the bed. Suction the oropharynx, nasopharynx, and upper esophagus frequently. Irrigate the tube at least every 2 hours. Maintain proper balloon pressures. Maintain proper positioning by verifying balloon placement by X-ray, as ordered, and maintaining traction on the balloon. Cut and remove the tube immediately if airway compromise occurs.	• Compression balloon tubes, such as the Sengstaken-Blakemore tube, are used to control hemorrhage in patients with esophageal varices. The balloon applies direct pressure against bleeding vessels, while the gastric tube permits continued decompression and aspiration. Elevating the head of the bed helps prevent esophageal reflux and associated irritation. When the tube is in place, the patient is unable to swallow salivary secretions. Also, nasal secretions may be increased because of local irritation from the tube. Irrigation ensures patency of the tube and prevents gastric distention. Excessive pressures may result in perforation, inflammation, or ulceration of the esophagus or gastric mucosal lining, whereas insufficient pressure may be ineffective or contribute to tube displacement. X-ray verification and maintenance of traction help ensure correct positioning. If the tube becomes displaced, it may cause airway obstruction. Cutting the tube deflates the gastric and esophageal balloons and permits immediate removal.
• administering vitamin K_1 (phytonadione [AquaMEPHYTON]) I.M., as ordered	• Patients who have been on I.V. feedings or multiple antibiotics for a prolonged period may develop vitamin K deficiency, because this catalyst for clotting factor production is either obtained through a normal diet or synthesized by intestinal bacteria. Replacement therapy may be necessary to restore normal clotting status.

Interventions	Rationales
• preparing the patient for surgery if bleeding remains uncontrolled for more than 24 hours, requires more than 6 to 8 units of blood, or results in severe hypovolemia, or if the hematocrit does not increase in response to administration of blood products.	• If bleeding does not stop or if the patient fails to respond to replacement therapy, surgery must be done to identify and correct the problem.
5. Administer medications to control gastric acidity, monitoring gastric aspirate pH, and adjusting dosage, as ordered, to maintain a pH >5.0. The following medications are commonly prescribed:	5. Gastric hyperacidity is a primary contributor to ulcer development. A low gastric pH level indicates hyperacidity.
• histamine blockers of H_2 receptors, such as cimetidine (Tagamet) or ranitidine (Zantac), usually I.V. during acute bleeding episodes.	• Cimetidine inhibits the action of histamine, thus raising the gastric pH. However, it must be used cautiously in patients who are receiving anticoagulant therapy because cimetidine can slow warfarin (Coumadin) absorption and further prolong prothrombin time.
• antacids, instilled via gastric tube.	• Antacids cause neutralization of gastric acid, thus removing a source of mucosal irritation and facilitating the healing process. If oral cimetidine is also being administered, antacids should not be given at the same time because they can decrease cimetidine absorption.
6. Prepare the patient and family for and assist with diagnostic procedures, as ordered, such as endoscopic examination, angiography, or other studies.	6. Identification of the site and cause of the bleeding is essential because delay in diagnosis is associated with a higher mortality.
7. Additional individualized interventions: ____________	7. Rationales: ____________

Target outcome criteria

Within 24 hours of detection of bleeding, the patient will:
- exhibit systolic blood pressure >90 mm Hg
- exhibit normal heart rate
- have urine output of at least 60 ml/hour
- show no orthostatic changes in vital signs
- have warm, dry skin
- exhibit gastric pH >5.0.

Nursing diagnosis: *Potential for injury: complications related to undetected bleeding, inadequate organ perfusion, accumulation of toxins, electrolyte imbalance, release of procoagulants, or perforation of ulcer*

NURSING PRIORITY: Prevent or promptly detect and treat complications.

Interventions	Rationales
1. Continue to perform guaiac tests on all gastric contents and stools at least daily, even after the patient's condition has stabilized.	1. As much as 200 ml of blood may be lost daily without detectable clinical signs. Early detection allows prompt treatment.
2. Immediately report and thoroughly investigate any complaint of chest pain, particularly in a patient with preexisting cardiac disease.	2. Blood loss reduces the level of circulating hemoglobin, thus compromising normal delivery of oxygen to tissues. If coronary circulation is already impaired, this reduction may precipitate ischemic changes or myocardial infarction.

(continued)

Interventions	Rationales
3. Monitor parameters of renal and hepatic function, including hourly urine outputs, daily BUN and creatinine levels, and daily weight. Note daily serum electrolyte values, including serum calcium, particularly if the patient has received multiple blood transfusions.	3. Hemorrhage and the resulting hypovolemia may cause renal and hepatic hypoperfusion, eventually leading to renal or liver failure. Portal hypertension, commonly associated with esophageal varices, contributes to elevated blood ammonia levels and can result in hepatic encephalopathy. Hypocalcemia is a common side effect of multiple transfusions because calcium binds with the preservative in stored blood.
4. Observe for bleeding from other sites, such as epistaxis or petechiae. See the "Disseminated Intravascular Coagulation" care plan, page 253.	4. Bleeding from other sites may signal the development of disseminated intravascular coagulation, a grave complication of hemorrhage. The care plan for this disorder contains detailed interventions.
5. Immediately report any complaint of sudden, severe abdominal pain or rigidity, and prepare the patient for surgery if these occur.	5. These signs and symptoms may indicate gastric perforation, which causes peritonitis, sepsis, and shock unless promptly treated. Immediate surgical intervention is warranted to remove gastric contents from the peritoneal cavity.
6. Additional individualized interventions: ____________	6. Rationales: ____________

Target outcome criteria

Throughout the stay in the critical care unit, the patient will:

- exhibit decreasing BUN and normal creatinine values
- display electrolytes within normal limits
- maintain urine output >60 ml/hour
- remain alert and oriented.

Nursing diagnosis: *Fear related to sight of blood and distressing physical symptoms*

NURSING PRIORITY: Reduce the patient's fear.

Interventions	Rationales
1. Provide care promptly, explaining all interventions to the patient in simple terms. Avoid expressing dismay or revulsion at the sight of bleeding; assume a calm, confident, matter-of-fact manner. Acknowledge the patient's fear by saying, for example, "I know it must be pretty scary to see all this blood, but we treat this condition often. We will be replacing your blood by giving you transfusions and extra fluids."	1. The sight of blood is normally extremely threatening to the patient, who justifiably may fear bleeding to death. Anxiety may interfere with the patient's ability to comprehend, but simple explanations about what is happening may help provide reassurance that he is receiving the care needed. Providing recognition of the normalcy of the patient's fear reduces the patient's sense of isolation. Patients often are quite concerned about bloody excreta and losing bowel control. Your calm acceptance may minimize shame related to these losses of bodily control.
2. Encourage verbalization of feelings by using active listening skills. See the "Ineffective Coping" care plan, page 26.	2. Verbalizing feelings helps the patient identify specific fears and begin to mobilize coping strategies. The "Ineffective Coping" care plan details interventions that may be helpful in promoting coping behaviors.
3. Accept expressions of anxiety related to the possibility of death. See the "Grieving and Dying" care plan, page 15.	3. Issues of death are always of acute importance for patients with critical conditions. The "Grieving and Dying" care plan contains specific interventions useful in caring for patients and families confronting issues of mortality.

Interventions

4. Additional individualized interventions: ___________

Rationales

4. Rationales: ___________

> **Target outcome criteria**
> After initial stabilization, the patient will verbalize feelings about his condition, if desired.

Nursing diagnosis: *Knowledge deficit related to potential recurrent bleeding*

NURSING PRIORITY: Teach assessment and preventive measures.

Interventions	Rationales
1. See the "Knowledge Deficit" care plan, page 45.	1. The "Knowledge Deficit" care plan contains detailed interventions related to patient and family teaching.
2. Defer detailed teaching until patient is alert and physiologically stable. Then, as indicated by condition, discuss with the patient:	2. Teaching in the critical care unit may be limited by the patient's condition, but abbreviated teaching may lay the groundwork for more detailed education before discharge.
• precipitating or contributing factors of bleeding episode, for example, alcohol consumption or medication use	• Awareness of contributing factors over which the patient has control may decrease the likelihood of a recurrence.
• signs and symptoms indicating possible recurrence, for example, melena, coffee-ground vomitus, weakness, or dizziness	• Early medical attention if bleeding recurs may avert the need for prolonged hospitalization.
• other causes of dark stools, for example, iron, beets, berries, or greens	• Knowing other causes may avert undue alarm.
• dietary recommendations, as ordered, for example, avoidance of caffeine.	• Careful dietary management may be the primary post-bleeding therapy for some conditions.
3. Additional individualized interventions: ___________	3. Rationales: ___________

> **Target outcome criteria**
> Before transfer, the patient will (as condition allows):
> • list any precipitating or contributing factors identified
> • describe signs and symptoms of possible recurrence of bleeding
> • verbalize understanding of dietary recommendations, if any.

Transfer planning

NURSING TRANSFER CRITERIA

Upon transfer, documentation shows evidence of:

- stable vital signs within normal limits for the patient
- urine output of at least 60 ml/hour
- decreasing BUN values
- normal serum electrolytes
- normal skin perfusion
- gastric pH of 5.0 or greater
- negative guaiac test of stools or vomitus
- level of consciousness stable for >12 hours
- balanced intake and output.

PATIENT-FAMILY TEACHING CHECKLIST

Document evidence that patient and family demonstrate understanding of:

__ cause and site of bleeding
__ precipitating or contributing factors
__ signs and symptoms indicating possible recurrence of bleeding
__ dietary recommendations, if any.

DOCUMENTATION CHECKLIST

Using outcome criteria as a guide, document:

__ clinical status on admission
__ significant changes in status
__ pertinent diagnostic test findings
__ bleeding episodes
__ fluid and blood replacement measures
__ intake and output
__ emotional response
__ pharmacologic interventions
__ procedures to stop bleeding
__ patient-family teaching
__ transfer planning.

ASSOCIATED CARE PLANS

Acute Renal Failure
Disseminated Intravascular Coagulation
Impaired Physical Mobility
Ineffective Coping
Knowledge Deficit
Liver Failure
Nutritional Deficit
Pancreatitis
Shock

REFERENCES

Amato, E. "A Nursing Reference: Gastrointestinal Tubes and Drains," Parts I and II, *Critical Care Nurse* 2(6):50-57, November/December 1982, and 3(1):46-48, January/February 1983.

Briones, T. "Nursing Care Plan for the Patient with Acute Gastrointestinal (GI) Bleeding," *Critical Care Nurse* 4(2):22-24, March/April 1984.

Broadwell, D. "Gastrointestinal System," in *Clinical Nursing*. Edited by Thompson, J., et al. St. Louis: C.V. Mosby Co., 1986.

Busby, H., and Seiffert, W. "Acute Gastrointestinal Bleeding," in *Critical Care Nursing: A Holistic Approach*, 4th ed. Edited by Hudak, C., Gallo, B., and Lohr, T. Philadelphia: J.B. Lippincott Co., 1986.

Dusek, J. "Iced Gastric Lavage Slows Bleeding in Gastric Hemorrhage—Fact or Myth?" *Critical Care Nurse* 4(4):8, July/August 1984.

Holloway, N., and Tueller, B. "Nutrition," in *Nursing the Critically Ill Adult*, 3rd ed. Edited by Holloway, N. Menlo Park, Calif.: Addison-Wesley Publishing Co., 1988.

Kneisl, C., and Ames, S.A. *Adult Health Nursing: A Biopsychosocial Approach*. Menlo Park, Calif.: Addison-Wesley Publishing Co., 1986.

Luckmann, J., and Sorensen, K. *Medical-Surgical Nursing: A Psychophysiologic Approach*, 3rd ed. Philadelphia: W.B. Saunders Co., 1987.

Van DeVelde-Coke, S. "The Gastrointestinal System," in *Core Curriculum for Critical Care Nursing*, 3rd ed. Edited by Alspach, J., and Williams, S. Philadelphia: W.B. Saunders Co., 1985.

Liver Failure

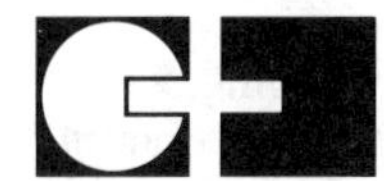

DRG information

DRG 205 Disorders of Liver Except Malignancy, Cirrhosis, or Alcoholic Hepatitis. With Complications or Comorbidity (CC).
Mean LOS = 6.7 days
Principal diagnoses include:
- acute or chronic liver failure
- various types of hepatitis
- hepatomegaly
- jaundice, unspecified etiology
- hepatic infarction.

DRG 206 Disorders of Liver Except Malignancy, Cirrhosis, or Alcoholic Hepatitis. Without CC.
Mean LOS = 4.2 days
Principal diagnoses include selected principal diagnoses listed under DRG 205. The distinction is that a case assigned DRG 206 has no complications or comorbidities.

Introduction

DEFINITION AND TIME FOCUS

In liver failure, which can result from almost all forms of liver disease, parenchymal cells are progressively destroyed and replaced with fibrotic tissue. Once chronically damaged, the liver will never regain normal structure. However, because liver cells retain an enormous regenerative capacity, functional compensation may be attained if precipitating factors are eliminated.

This clinical plan focuses on the patient presenting with acute symptoms of liver failure that require admission to a critical care unit. These symptoms include hepatic encephalopathy, fluid and electrolyte imbalance from ascites, and related potential complications of liver failure. The liver is an essential organ for life. Its functions are metabolic, secretory, excretory, and vascular. Metabolic functions include glycogen formation, storage, and breakdown; glucose formation; fat storage, breakdown, and synthesis; amino acid deamination; ammonia conversion; and synthesis of plasma proteins, including clotting factors. Secretory functions include bile production and bilirubin conjugation. Excretory functions include detoxification of hormones and drugs. Vascular functions include blood storage and filtration.

ETIOLOGY AND PRECIPITATING FACTORS

- Laënnec's (alcoholic) cirrhosis with an acute episode of alcohol ingestion, hypovolemia from rapid diuresis or shock, gastrointestinal bleeding, or infection
- acute hepatic failure caused by fulminant hepatitis, hepatotoxic chemicals, or biliary obstruction

Focused assessment guidelines

NURSING HISTORY (Functional health pattern findings)

Health perception–health management pattern

- complains most commonly about weakness and fatigue
- may have been under treatment for chronic alcoholism, hepatitis, or biliary obstructive disease

Nutritional-metabolic pattern

- commonly has diet history that includes excessive alcohol consumption and fat intolerance
- usually reports anorexia and resulting weight loss
- may report ingestion of certain drugs, such as large doses of acetaminophen, tetracycline, or antituberculosis drugs (isoniazid)

Elimination pattern

- may report clay-colored stools or dark urine resulting from jaundice

Activity-exercise pattern

- may report psychomotor defects

Sleep-rest pattern

- may report increased drowsiness

Cognitive-perceptual pattern

- patient's family commonly report intellectual deterioration and slurred speech in beginning stages of hepatic encephalopathy
- patient's family may report personality changes or altered moods

Sexuality-reproductive pattern

- male patient may be impotent because of endocrine changes
- female patient may report erratic menstruation

Role-relationship pattern

- may have job involving hepatotoxic chemicals such as vinyl chloride

PHYSICAL FINDINGS

General appearance

- fever unaffected by antibiotics; reason for fever is unknown

Cardiovascular

- hyperkinetic circulation: flushed extremities, bounding pulse, and capillary pulsations that result primarily from liver cell failure but also may occur with the opening of many normally present but functionally inactive arteriovenous anastomoses

Pulmonary
• cyanosis

Neurologic
• hyperactive reflexes, positive Babinski's reflex
• various stages of encephalopathy with resultant altered level of consciousness

Gastrointestinal
• fetor hepaticus: sweetish, slightly fecal breath smell, presumably intestinal in origin
• hepatomegaly, splenomegaly
• ascites
• distant bowel sounds and muffled percussion notes

Endocrine
• male: hypogonadism, gynecomastia
• female: gonadal atrophy

Integumentary
• jaundiced skin, sclera, and mucous membranes from failure to metabolize bilirubin
• vascular spiders: consist of central arteriole with radiating small vessels; usually in vascular territory of superior vena cava (above nipple line)
• palmar erythema: hands are warm and palms are bright red; attributable to estrogen excess
• easy bruising from inadequate clotting factors
• "paper money skin": numerous small blood vessels which resemble silk threads in a dollar bill

DIAGNOSTIC STUDIES
• complete blood count—may reveal decreased hematocrit and hemoglobin values, which reflect the liver's inability to store hematopoietic factors (such as iron, folic acid, and vitamin B_{12}); decreased white blood cell (WBC) and thrombocyte levels, which appear with splenomegaly; and elevated WBC count, which may indicate infection.
• increased prothrombin time—reflects decreased synthesis of prothrombin, impaired vitamin K absorption, or both.
• enzyme tests—may show elevated serum glutamic-oxaloacetic transaminase (SGOT), serum glutamic-pyruvic transaminase (SGPT), alkaline phosphatase, and lactic dehydrogenase values, which reflect hepatocellular or biliary tissue dysfunction and necrosis.
• protein metabolite tests (serum albumin and total protein levels)—may reflect impaired protein synthesis.
• lipid and carbohydrate tests—may reveal decreased serum cholesterol levels, reflecting impaired hepatic synthesis, or increased levels, reflecting obstructive pathology; elevated serum ammonia values, reflecting impaired hepatic synthesis of urea; and decreased serum glucose levels, which accompany malnutrition.
• bilirubin levels (total and direct)—increased in liver disease.
• urine and stool tests—may reveal increased urine urobilinogen and reduced fecal urobilinogen values, which accompany jaundice.
• testosterone level—reduced.
• abdominal ultrasound—may be performed if biliary obstruction is suspected.
• abdominal X-rays—may reveal liver enlargement.
• angiography or superior mesenteric arteriography—important for evaluation of portal hypertension.
• liver scan—reveals abnormalities in hepatic structure.
• liver biopsy—indicates extent of hepatic tissue changes.
• electroencephalography (EEG)—may show generalized slowing of frequency, which substantiates encephalopathy.
• endoscopy—helps locate gastrointestinal bleeding site.

POTENTIAL COMPLICATIONS
• hepatorenal failure
• disseminated intravascular coagulation
• bleeding esophageal varices

Collaborative problem: *Deteriorating neurologic status related to hepatic encephalopathy syndrome*

NURSING PRIORITIES: (a) Monitor changes in psychomotor skills, mental status, and speech, and (b) eliminate precipitating factors that decrease hepatocellular function.

Interventions	Rationales
1. Assess neurologic status hourly. Describe the changes observed, typically: • Stage 1: confusion, altered mood or behavior, psychomotor deficits • Stage 2: drowsiness, inappropriate behavior • Stage 3: stupor, marked confusion, and inarticulate speech (although patient may speak or obey simple commands) • Stage 4: coma, but response to painful stimuli still present • Stage 5: deep coma; no response to painful stimuli.	1. Symptoms vary; therefore, close monitoring is important. The encephalopathy syndrome results from impaired nitrogen metabolism, passage of toxic substances of intestinal origin (ammonia, active amines, and short-chain fatty acids) to the brain, and numerous other metabolic abnormalities occurring in hepatocellular failure. The toxic substances are thought to interfere with glucose metabolism and cerebral blood flow. Chronic exposure of brain cells to these substances through repeated bouts of encephalopathy results in irreversible brain cell damage.
2. Assess for asterixis (flapping tremor of the wrist).	2. This sign, caused by impaired flow of proprioceptive information to the brain stem reticular formation, indicates that patient is in early stages of encephalopathy.
3. Auscultate the chest and assess respiratory rate hourly. Administer oxygen therapy via nasal prongs, as ordered. Anticipate more aggressive measures, such as intubation, if the encephalopathy progresses to coma.	3. The patient with long-standing liver disease will have developed decreased oxygen saturation and decreased diffusing capacity before the onset of encephalopathy. Therefore, respiratory support measures are commonly required.
4. Stop intake of dietary protein. Also stop administration of all drugs containing nitrogen, such as ammonium chloride, urea, and methionine, as ordered.	4. Intake of dietary protein and drugs containing nitrogen increase the accumulation of nitrogenous substances that cannot be broken down by the liver.
5. Administer neomycin via nasogastric tube, if ordered. The usual dose is 1 g.	5. Neomycin is effective in decreasing the intestinal bacterial organisms that produce ammonia.
6. Administer lactulose via nasogastric tube, if ordered. The usual dose is 10 to 30 ml. Monitor for diarrhea; if it occurs, consult with the doctor about reducing the dose.	6. Although lactulose's exact mechanism of action is unclear, it may be instrumental in chelating ammonia (NH_3), acting as an osmotic agent for inducing diarrhea, changing gut pH resulting in excretion of ammonium (NH_4^+), or changing gut flora to decrease the growth of ammonia-forming bacteria. Diarrhea is a sign of excessive dosage.
7. Stop any diuretic therapy, as ordered.	7. If patient has hepatic cirrhosis, the most common cause of hepatic encephalopathy is excessive diuresis from diuretic therapy. The resulting hypovolemia further reduces hepatic perfusion, precipitating the encephalopathy.
8. Administer enema solutions that are neutral and free of acid, as ordered.	8. Purging the intestines reduces ammonium absorption and may result in improvement of clinical symptoms and EEG readings.

(continued)

Interventions	Rationales
9. Avoid all sedatives metabolized primarily by the liver. If the patient is uncontrollable, administer half the usual dose of barbiturate, as ordered. Morphine and paraldehyde are absolutely contraindicated.	9. Patients in impending coma are extremely sensitive to sedatives. Drugs metabolized primarily by the liver are particularly dangerous because toxic accumulations can occur rapidly from the impaired hepatic perfusion. Some sedation may be necessary, however, if the patient becomes agitated as hepatic failure worsens and toxic metabolic substances accumulate. Long-acting, short-chain barbiturates that are excreted largely by the kidney are advocated. Morphine and paraldehyde may precipitate coma.
10. Provide patient-family teaching associated with above interventions, as appropriate. Emphasize causes of changes in neurologic status and rationales for methods to reduce encephalopathy.	10. Although patient teaching may be of limited success because of altered level of consciousness, brief and repeated explanations may help the patient feel more secure psychologically. Teaching family members may help them understand mood swings and behavior changes.
11. Additional individualized interventions: ________	11. Rationales: ________

Target outcome criteria
Within 24 to 48 hours of admission, the patient will:
- awaken and display improved neurologic status
- display a decreased need for respiratory support.

Collaborative problem: *Potential fever related to liver disease or infection*

NURSING PRIORITY: Assist in determining the differential diagnosis of fever.

Interventions	Rationales
1. Assess the temperature every 4 hours. If elevated, assess more frequently.	1. Continuous low-grade fever rarely exceeding 100.4° F. (38° C.) is seen in about one third of patients with liver disease. This fever is unaffected by antibiotics and attributable to liver disease alone, although the reason for it is unknown. However, patients may have fever from infection. The liver normally is bacteriologically sterile and filters bacteria from the bloodstream. Cirrhosis allows bacteria to pass through into the circulation. Differentiation of possible causes of fever is necessary to institute effective treatment modalities.
2. Observe for cloudy, concentrated urine and pain upon urination, if a catheter is not in place. Avoid catheterization, if possible.	2. These signs indicate urinary tract infection. Avoiding catheterization reduces the risk of infection. Remember, urine may be dark amber because of jaundice.
3. Auscultate lung fields at least every 2 hours. Also assess respiratory rate, skin color, and level of cyanosis.	3. Respiratory difficulties may indicate aspiration pneumonia. Pulmonary arteriovenous shunting from liver disease and the resultant decreased oxygen saturation place patient at increased risk for pneumonia.
4. Auscultate bowel sounds at least every 4 hours. Observe for abdominal rigidity, increased size of abdominal girth, or vomiting.	4. Spontaneous peritonitis is known to occur in patients with liver disease.

Interventions	Rationales
5. If infection is diagnosed, assist with treatment, as ordered; for example, administer antibiotics. If the fever stems solely from liver disease, provide symptomatic care, such as frequent linen changes.	5. Infection requires prompt, aggressive treatment because it promotes protein accumulation from tissue catabolism. Low-grade fever may remain if fever results solely from liver disease. Frequent liver changes reduce discomfort from diaphoresis.
6. Additional individualized interventions: ________	6. Rationales: ________

Target outcome criteria
Within 24 to 48 hours, the patient will:
- have the cause of fever determined
- have appropriate therapy initiated.

Collaborative problem: *Fluid and electrolyte imbalance related to ascites*

NURSING PRIORITY: Restore a more normal fluid balance.

Interventions	Rationales
1. Maintain close monitoring of fluid and electrolyte status, including strict intake and output measurements, hourly determination of urine specific gravity, daily weights, and assessment of lung fields at least every 2 hours for crackles or rhonchi.	1. Close monitoring of fluid status is necessary to judge the degree of cardiovascular and pulmonary compromise imposed by ascites. In liver failure, ascites develops from lowered plasma oncotic pressure, portal venous hypertension, and sodium and water retention. The lowered plasma oncotic pressure results from the liver's failure to synthesize albumin. This lowered oncotic pressure, combined with increased hydrostatic pressure from portal hypertension, causes fluid to shift into interstitial spaces (third spacing) in the peritoneal cavity. The resulting depletion of effective intravascular volume causes the renal tubules to retain sodium and water via the aldosterone effect.
2. Percuss and palpate the abdomen every 4 hours. Do not rely solely on abdominal girth measurements.	2. Percussion and palpation allow evaluation of changes in the ascitic process. Dullness on percussion in the flanks is the earliest sign of ascites and indicates approximately 2 liters of fluid. The liver and spleen may be palpated if only moderate amounts of fluid are present; with tense ascites, it is difficult to palpate abdominal viscera. A fluid thrill means the presence of a large amount of free fluid. It is a very late sign of fluid under tension. Abdominal girth measurements are unreliable as gaseous distention is common.
3. Maintain strict bed rest.	3. Recumbency increases renal perfusion and the kidneys' ability to excrete excess fluid.
4. Implement dietary restrictions, as ordered. Typically, restrict sodium intake to 0.5 g/day and fluid intake to 1 liter/day.	4. The rate of ascitic fluid reabsorption is limited to 700 to 900 ml a day. Limiting sodium and water intake restricts the rate of ascitic fluid production.
5. Provide patient-family teaching about above measures, as appropriate.	5. Understanding the effects of ascites and treatment methods improves the patient's and family's cooperation with the treatment plan, increasing the likelihood of its effectiveness.
6. Additional individualized interventions: ________	6. Rationales: ________

Target outcome criteria
Within 4 days, the patient will:
- manifest urine output of 60 ml/hour or above
- display urinary sodium excretion >10 mEq/24 hours
- show lessened ascites and edema, as evidenced by decreased weight and improved respiratory status.

Collaborative problem: *Potential gastrointestinal hemorrhage related to esophageal varices*

NURSING PRIORITY: Monitor for, prevent, or promptly treat hemorrhage.

Interventions	Rationales
1. Observe for and report signs of esophageal bleeding, such as hematemesis. See the "Gastrointestinal Hemorrhage" care plan, page 191, for specific nursing interventions.	1. The mechanism of esophageal varices formation is unclear; they are thought to be caused by excessive portal venous backflow into the esophageal vasculature. Hematemesis of frank red blood indicates active bleeding. The "Gastrointestinal Hemorrhage" care plan contains detailed information on detecting and treating bleeding varices.
2. Additional individualized interventions: ______	2. Rationales: ______

Target outcome criteria
Within 24 hours of detection of bleeding, the patient will:
- exhibit vital signs within normal limits
- have warm, dry skin.

Nursing diagnosis: *Nutritional deficit related to catabolism from liver disease*

NURSING PRIORITY: Restore nutritional metabolism to an anabolic state.

Interventions	Rationales
1. Implement dietary prescriptions, as ordered. Maintain high-caloric intake, usually 1,600 calories/day, by administering high-carbohydrate I.V. infusions, as ordered. If jaundice is present, do not administer oral fat or fat infusions.	1. Dietary control of precursors to toxic metabolites plays an important role in the control of symptoms. High-caloric intake is necessary to meet energy needs. Jaundice indicates decreased bile salt levels, which impair fat absorption.
2. If encephalopathy is present, do not administer protein. Once encephalopathy has subsided, begin protein intake at 20-g/day increments. Monitor closely for recurrence of encephalopathy.	2. Inability to metabolize protein causes the blood ammonia level to rise, producing encephalopathy. Restricting protein intake helps eliminate symptoms. Gradual reintroduction of protein allows careful determination of the amount the patient can metabolize safely. Recurrence of symptoms would indicate the need for permanent restriction of protein intake.
3. Emphasize to the patient and family the importance of dietary control.	3. The necessary dietary restrictions may make the diet unpalatable and difficult to accept. Understanding their rationale increases the patient's motivation to follow recommendations and the likelihood of family reinforcement of motivation.

Interventions	Rationales
4. Additional individualized interventions: ________	4. Rationales: ________

Target outcome criteria
Within 96 hours, the patient will tolerate protein intake.

Nursing diagnosis: *Potential impaired skin integrity related to jaundice, increased bleeding tendencies, malnutrition, and ascites*

NURSING PRIORITY: Maintain or restore skin integrity.

Interventions	Rationales
1. Monitor skin condition. Particularly note the presence of vascular spiders.	1. Careful monitoring of skin status, commonly overlooked when the patient is in the critical care unit, is important because it allows early detection of skin problems to which liver failure patients are particularly susceptible. Vascular spiders can bleed profusely.
2. Monitor prothrombin time, as ordered.	2. Liver failure impairs the synthesis of clotting factors. A prolonged prothrombin time increases the risk of skin bruising and breakdown.
3. Turn the patient and rub body prominences every 2 hours. Implement additional measures in the "Impaired Physical Mobility" care plan, page 33, as appropriate.	3. Malnutrition and ascites predispose the patient to decubitus ulcer formation. The "Impaired Physical Mobility" care plan itemizes detailed information on potential skin problems.
4. Provide symptomatic treatment of pruritus, as necessary; for example, bathe the skin with cool water.	4. Pruritus, which results from jaundice, can be a maddening symptom that bedevils the patient. Treatment may be limited because phenothiazides and antihistamines are contraindicated if the patient has encephalopathy.
5. Additional individualized interventions: ________	5. Rationales: ________

Target outcome criteria
Within 48 hours, the patient will have no apparent skin breakdown.

Transfer planning

NURSING TRANSFER CRITERIA

Upon transfer, documentation shows evidence of:
- improved neurologic status
- absence of respiratory complications
- adequate urine output
- reduction of ascites and weight
- normal temperature or maintenance of only low-grade fever
- resumption of protein and fat intake, either I.V. or oral.

PATIENT-FAMILY TEACHING CHECKLIST

Document evidence that patient and family demonstrate understanding of:

__ relationship between alcohol consumption and exacerbation of liver disease
__ causes of changes in neurologic status and relationship to liver disease
__ effects of ascites and methods of treatment
__ importance of diet in liver disease.

DOCUMENTATION CHECKLIST

Using outcome criteria as a guide, document:
__ clinical status on admission
__ significant changes in status
__ pertinent laboratory and diagnostic test findings
__ weight
__ intake and output measurements
__ fluctuations in fever and associated symptoms
__ skin integrity
__ any signs of GI bleeding
__ patient-family teaching
__ transfer planning.

ASSOCIATED CARE PLANS

Gastrointestinal Hemorrhage
Impaired Physical Mobility
Nutritional Deficit
Sensory-Perceptual Alteration

REFERENCES

Alspach, J., and Williams, S. *Core Curriculum for Critical Care Nursing.* Philadelphia: W.B. Saunders Co., 1985.

Gastrointestinal Disorders. Nurse's Clinical Library Series. Springhouse, Pa.: Springhouse Corp., 1985.

Luckmann, J., and Sorensen, K. *Medical-Surgical Nursing: A Psychophysiologic Approach,* 3rd ed. Philadelphia: W.B. Saunders Co., 1987.

Sherlock, S. *Diseases of the Liver and Biliary System.* Boston: Blackwell Scientific Publications, 1987.

Pancreatitis

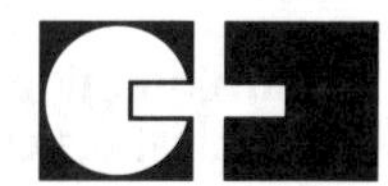

DRG information

DRG 204 Disorder of Pancreas Except Malignancy.
Mean LOS = 6.1 days
Principal diagnoses include:
- pancreatitis
- benign neoplasm of pancreas, except islets of Langerhans
- injury to any portion of the pancreas.

Introduction

DEFINITION AND TIME FOCUS

Pancreatitis (inflammation of the pancreas) represents an autodigestive disorder in which premature activation of pancreatic proteolytic enzymes damages the organ itself. The exact physiologic mechanism is unknown, but theoretically, duodenal reflux or spasm, or blockage of pancreatic ducts by gallstones or edema, may result in the backup of pancreatic secretions. Pancreatitis may be a complication of surgical treatment of other biliary tract or gastrointestinal disease; numerous other causative factors have also been implicated.

Depending on the nature and severity of the disorder, significant edema, tissue necrosis, and life-threatening hemorrhage may result. Pancreatitis may be either acute or chronic. Chronic pancreatitis causes progressive loss of pancreatic function and may be associated with repeated bouts of acute pancreatitis. This care plan focuses on the care of the patient who is admitted to the critical care unit for diagnosis and management of an episode of acute pancreatitis.

ETIOLOGY AND PRECIPITATING FACTORS

- alcohol abuse
- cholecystitis or cholelithiasis
- abdominal surgical procedures
- trauma
- peptic or duodenal ulcer
- hyperparathyroidism
- viral hepatitis
- mumps
- hyperlipidemia
- anorexia nervosa
- ischemia related to shock
- metabolic disorders
- use of certain medications: thiazide diuretics, steroids, sulfonamides, oral contraceptives, tetracycline, acetaminophen (in excessive doses).

Focused assessment guidelines

NURSING HISTORY (Functional health pattern findings)

Health perception–health management pattern

- commonly complains of severe abdominal pain in epigastric or umbilical region that radiates into back or flank
- may note that pain increases when supine or when food is taken and after administration of certain narcotics
- may have history of gallbladder disease or alcoholism with recent dietary indiscretion or drinking binge

Nutritional-metabolic pattern

- commonly describes nausea or vomiting
- may complain of anorexia
- may note recent weight loss

Elimination pattern

- may note increased flatus
- may describe steatorrhea (associated with chronic disease)

Activity-exercise pattern

- may prefer hunched, sitting position because of pain
- may become dizzy or faint when standing

Cognitive-perceptual pattern

- may complain of shoulder pain or frequent hiccups (if diaphragmatic irritation is present)
- may complain of pleuritic-like pain that increases with deep inspiration

Coping–stress tolerance pattern

- may habitually use unhealthy coping mechanisms (such as alcoholism)

PHYSICAL FINDINGS

General appearance

- hunched posture
- restlessness

Cardiovascular

- fever
- tachycardia
- hypotension

Pulmonary

If pleural effusion is present:
- reduced chest excursion
- crackles
- tachypnea

Gastrointestinal
- abdominal distention
- guarding
- reduced or absent bowel sounds
- ascites

Neurologic
- seizures
- stupor
- neuromuscular irritability

Integumentary
- jaundice
- pallor
- diaphoresis
- Cullen's sign (ecchymosis around umbilicus)
- Grey Turner's sign (ecchymosis in flank, retroperitoneal, and groin area)
- cool extremities
- cyanosis (if advanced shock)

Musculoskeletal
If hypocalcemia is present:
- tetany
- positive Chvostek's sign
- positive Trousseau's sign

Renal
- oliguria (if acute tubular necrosis)

DIAGNOSTIC STUDIES
- serum amylase level—elevated in acute pancreatitis, usually >500 units/dl, and peaks 2 to 24 hours after onset of symptoms. Although not specific for pancreatitis, increased enzyme levels occur during pancreatic inflammation.
- amylase-creatinine clearance ratio—indicates acute pancreatitis if >5%.
- urine amylase level—elevated for the first 3 to 5 days of illness; it reflects pancreatic secretion better than serum value. In acute pancreatitis, renal clearance of amylase is markedly increased.
- serum calcium level—decreased, usually <8 mg/dl (unless hyperparathyroidism is present, in which instance value may be normal).
- complete blood count (CBC)—likely to reveal leukocytosis. Hemoglobin and hematocrit values vary depending on fluid status, hemorrhage, or degree of compensation.
- serum and urine glucose levels—may be elevated because of altered insulin production.
- serum lipase level—elevated.
- serum and urine bilirubin levels—elevated.
- serum albumin value—usually <3.2 g/dl.
- serum triglyceride levels—may be elevated.
- serum electrolyte levels—may reveal hypokalemia or hyponatremia.
- abdominal ultrasound—may provide evidence of inflammation, edema, gallstones, calcified pancreatic ducts, abscess, organ enlargement, or hematoma, or pseudocyst (cavities of exudate, blood, and pancreatic products that may expand and compress other organs).
- computed tomography (CT) scan—visualizes tumors, dilated pancreatic ducts, calcification, or pseudocyst.
- abdominal X-rays—may reveal areas of calcification or adhesions, or identify indicators of reduced bowel motility.
- upper GI X-rays—may show enlarged pancreas or may reveal stomach displacement from pseudocyst formation.
- chest X-ray—may reveal diaphragmatic elevation if abscess formation or peritonitis is present; it may identify areas of atelectasis or effusion.
- I.V. cholangiography—used to rule out acute cholecystitis as cause of symptoms.
- paracentesis—may reveal elevated amylase levels or blood, both associated with acute pancreatitis.

POTENTIAL COMPLICATIONS
- hypovolemic shock
- hemorrhage
- adult respiratory distress syndrome
- renal failure
- pulmonary edema
- myocardial infarction
- peritonitis or sepsis
- pleural effusion
- abscess formation
- hyperglycemia or diabetes mellitus
- paralytic ileus
- pseudocyst formation (cavities of exudate, blood, and pancreatic products which may expand and compress other organs)

Collaborative problem: *Potential hypovolemic shock related to hemorrhage, fluid shifts, hyperglycemia, or vomiting*

NURSING PRIORITY: Maintain fluid volume.

Interventions / Rationales

1. Monitor vital signs, intake and output, hemodynamic pressures, and EKG findings according to "Monitoring Standards" appendix, page 314, or unit protocol. Immediately report any findings indicating hypovolemia.

Rationale: 1. The damaged pancreas releases several substances that have systemic vasoactive effects. Kinins increase vascular permeability and cause vasodilation, increasing the likelihood of shock. Elastase and chymotrypsin cause necrosis and damage blood vessels, which may precipitate hemorrhage. In addition, pancreatic fluid and blood entering the peritoneum may cause chemical irritation of the bowel and bowel atony, resulting in fluid shift into interstitial spaces (third spacing) as fluid leaks out of the damaged intestine. Reduced renal blood flow may lead to acute tubular necrosis.

2. Maintain I.V. access through peripheral or central lines. Monitor I.V. fluid replacement, usually with lactated Ringer's solution or dextrans or albumin. If hemorrhage is suspected, anticipate and monitor transfusion, as ordered.

Rationale: 2. Rapid I.V. infusion of large volumes of fluid or blood is the primary immediate treatment indicated for hypovolemia. Untreated, hypovolemia quickly results in circulatory collapse and tissue death.

3. Assess blood glucose or urine glucose and ketone levels at least every 4 to 6 hours or more frequently if severe hyperglycemia is present. Administer regular insulin, as ordered, and monitor and document effects.

Rationale: 3. Injury to the insulin-producing islet cells of the pancreas commonly decreases insulin production and causes at least transient hyperglycemia. If damage is severe, particularly if chronic pancreatitis is also present, overt diabetes mellitus may develop. Hyperglycemia may contribute further to functional hypovolemia as the body responds to the hyperosmolar state with further fluid shifts.

4. Monitor serum electrolytes daily, as ordered, including serum calcium. See "Fluid and Electrolyte Imbalances" appendix, page 317. Stay alert for characteristic signs of severe hypocalcemia: neuromuscular irritability and tetany.

Rationale: 4. Fluid shifts associated with acute pancreatitis may result in any of various electrolyte imbalances, including hypokalemia and hyponatremia. Hypocalcemia is a common finding, possibly from the bonding of calcium with fatty substances. Clinically significant hypocalcemia is associated with a poorer prognosis.

5. Maintain continuous gastric drainage with low suction, as ordered, preferably with a double-lumen tube. Administer anticholinergic medications, if ordered. Test gastric drainage for blood at least every 8 hours. Withhold food and fluids.

Rationale: 5. Draining gastric secretions removes a stimulus for pancreatic secretions, thus reducing the release of vasoactive substances and allowing the damaged pancreas to rest. A double-lumen tube is preferable for continuous suction because the air vent minimizes possible damage to the gastric mucosa. Anticholinergic use is controversial because such medication may contribute to ileus; some practitioners believe anticholinergics are effective in reducing pancreatic secretions, but this is unproven. Withholding food and fluids prevents stimulation of gastric secretions from food.

6. Administer I.V. dopamine (Intropin) or other vasopressor, as ordered, if hypotension persists.

Rationale: 6. In acute pancreatitis, the release of myocardial depressant factor from the pancreas is thought to reduce cardiac output. Dopamine has a positive inotropic effect on the heart, increasing cardiac output, and a dopaminergic effect on the kidneys, improving renal blood flow.

(continued)

Interventions

7. Administer I.V. histamine (H_2)-receptor antagonists, such as cimetidine (Tagamet) or ranitidine (Zantac), as ordered. Monitor gastric pH.

Rationales

7. H_2-receptor antagonists reduce gastric acid secretion. Because gastric acid release may stimulate increased pancreatic activity, these medications are helpful in controlling hemorrhage. H_2-receptor antagonists also decrease the risk of pneumonitis, if the patient aspirates gastric secretions. The gastric pH should be maintained at >5.0; medication dosage may require adjustment to achieve this.

8. Prepare for surgery if hemodynamic parameters do not stabilize in response to therapeutic interventions.

8. Persistent shock indicates the need for surgical intervention to stop bleeding, relieve duct obstruction, drain abscess or pseudocyst, or evaluate other possible intra-abdominal pathology.

9. Additional individualized interventions: ____________

9. Rationales: ____________

Target outcome criteria

Within 24 hours of admission and then continuously, the patient will:
- have vital signs within normal limits for patient
- display serum glucose and urine glucose and ketone levels returning to normal
- have serum electrolyte levels returning to normal.

Nursing diagnosis: *Pain related to edema, necrosis, autodigestive processes, abdominal distention, abscess formation, ileus, or peritonitis*

NURSING PRIORITIES: (a) Monitor, evaluate, and relieve pain, and (b) treat underlying cause(s) of pain.

Interventions

1. Assess pain, noting location, character, severity, radiation, frequency, and any accompanying symptoms. Immediately report changes in pain quality or location, particularly if abdominal rigidity, reduced or absent bowel sounds, palpable abdominal mass, or other indications of generalized peritonitis or abscess occur. See the "Acute Pain" care plan, page 10.

Rationales

1. Evaluation of the type of pain the patient is experiencing is essential for early detection of possible complications. Typically, the pain accompanying acute pancreatitis is severe, steady, and felt across the entire abdomen, and it commonly radiates to the back or flank. Tenderness to deep palpation is not uncommon; however, the abdomen usually remains soft. Abdominal rigidity and reduced bowel sounds may indicate development of peritonitis; a mass may indicate abscess or pseudocyst. Prompt surgical intervention is warranted if these occur. The "Acute Pain" care plan contains general interventions for any patient in pain.

2. Ensure that blood samples for serum amylase and lipase levels are obtained before administering analgesics.

2. Many analgesics, including meperidine (Demerol) and morphine, may cause elevations in serum amylase and lipase levels, obscuring accurate use of these findings for diagnosis.

3. Medicate, as ordered, with narcotic analgesics, usually meperidine (Demerol) or pentazocine (Talwin). Observe for increased pain following narcotic administration and collaborate with doctor to adjust pain control regimen, as indicated.

3. The severity of pain associated with acute pancreatitis generally warrants narcotic analgesia. Morphine is thought to cause increased spasm of Oddi's sphincter and thus is usually avoided for these patients. However, other analgesics, including meperidine, may also have such effects to some degree.

4. Administer antacids, as ordered, clamping the gastric tube for 30 minutes after administration. When oral intake is resumed, avoid simultaneous administration of antacids with oral cimetidine.

4. Antacids reduce gastric acidity and associated discomfort; some products may also act to relieve flatulence and distention. Cimetidine absorption may be impaired if antacids are given at the same time.

Interventions	Rationales
5. If the patient's condition permits, begin teaching dietary and life-style measures that reduce discomfort and help avert recurrence of acute attacks. Include family members in all teaching. Address the following considerations: • need for lifelong avoidance of alcohol • low-fat diet, depending upon presence of gallbladder disease • avoidance of caffeine or other substances linked to increased gastric secretions.	5. Teaching in the critical care setting may be limited by the patient's condition, but introductory material can lay the groundwork for more thorough discussion after the patient has stabilized. Alcohol is a common precipitating factor in the recurrence of acute pancreatitis, although the exact physiologic mechanism is not known. Gallbladder disease may indicate the need for low-fat diet to avoid exacerbating symptoms. Caffeine causes increased gastric acid secretion and thus increases pancreatic activity.
6. Additional individualized interventions: ____________	6. Rationales: ____________

Target outcome criteria
Within 2 hours of the onset of pain, the patient will verbalize pain relief.

Nursing diagnosis: *Potential for injury: complications related to pulmonary insults, hypovolemia, alcoholism, or other factors*

NURSING PRIORITY: Prevent or detect and promptly treat complications.

Interventions	Rationales
1. Assess lung sounds, sputum production, skin color, and respiratory rate and effort frequently, at least every 2 hours. Report decreased breath sounds, crackles, productive cough, increased respiratory rate or effort or other signs of respiratory complications immediately. Monitor arterial blood gas levels daily or as ordered, and report abnormal results.	1. Patients with acute pancreatitis are at increased risk for pulmonary complications from edema, fluid shifts, diaphragmatic irritation, and possible decreased myocardial contractility. Adult respiratory distress syndrome, pulmonary edema, pleural effusion, or pneumonia may occur. Endotracheal intubation and mechanical ventilation may be required for adequate oxygenation if respiratory impairment is a factor. Early intervention reduces the risk of significant hypoxic damage.
2. Encourage deep breathing, coughing, use of incentive spirometer, and position changes at least every 2 hours.	2. Abdominal distention, pain, and the use of narcotic medications may contribute to reduced chest expansion, predisposing the patient to pulmonary abnormalities. These measures help re-expand atelectatic areas and improve clearance of pulmonary secretions.
3. Assess for indicators of paralytic ileus, perforated viscus, or peritonitis, such as reduced or absent bowel sounds, vomiting, increased abdominal distention, rigid or boardlike abdomen, and tympany.	3. These conditions may arise as a result of chemical irritation of the bowel, necrosis, and abscess formation associated with acute pancreatitis. Unless immediate surgical intervention ensues, sepsis may develop.
4. Monitor for signs and symptoms of pseudocyst development, such as increasing tenderness, palpable mass, upper abdominal pain, diarrhea, and worsening of general condition despite interventions.	4. Pseudocysts are pockets left in the pancreas after tissue necrosis occurs in which blood, tissue debris, and pancreatic secretions accumulate. They may resolve spontaneously, but may rupture and cause chemical peritonitis or grow so large that they cause compression of other organs. Intervention may include surgical resection or drainage.

(continued)

Interventions	Rationales
5. Assess for and report indications of disseminated intravascular coagulation (DIC), such as bleeding or oozing from wounds, drains, or puncture sites; purpura of the chest or abdomen; petechiae; hematuria; melena; or epistaxis. Guaiac-test all drainage. See the "Disseminated Intravascular Coagulation" care plan, page 253, for details.	5. DIC is a major potential complication associated with acute pancreatitis, possibly from release of tissue fragments, toxins associated with the shock state, or other physiologic mechanisms. Early detection allows prompt treatment. The "Disseminated Intravascular Coagulation" care plan contains interventions for the care of patients who develop this disorder.
6. Assess for early indications of renal impairment, such as oliguria or anuria, increased urine osmolality, and elevated blood urea nitrogen level.	6. Hypovolemia may decrease renal perfusion and lead to acute renal failure. Renal impairment may also occur in acute pancreatitis when volume status is normal; the mechanism involved is unclear, but may involve DIC.
7. Be alert for indications of alcohol withdrawal syndrome, such as agitation, tremors, insomnia, hypertension, and anxiety. If alcoholism is a likely contributing factor to the patient's condition, consult with doctor regarding measures to prevent or minimize alcohol withdrawal syndrome.	7. Because excessive alcohol intake is a common precipitating factor in acute pancreatitis, the possibility of overt or hidden alcoholism must always be considered. Untreated, the withdrawal syndrome may progress rapidly to seizures, hallucinations, hyperthermia, other severe complications, or death.
8. Additional individualized interventions: ______	8. Rationales: ______

Target outcome criteria
Throughout unit stay, the patient will:
- perform pulmonary hygiene measures as instructed
- manifest no evidence of complications
- receive prompt treatment if complications develop.

Nursing diagnosis: *Nutritional deficit related to vomiting, pain, gastric suction, NPO (nothing by mouth) status, and impaired digestion of nutrients*

NURSING PRIORITY: Maintain or restore adequate nutritional intake.

Interventions	Rationales
1. Assess nutritional status. See the "Nutritional Deficit" care plan, page 53, for details.	1. Baseline assessment of nutritional status is essential for planning appropriate maintenance or replacement therapy. The "Nutritional Deficit" care plan provides details on evaluating patients' nutritional status.
2. Administer I.V. hyperalimentation (IVH), also called total parenteral nutrition, as ordered, and monitor patient response, including careful monitoring of glucose levels.	2. Oral nutrient intake during an acute pancreatitis episode tends to exacerbate pain and increase pancreatic activity. In patients requiring prolonged NPO status, IVH may be indicated to avert malnutrition. Increased protein and calories are necessary for healing and for maintenance of the body's immunologic defenses. In pancreatitis, glucose levels may be elevated because of damage to the insulin-producing islet cells in the pancreas; if hyperglycemia has been present, the additional glucose load of IVH will necessitate readjustment of insulin dosage.
3. As the patient's condition permits, institute dietary teaching, as indicated, including: • diabetic diet • use of pancreatic enzymes, if recommended • avoidance of alcohol and caffeine.	3. Careful dietary teaching may help the patient avert recurrences. A diabetic diet may be necessary because of reduced pancreatic insulin production. Oral intake of pancreatic enzymes helps replace deficient enzymes. Alcohol and caffeine avoidance eliminates common triggers of acute pancreatitis.

Interventions	Rationales
4. Additional individualized interventions: ________	4. Rationales: ________

Target outcome criteria
Throughout unit stay, the patient will maintain adequate nutritional intake. (See the "Nutritional Deficit" care plan for specific criteria.)

Transfer planning

NURSING TRANSFER CRITERIA

Upon transfer, documentation shows evidence of:
- stable vital signs
- normal electrolyte values
- serum glucose controlled by medication, as needed
- pain controlled by medication
- absence of pulmonary or cardiovascular complications
- normal bowel sounds and elimination
- normal urine output
- adequate nutritional intake.

PATIENT-FAMILY TEACHING CHECKLIST

Document evidence that patient and family demonstrate understanding of:

__ disease process, precipitating factors, and prognosis
__ dietary considerations
__ diabetic teaching, as required by condition
__ signs and symptoms indicating recurrence or complications
__ pain relief measures.

DOCUMENTATION CHECKLIST

Using outcome criteria as a guide, document:

__ clinical status on admission
__ significant changes in status
__ pertinent laboratory and diagnostic test findings
__ fluid intake and output
__ bowel function
__ patient-family teaching
__ transfer planning.

ASSOCIATED CARE PLANS

Acute Pain
Adult Respiratory Distress Syndrome
Diabetic Ketoacidosis
Disseminated Intravascular Coagulation
Ineffective Coping
Knowledge Deficit
Nutritional Deficit
Pulmonary Embolism

REFERENCES

Kneisl, C.R., and Ames, S.W. *Adult Health Nursing: A Biopsychosocial Approach*. Menlo Park, Calif.: Addison-Wesley Publishing Co., 1986.

Luckmann, J., and Sorensen, K.C. *Medical-Surgical Nursing: A Psychophysiologic Approach*, 3rd ed. Philadelphia: W.B. Saunders Co., 1987.

Strasen, L. "Acute Alcohol Withdrawal Syndrome in the Critical Care Unit," *Critical Care Nurse* 2(6):24-31, November/December 1982.

Thompson, J.M., et al. *Clinical Nursing*. St. Louis: C.V. Mosby Co., 1986.

Wills, S.L., and Trembley, S.F. *Critical Care Review for Nurses*. Belmont, Calif.: Wadsworth Publishing Co., 1984.

Diabetic Ketoacidosis

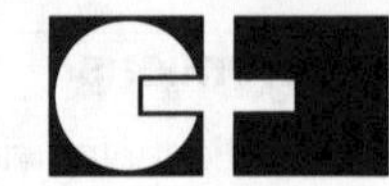

DRG information

DRG 294 Diabetes. Age >35.
Mean LOS = 6.1 days
Principal diagnoses include:
- diabetes without mention of complication
- diabetes with coma
- diabetes with ketoacidosis
- diabetes with other specified manifestations
- diabetes with unspecified complications
- glycosuria.

DRG 295 Diabetes. Age 0 to 35.
Mean LOS = 4.5 days
Principal diagnoses include selected principal diagnoses listed under DRG 294.

Introduction

DEFINITION AND TIME FOCUS

Diabetic ketoacidosis (DKA) is an endocrine emergency precipitated by a relative or absolute insulin scarcity. Diabetes mellitus (DM), the disease of insulin deficiency, provokes unbalanced metabolism of carbohydrates, fats, and proteins, which results in various physiologic derangements that may become life-threatening. Insulin, an anabolic hormone secreted by pancreatic islet cells, facilitates glucose transport across cell membranes. It thus promotes glucose uptake and metabolism and deposition of glycogen, the storage form of glucose. Insulin also promotes fatty acid synthesis and amino acid transport while inhibiting excessive breakdown of fats and proteins. In Type I (insulin-dependent) diabetes, the basic defect is thought to be inadequate or absent insulin secretion, whereas in Type II (non-insulin-dependent) diabetes, inadequate insulin secretion or insulin resistance or both are thought to be responsible.

This care plan focuses on the diabetic patient admitted to the intensive care unit with ketoacidosis, an ominous manifestation of Type I DM that results in hyperosmolality and severe volume depletion.

ETIOLOGY AND PRECIPITATING FACTORS

- undiagnosed DM
- reduced or missed insulin dose
- increased insulin need, for example, from infection (the most common cause), trauma, surgery, or emotional stress
- medications that impair insulin metabolism, for example, thiazide diuretics or phenytoin (Dilantin)
- no identifiable precipitating factor

Focused assessment guidelines

NURSING HISTORY (Functional health pattern findings)

Health perception–health management pattern
- reports or displays acute onset of symptoms
- is likely to have family history of DM

Nutritional-metabolic pattern
- reports or displays increased thirst (polydipsia)
- reports or displays increased hunger (polyphagia)

Elimination pattern
- may complain of excessive urination (polyuria)

Activity-exercise pattern
- may complain of weakness, lethargy, or fatigue

Sleep-rest pattern
- may report disturbed sleep (from nocturia)

Cognitive-perceptual pattern
- may report or display dizziness or confusion
- may complain of abdominal pain

PHYSICAL FINDINGS

Neurologic
- decreased level of consciousness, ranging from confusion to coma

Pulmonary
- tachypnea
- Kussmaul's respirations
- acetone breath odor

Cardiovascular
- tachycardia
- hypotension
- weak peripheral pulses
- capillary refill time >3 seconds

Gastrointestinal
- dry mucous membranes
- vomiting

Integumentary
- warm, dry, flushed skin
- poor skin turgor

Musculoskeletal
- weakness
- decreased or absent deep tendon reflexes

Renal
• polyuria (early)
• oliguria (late)

DIAGNOSTIC STUDIES
• blood glucose level—elevated, typically to as much as 500 mg/dl, but may be 1,000 to 1,500 mg/dl if severe volume depletion or impaired renal function is present.
• serum ketone measurement—positive.
• urine glucose level—positive.
• urine ketone level—positive.
• serum osmolality—increased but usually <330 mOsm/liter.
• serum electrolyte levels—may reveal abnormalities that may vary depending upon preexisting electrolyte levels, volume depletion, and length of time since DKA onset; typically, hyperkalemia early, hypokalemia late; hyponatremia early, hypernatremia late.
• arterial blood gas (ABG) levels—usually reveal pH <7.3, indicating severe metabolic acidosis.
• anion gap >14 mEq/liter, indicating abnormal increase in organic acids.
• blood urea nitrogen and creatinine values—may be elevated, reflecting decreased renal perfusion.
• cardiac enzyme test—used to rule out myocardial infarction as source of symptoms.
• serum amylase—used to rule out pancreatitis as source of symptoms.
• blood, urine, and sputum cultures—used to detect infection, a common precipitator of DKA.
• 12-lead EKG—used to rule out myocardial infarction.
• chest X-ray—used to rule out infection, a common precipitator of DKA.

POTENTIAL COMPLICATIONS
• respiratory failure
• hypovolemic shock
• renal failure
• hypoglycemia
• pulmonary edema
• cerebral edema
• infection

Collaborative problem: *Hypovolemia related to osmotic diuresis or vomiting, or both*

NURSING PRIORITY: Restore fluid volume rapidly.

Interventions	Rationales
1. Monitor for signs and symptoms of dehydration and shock, such as tachycardia; hypotension; weak peripheral pulses; capillary refill time >3 seconds; warm, dry, flushed skin; poor skin turgor; and polyuria or oliguria. Continuously monitor blood pressure and cardiac rate and rhythm.	1. In DKA, the blood glucose level rockets because of decreased cellular uptake and use of glucose. The resulting hyperglycemia increases serum osmolality and triggers a fluid shift from the intracellular to the extracellular space, producing intracellular dehydration. Compensatory renal glucose spillage, a powerful control mechanism to prevent excessive hyperglycemia, produces an intense, obligatory osmotic diuresis resulting in extracellular dehydration. Eventually, severe dehydration decreases glomerular filtration. The resulting oliguria aggravates the hyperglycemia and hyperosmolality. Signs and symptoms indicate the severity of the deficit and the adequacy of fluid replacement. As volume is restored, signs and symptoms should gradually resolve; failure to do so indicates inadequate fluid replacement or continuing fluid losses.
2. Observe for signs and symptoms of electrolyte imbalances (see the "Fluid and Electrolyte Imbalances" appendix, page 317, for details):	2. Electrolyte status may change rapidly, so observe closely to identify any imbalances present.
• hyperkalemia in the first 1 to 4 hours of treatment	• Buffering of excess hydrogen ions released in acidosis displaces intracellular potassium into the serum.
• hypokalemia after 1 to 4 hours of treatment	• Renal excretion of potassium accelerates because of hyperkalemia, producing a deficit of total body potassium that is masked by the high serum level. As therapy reduces acidosis, potassium ions move back from the serum into the cells, unmasking the underlying deficit.
• hyponatremia early in treatment	• Hyponatremia results from urinary sodium losses caused by diuresis and from ketone excretion.

(continued)

Interventions	Rationales
• hypernatremia later in treatment.	• As metabolic control is restored, the kidneys begin to conserve sodium. This sodium retention, added to sodium administration in I.V. fluids, may produce hypernatremia.
3. Monitor serum osmolality and electrolyte values, as ordered. Report abnormal values to the doctor.	3. Laboratory values provide objective data on the type and degree of physiologic derangements present. They also provide a rational basis for therapy: Serum osmolality values guide fluid replacement, whereas electrolyte values guide electrolyte repletion.
4. On admission, establish and maintain one or more I.V. lines in large peripheral veins.	4. Dehydration is the most immediately life-threatening aspect of DKA. Large veins permit the rapid administration of large amounts of fluid necessary to reverse the severe dehydration.
5. Insert an indwelling urinary catheter, as ordered. Monitor intake and output (I&O) and specific gravity meticulously. Weigh the patient daily, and document findings.	5. An indwelling catheter facilitates accurate measurement of urinary fluid loss. I&O, specific gravity, and weight records provide data on the degree of fluid imbalance and therapeutic effectiveness. Initially, output will exceed intake markedly, unless severe dehydration and oliguria are present. As the patient is rehydrated, fluid losses continue for the first several hours until glycosuria and osmotic diuresis are controlled.
6. Administer I.V. solutions, as ordered, typically:	6. The selection of the appropriate type of I.V. fluid depends on the blood glucose and electrolyte levels, whereas the amount depends on the degree of preexisting fluid deficit and ongoing fluid losses. The average fluid deficit on admission is 6 liters. Volume repletion is essential in reversing hypovolemia and allowing continued renal glucose excretion, an important compensatory mechanism in restoring glucose levels to normal range.
• normal saline solution, 1 to 2 liters in the first 2 hours	• Normal saline solution replaces volume and sodium lost in DKA without increasing blood glucose.
• plasma volume expanders, such as albumin, if dehydration is severe (administer only after normal saline solution administration is underway)	• Usually, normal saline administration is sufficient to reverse volume depletion. In severe dehydration, plasma volume expanders may be necessary. If they are administered before normal saline solution, however, their hypertonicity increases cellular dehydration.
• 0.45% sodium chloride, after the first few hours, or 0.45% sodium chloride with 5% dextrose in water when blood glucose level reaches 250 mg/dl or urinary glucose level is <1%.	• As the serum sodium level returns to normal, the saline concentration in I.V. solutions is reduced to prevent sodium overload. A solution containing glucose may be used as the blood glucose level returns to normal to prevent hypoglycemia (as described in the next problem).
7. Administer therapy for electrolyte imbalances, as ordered.	7. Hyperkalemia, hyponatremia, and hypernatremia usually resolve with appropriate fluid administration and control of hyperglycemia. Hypokalemia usually requires I.V. administration of supplemental potassium.
8. For at least 24 hours after rapid fluid repletion, observe for signs and symptoms of pulmonary edema, such as crackles, dyspnea, cough, or frothy sputum. If any are present, alert the doctor immediately.	8. Rapid fluid repletion causes hemodilution. Lowered plasma oncotic pressure may allow fluid to leak into the pulmonary interstitial space, producing pulmonary edema. Pulmonary edema requires prompt aggressive medical intervention.
9. Additional individualized interventions: ______	9. Rationales: ______

Target outcome criteria

Within 12 hours after the onset of therapy, the patient will:
- have blood pressure and cardiac rate and rhythm within normal limits
- display adequate peripheral perfusion, as manifested by strong peripheral pulses and capillary refill time <3 seconds.

Within 24 hours after the onset of therapy, the patient will:
- have urine output of 60 to 100 ml/hour
- have a balanced I&O
- have normal skin turgor, mucous membrane moisture, and other clinical signs of adequate hydration
- show no signs or symptoms of electrolyte imbalances.

Collaborative problem: *Hyperglycemia related to decreased cellular glucose uptake and utilization*

NURSING PRIORITY: Restore glucose control gradually.

Interventions	Rationales
1. Assess blood glucose levels on admission and as ordered. Perform bedside fingerstick monitoring of blood glucose every hour until normal, then every 6 hours or as ordered. Monitor urine glucose levels only if bedside blood glucose monitoring is unavailable.	1. Blood glucose levels provide the most direct indication of the degree of deranged glucose metabolism and are used to determine therapy. As glomerular filtration of glucose exceeds the transport maximum, glucose spills into the urine. Because blood glucose levels are much more accurate than urine glucose levels, urine checks are being phased out in favor of fingerstick bedside monitoring of glucose levels.
2. Assess blood ketone level on admission and as ordered. Perform bedside urine ketone monitoring every hour until stable, then every 6 hours.	2. When carbohydrate metabolism is impaired, the body uses fat as an alternate energy source. Lipolysis produces free fatty acids, which when oxidized produce ketone bodies. Blood ketone levels directly reflect the degree of ketogenesis occurring. The body initially compensates for ketogenesis by buffering ketoacids with bicarbonate. When ketoacid production exceeds buffering, ketoacids accumulate in the blood, producing acidosis. Some of the excess ketoacids are excreted in the urine (largely as sodium salts). Urine ketone levels measure ketone excretion.
3. Administer insulin, as ordered, typically an initial I.V. bolus of regular insulin followed by periodic boluses or a continuous I.V. infusion.	3. Administration of exogenous insulin controls the gluconeogenesis and ketogenesis occurring and increases cellular glucose uptake. In profound dehydration, tissue absorption of medications may be erratic, so subcutaneous and intramuscular routes are not preferred; the intravenous route is most reliable. The optimal dose and type of I.V. administration are controversial. High-dose insulin therapy, although effective, increases the risks of hypoglycemia and cerebral edema from lowering the blood glucose level too rapidly, as explained in the next problem. Low-dose therapy, although equally as effective as high-dose therapy in many cases, carries the risk of undertreatment. Periodic boluses may allow swings in blood glucose. Continuous infusion may allow delivery of unexpectedly low dosage because insulin binds to I.V. tubing and bottle or bag of solution.

(continued)

Interventions	Rationales
4. Alert the doctor when the blood glucose level reaches 250 mg/dl or urinary glucose level is <1%.	4. As metabolic control is reestablished, blood glucose level may drop precipitously from the combined effects of therapy and the body's continuing glycosuria. At 250 mg/dl, the intravenous fluids should be changed from normal saline solution to one containing glucose, or the insulin dose should be reduced to avoid hypoglycemia. A urine glucose level below 1% could indicate normoglycemia; however, it also is found in hypoglycemia, a threat to survival. For this reason, urine glucose levels should not be allowed to drop below 1%; doing so negates their value in detecting hypoglycemia.
5. Observe for signs and symptoms of medication-induced hypoglycemia, such as headache, confusion, irritability, restlessness, trembling, pallor, diaphoresis, and stupor. If these signs and symptoms are present, notify the doctor, obtain a blood glucose level without delay, and treat immediately with I.V. glucose, glucagon, or oral glucose, depending upon unit protocol and the patient's level of consciousness.	5. The brain depends on glucose almost exclusively for energy. Hypoglycemia produces dramatic cerebral dysfunction and a profound stress response. The longer hypoglycemia persists, the greater the chance of transient or permanent neurologic damage. Hypoglycemic reactions may be fatal if left untreated.
6. Additional individualized interventions: ______	6. Rationales: ______

Target outcome criteria

Within 2 hours of the onset of therapy, the patient will display a blood glucose level returning to normal.

Within 24 hours of the onset of therapy, the patient will:
- display a blood glucose level <250 mg/dl
- have urine negative for ketones.

Nursing diagnosis: *Sensory-perceptual alteration related to cerebral dehydration, decreased perfusion, hypoxemia, or acidosis*

NURSING PRIORITIES: (a) Ensure patient safety, and (b) monitor return to the patient's usual level of consciousness (LOC).

Interventions	Rationales
1. Implement standard safety precautions, such as keeping side rails up, for critically ill patients.	1. A decreased LOC makes patients unable to protect themselves from accidental injury.
2. Observe LOC constantly. Alert the doctor if LOC does not return to normal within 2 hours of the onset of therapy.	2. Decreased LOC in early DKA may result from hyperosmolality, marked cellular dehydration produced by osmotic diuresis, altered cellular function from anaerobic metabolism, or acidotic cerebrospinal fluid. Persistently decreased or worsening LOC may result from cerebral edema caused by a precipitous lowering of the blood glucose level. Rapid lowering creates a substantial difference between blood glucose concentration and the concentration of glucose metabolites in the brain. The resulting osmotic gradient draws water into the brain, producing cerebral edema. LOC should return to normal with therapy; failure to do so suggests the possibility of other disorders and requires further medical evaluation.
3. Additional individualized interventions: ______	3. Rationales: ______

Target outcome criteria
Within 24 hours of the onset of therapy, the patient will display his normal LOC.

Collaborative problem: *Acidosis related to altered LOC, ketosis, and decreased tissue perfusion*

NURSING PRIORITIES: (a) Maintain optimal ventilation and oxygenation, and (b) restore normal acid-base balance.

Interventions	Rationales
1. Maintain a patent airway.	1. Decreased LOC increases aspiration risk.
2. Monitor respiratory status every hour, including:	2. Serial assessments allow timely detection of respiratory abnormalities.
• respiratory rate and depth	• The body responds to ketoacidosis, a form of metabolic acidosis, by increasing the rate and depth of ventilation to blow off carbon dioxide and induce a compensatory respiratory alkalosis. The presence of Kussmaul's breathing indicates severe acidosis.
• breath odor	• Acetone breath indicates respiratory excretion of ketones.
• breath sounds.	• Breath sounds indicate the adequacy of ventilation and may indicate pneumonia (an infection that may have precipitated DKA) or fluid overload.
3. Anticipate intubation and mechanical ventilation if increasing respiratory distress is present.	3. These measures may be necessary for some patients to maintain airway patency and ventilatory adequacy.
4. Administer oxygen, as ordered.	4. Acidosis impairs oxygen delivery to tissues. Hypoxia provokes anaerobic metabolism, which produces lactic acid and further worsens the metabolic acidosis. Supplemental oxygen elevates arterial oxygen tension, reducing the need for anaerobic metabolism.
5. Monitor ABG levels, as ordered.	5. ABG levels document the type and degree of acid-base imbalances present and the effectiveness of therapy for DKA. Abnormalities normally resolve with fluid and electrolyte replacement and insulin therapy.
6. Administer I.V. sodium bicarbonate, as ordered, typically if pH is <7.1 or bicarbonate <10 mEq/liter.	6. These parameters indicate severe acidosis. Bicarbonate administration replenishes bicarbonate ions, which buffer excessive hydrogen ions, thus returning pH to normal.
7. While the patient is acutely ill, withhold food and fluids, even if the patient is extremely thirsty. Insert a gastric tube, as ordered, and connect to suction. Auscultate bowel sounds every 8 hours. Remove the gastric tube and allow oral intake of food and fluids only after LOC and bowel sounds return to normal.	7. Intense thirst is a compensatory mechanism for volume depletion, but oral fluid intake can be dangerous. Because hyperglycemia decreases bowel motility, patients commonly suffer from abdominal pain, nausea, and vomiting. Vomiting increases the risk of aspiration. Bowel sounds reflect gastrointestinal motility. Allowing oral intake only after bowel sounds and LOC are normal reduces the risk of aspiration.

(continued)

Interventions	Rationales
8. Additional individualized interventions: ______	8. Rationales: ______

Target outcome criteria

Within 24 hours of the onset of therapy, the patient will:
- breathe at a rate of 12 to 24 respirations per minute
- display eupnea.

Within 36 hours of the onset of therapy, the patient will:
- have ABG levels within normal limits
- have normal bowel sounds
- be able to take oral food and fluids safely.

Nursing diagnosis: *Knowledge deficit related to complex disease and therapy*

NURSING PRIORITY: Identify and meet immediate learning needs.

Interventions	Rationales
1. Refer to the "Knowledge Deficit" care plan, page 45.	1. The "Knowledge Deficit" care plan provides general guidelines for patient teaching.
2. When the patient's condition allows, determine learning needs. Ascertain whether DM is a new or previously identified diagnosis. If the patient is a known diabetic, assess for possible precipitators of DKA, for example, a missed insulin dose or overlooked signs of infection.	2. Learning needs vary depending upon whether the patient is a new or known diabetic. If the patient is newly diabetic, extensive teaching is necessary. With a known diabetic, DKA episodes are usually preventable, and instruction may focus on previously unmet teaching needs or areas needing reinforcement.
3. When the patient's condition allows, begin a teaching program.	3. Although teaching is crucial to successful management of DM, physiologic needs take precedence in the critical care unit (CCU) phase, and extensive teaching may need to be deferred until after the patient is stabilized.
• Use the patient's symptomatic episode as a teaching tool. Involve the family members in all teaching sessions.	• The immediacy of the DKA episode makes it a powerful teaching tool for actively involving the patient and family.
• As appropriate, initiate teaching about the cause of diabetes, signs and symptoms, significance of insulin, injection techniques, factors affecting medication needs (such as food intake and exercise), therapeutic diet, blood and urine testing, importance of consistent level of daily exercise, increased susceptibility to infections, recognition and management of hyperglycemic and hypoglycemic episodes, and long-range complications, such as neuropathy and retinopathy. Refer to the "Diabetes Mellitus" care plan in *Medical-Surgical Care Plans* edited by Nancy Holloway (Springhouse, 1988) for details.	• Although the patient's and family's knowledge of all the facets identified are essential for appropriate ongoing home management of DM, only initial teaching is feasible in the CCU. The "Diabetes Mellitus" care plan contains detailed information on each of these aspects.
4. Document learning needs and teaching. When the patient is transferred out of the CCU, communicate learning needs and arrange with colleagues for continuation of the teaching plan.	4. The patient's condition, extensiveness of learning needs, and the hectic CCU atmosphere may mean that the patient is likely to be transferred before completing all teaching. Documentation and communication enhance continuity of care.
5. Additional individualized interventions: ______	5. Rationales: ______

Target outcome criteria
By the time of transfer, the patient and family will:
• identify learning needs
• show beginning involvement in the teaching-learning process, if appropriate.

Transfer planning

NURSING TRANSFER CRITERIA

Upon transfer, documentation shows evidence of:
• stable vital signs within normal limits
• blood glucose level within normal limits without I.V. insulin
• return to premorbid LOC—ideally, alert and oriented
• ABG levels within normal limits.

PATIENT-FAMILY TEACHING CHECKLIST

Document evidence that patient and family demonstrate understanding of initial teaching related to:
__ cause and implications of DM
__ precipitators of DKA, including signs and symptoms and appropriate responses
__ significance of insulin
__ signs, symptoms, and interventions for hyperglycemia and hypoglycemia
__ dietary management
__ exercise plan
__ blood and urine testing
__ plan for completing unmet learning needs.

DOCUMENTATION CHECKLIST

Using outcome criteria as a guide, document:
__ clinical status on admission
__ significant changes in status
__ pertinent diagnostic test findings
__ I.V. fluid therapy
__ pharmacologic intervention
__ oxygen administration
__ patient and family teaching
__ transfer planning.

ASSOCIATED CARE PLANS

Acute Renal Failure
Grieving and Dying
Hyperglycemic Hyperosmolar Nonketotic Coma
Knowledge Deficit
Sensory-Perceptual Alteration
Shock

REFERENCES

Carroll, P., and Matz, R. "Uncontrolled Diabetes Mellitus in Adults: Experience in Treating Diabetic Ketoacidosis and Hyperosmolar Nonketotic Coma with Low-Dose Insulin and a Uniform Treatment Regime," *Diabetes Care* 6:6, 1983.

Davidoff, F. "Diabetic Emergencies," in *Critical Care Nursing: A Holistic Approach*, 4th ed. Edited by Hudak, C., Gallo, B., and Lohr, T. Philadelphia: J.B. Lippincott Co., 1986.

Foster, D., and McGarry, J. "The Metabolic Derangements and Treatment of Diabetic Ketoacidosis," *New England Journal of Medicine* 309:159-69, 1983.

Kriesberg, R. "Diabetic Ketoacidosis, Alcoholic Ketosis, Lactic Acidosis, and Hyporeninemic Hypoaldosteronism," in *Diabetes Mellitus: Theory and Practice*, 3rd ed. Edited by Ellinberg, M., and Pitkin, H. New York: Medical Publishing Co., 1983.

Malone, R. "Diabetes Mellitus," in *Medical-Surgical Care Plans*. Edited by Holloway, N. Springhouse, Pa.: Springhouse Corp., 1988.

Tueller, B. "Endocrine-Metabolic Imbalances," in *Nursing the Critically Ill Adult*, 3rd ed. Edited by Holloway, N. Menlo Park, Calif.: Addison-Wesley Publishing Co., 1988.

Hyperglycemic Hyperosmolar Nonketosis

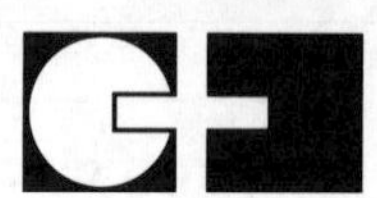

DRG information

DRG 294 Diabetes. Age > 35.
Mean LOS = 6.1 days
Principal diagnosis includes diabetes with hyperosmolar nonketotic coma

DRG 295 Diabetes. Age 0 to 35.
Mean LOS = 4.5 days

Introduction

DEFINITION AND TIME FOCUS

Hyperglycemic hyperosmolar nonketosis (HHNK) is an endocrine emergency with a mortality rate as high as 50%, if left untreated. Like diabetic ketoacidosis (DKA), it produces profound hyperglycemia and hyperosmolality, but unlike DKA, ketosis and acidosis are absent. It presents a diagnostic puzzle because its clinical picture is similar to both DKA and cerebrovascular accidents. It may occur in Type I or Type II diabetes mellitus (DM) but is more common in Type II.

The basic defect in HHNK is a relative insulin deficiency in which enough insulin is secreted to prevent ketoacidosis but not enough to prevent hyperglycemia. Failure to recognize or respond to the thirst mechanism, which signals developing dehydration, exacerbates the problem. This care plan focuses on the patient admitted to the critical care unit with HHNK.

ETIOLOGY AND PRECIPITATING FACTORS

- undiagnosed DM
- previously stable DM that now requires increased insulin because of trauma, surgery, infection, or other conditions
- pharmacologic agents that impair insulin release or accelerate glucose production, such as thiazide diuretics, phenytoin (Dilantin), or glucocorticoids
- prolonged high-carbohydrate enteral or parenteral nutrition
- dialysis with hyperosmolar glucose solutions

Focused assessment guidelines

NURSING HISTORY (Functional health pattern findings)

Health perception–health management pattern

Note: History usually is obtained from a family member or friend because the patient's level of consciousness is decreased.

- underlying major illness, usually cardiovascular, pulmonary, renal, or endocrine
- usual age, 50 or older
- slow onset of symptoms, typically over days to weeks

Nutritional-metabolic pattern

- typically does not seem thirsty in response to developing dehydration

Elimination pattern

- may have complained of polyuria (early stage)

Cognitive-perceptual pattern

- may have complained of or displayed increasing drowsiness or confusion

PHYSICAL FINDINGS

Neurologic

- decreased level of consciousness, ranging from confusion to coma
- seizures

Pulmonary

- tachypnea
- absence of Kussmaul's breathing (differential finding from DKA)
- absence of acetone breath (differential finding from DKA)

Cardiovascular

- tachycardia
- hypotension
- capillary refill time >3 seconds

Renal

- polyuria (early stage)
- oliguria (late stage)

Integumentary

- dry skin
- poor skin turgor
- dry mucous membranes

Gastrointestinal

- decreased or absent bowel sounds

DIAGNOSTIC STUDIES

- blood glucose levels—markedly elevated, typically 600 to 1,800 mg/dl (higher than DKA).
- serum osmolality levels—elevated, typically >350 mOsm/kg.
- serum ketone test—negative (differential finding from DKA).
- urine glucose levels—positive.

• urine ketone test—negative (differential finding from DKA).
• blood urea nitrogen and creatinine levels—elevated, reflecting decreased renal perfusion.
• serum electrolyte levels—variable, typically marked hypernatremia and hypokalemia.
• arterial blood gas (ABG) values—show slight metabolic acidosis.
• blood, urine, wound, or sputum cultures— used to identify infection.
• 12-lead EKG—may reveal dysrhythmias.
• chest X-ray—used to identify pulmonary infection, a common precipitator of HHNK.

POTENTIAL COMPLICATIONS
• hypovolemic shock
• acute renal failure
• congestive heart failure
• disseminated intravascular coagulation
• pulmonary edema
• cerebral edema

Collaborative problem: *Hypovolemia related to osmotic diuresis*

NURSING PRIORITY: Restore fluid volume.

Interventions	Rationales
1. Monitor for signs and symptoms of dehydration and shock, such as tachycardia; hypotension; weak peripheral pulses; capillary refill time >3 seconds; warm, dry, flushed skin; poor skin turgor; polyuria or oliguria; increased hematocrit; increased urine specific gravity; and increased serum osmolality. Monitor blood pressure and cardiac rate and rhythm continuously.	1. Impaired insulin release or peripheral insulin resistance causes hyperglycemia, which in turn causes hyperosmolality. To compensate for the hyperosmolality, fluid shifts from the intracellular to the extracellular space, dehydrating cells. Renal glucose spillage, an important compensatory mechanism for hyperglycemia, triggers an intense osmotic diuresis. This diuresis causes obligatory fluid and electrolyte losses, reflected in an elevated hematocrit and increased serum osmolality. Severe hypovolemia decreases glomerular filtration, aggravating the hyperglycemia and hyperosmolality and eventually producing oliguria and increased specific gravity. HHNK patients usually have a greater fluid loss than in DKA. As volume is restored, signs and symptoms should resolve gradually; failure to do so indicates inadequate fluid replacement or continuing losses.
2. Observe for signs and symptoms of electrolyte imbalances, particularly hypernatremia and hypokalemia (see the "Fluid and Electrolyte Imbalances" appendix, page 317, for details). Monitor serum electrolyte levels, as ordered, and report abnormal values to the doctor. Administer electrolyte replacements, as ordered.	2. Electrolyte status may change rapidly in response to fluid shifts, so close observation for signs and symptoms of imbalances is essential. Hypernatremia results from the large water deficit. In contrast to DKA patients, whose acidosis causes hyperkalemia that commonly masks a low total body potassium, HHNK patients develop hypokalemia, reflecting urinary losses. Hypernatremia usually resolves with fluid administration, whereas hypokalemia usually requires earlier potassium replacement than with DKA. Potassium doses depend on serum potassium levels.
3. Monitor serum osmolality, as ordered. Report levels >295 mOsm/kg.	3. Laboratory values document the extent of hyperosmolality, which usually is more marked than in DKA because of the failure of the thirst mechanism and the intense osmotic diuresis, as previously described.
4. Implement standard measures for hypovolemia, as ordered: Maintain patency of one or more I.V. lines, insert an indwelling (Foley) urinary catheter, and monitor intake and output and daily weights. Refer to the "Diabetic Ketoacidosis" care plan, page 214, for details.	4. These measures are the same as with DKA. The "Diabetic Ketoacidosis" care plan describes these interventions and associated rationales in detail.
5. Administer I.V. solutions, as ordered, typically 6 to 8 liters in the first 12 hours:	5. Aggressive fluid repletion is necessary because of the large fluid volume deficit in HHNK.

(continued)

Interventions	Rationales
• normal saline solution if serum sodium level is <130 mEq/liter	• A very low serum sodium level reflects large urinary sodium losses. Isotonic saline solution replaces sodium and replenishes volume.
• 0.45% saline solution if serum sodium level is >145 mEq/liter	• An elevated serum sodium reflects decreased glomerular filtration and avid sodium retention in severe hypovolemia. Hypotonic fluid provides free water to reverse hyperosmolality.
• dextrose in water when blood glucose levels reach 250 mg/dl or serum osmolality reaches 300 mOsm/liter.	• As blood glucose or serum osmolality approaches normal level, changing to a glucose-containing solution prevents hypoglycemia.
6. During fluid replacement, monitor closely for signs and symptoms of fluid overload, including crackles, S_3 heart sound, neck-vein distention, dyspnea, or persistently depressed level of consciousness. If any indicators are present, notify the doctor.	6. Because HHNK patients usually are elderly and have significant preexisting disease, they are more prone to develop congestive heart failure, pulmonary edema, or cerebral edema than are DKA patients. These signs and symptoms require medical evaluation.
7. Additional individualized interventions: ____________	7. Rationales: ____________

Target outcome criteria
Within 24 hours of the onset of therapy, the patient will:
- have blood pressure, cardiac rate and rhythm, and peripheral perfusion within normal limits
- display a urine output of 60 to 100 ml/hour
- manifest serum osmolality levels within normal limits
- manifest serum electrolyte levels within normal limits.

Collaborative problem: *Hyperglycemia related to inadequate insulin secretion, or peripheral insulin resistance, or both*

NURSING PRIORITY: Lower blood glucose.

Interventions	Rationales
1. Implement measures for this problem contained in the "Diabetic Ketoacidosis" care plan, page 214, but with the following modifications:	1. Care for this problem is similar for HHNK patients and DKA patients, but with different emphasis on two points.
• Administer low-dose insulin judiciously, as ordered.	• Because patients have some endogenous insulin production, they are more sensitive to exogenous insulin than are DKA patients, and lower insulin doses are usually needed.
• Monitor very closely for medication-induced hypoglycemia.	• Because HHNK patients retain some control of glucose metabolism, they are especially vulnerable to developing hypoglycemia in response to measures that lower blood glucose.
2. If the patient has developed HHNK while on high-carbohydrate enteral nutrition or hyperosmolar dialysis, consult with the doctor about revising orders for these therapies.	2. Modifying or discontinuing these precipitators of HHNK removes an unnecessary glucose load for the patient.
3. Additional individualized interventions: ____________	3. Rationales: ____________

Target outcome criteria
Within 24 hours of the onset of therapy, the patient will display a blood glucose level <250 mg/dl.

Nursing diagnosis: *Sensory-perceptual alteration related to cerebral dehydration, decreased perfusion, hypoxemia, glucose deprivation, or cerebral edema during rapid rehydration*

NURSING PRIORITIES: (a) Restore the patient's level of consciousness, and (b) protect the patient from injury.

Interventions	Rationales
1. Evaluate neurologic status every 1 to 4 hours, as indicated by the rapidity of other changes in the patient's condition. Alert the doctor to deepening coma or other indications of deteriorating neurologic functioning.	1. Neurologic changes, which are characteristic of this disorder, correlate closely with the degree of hyperosmolality. Deteriorating neurologic function may indicate explosive pathophysiologic derangements, other previously undetected disorders, or inadequate therapy, and it requires medical evaluation.
2. Institute seizure precautions. Report any seizure activity to the doctor promptly.	2. Seizures occur commonly with HHNK, as a result of cerebral dehydration, cerebral edema (during rehydration), or glucose deprivation (if hypoglycemia occurs).
3. Additional individualized interventions: ______	3. Rationales: ______

Target outcome criteria
Within 24 hours, the patient will display his usual neurologic status; ideally, alert, oriented, and able to move all extremities.

Nursing diagnosis: *Knowledge deficit related to complex disease process*

NURSING PRIORITY: Teach the patient and family to avoid recurrence of HHNK, if appropriate.

Interventions	Rationales
1. Identify cause of HHNK. If it is DM, implement measures for this problem contained in the "Diabetic Ketoacidosis" care plan, page 214, as appropriate.	1. The "Diabetic Ketoacidosis" care plan details measures that also apply to teaching some HHNK patients. It is pertinent to patients with uncontrolled DM whose pathophysiologic process is ongoing and in whom HHNK may recur. It is inappropriate for patients whose HHNK resulted from high-carbohydrate nutrition or hyperosmolar dialysis; their HHNK should not recur once the cause has been removed.
2. Additional individualized interventions: ______	2. Rationales: ______

Target outcome criteria
By the time of transfer, the patient and family will:
• identify learning needs
• show beginning involvement in the teaching-learning process, if appropriate.

Transfer planning

NURSING TRANSFER CRITERIA

Upon transfer, documentation shows evidence of:
• stable vital signs within normal limits
• blood glucose level within normal limits without I.V. insulin
• return to usual LOC
• ABG levels within normal limits.

PATIENT-FAMILY TEACHING CHECKLIST

Document evidence that patient and family demonstrate understanding of:
___ cause and significance of HHNK
___ precipitators of HHNK and methods to decrease risk.
If the patient has DM, also document understanding of the following items:
___ oral hypoglycemic agents, if appropriate
___ signs, symptoms, and interventions for hyperglycemia and hypoglycemia
___ dietary management
___ exercise plan
___ blood and urine testing
___ learning needs at time of transfer.

DOCUMENTATION CHECKLIST

Using outcome criteria as a guide, document:
___ clinical status on admission
___ significant changes in status
___ pertinent laboratory and diagnostic test findings
___ I.V. fluid therapy
___ pharmacologic intervention
___ patient-family teaching
___ transfer planning.

ASSOCIATED CARE PLANS

Acute Renal Failure
Diabetic Ketoacidosis
Disseminated Intravascular Coagulation
Grieving and Dying
Knowledge Deficit
Shock

REFERENCES

Malone, R. "Diabetes Mellitus," in *Medical-Surgical Care Plans.* Edited by Holloway, N. Springhouse, Pa.: Springhouse Corp., 1988.

Tueller, B. "Hyperosmolar Hyperglycemic Nonketotic Coma," in *Nursing the Critically Ill Adult,* 3rd ed. Edited by Holloway, N. Menlo Park, Calif.: Addison-Wesley Publishing Co., 1988.

Acute Renal Failure

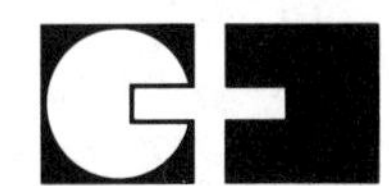

DRG information

DRG 316 Renal Failure.
Mean LOS = 6.2 days
Principal diagnoses include:
• chronic or unspecified renal failure
• acute renal failure (unspecified, with renal cortical necrosis, renal medullary necrosis, or tubular necrosis, or with other specified pathologic lesion in kidney)
• oliguria or anuria.
Additional DRG information: Renal failure accompanied by any operative procedure will not be classified under DRG 316.

DRG 317 Admit for Renal Dialysis.
Mean LOS = 1.8 days
Principal diagnoses include aftercare involving intermittent dialysis.

Additional DRG information: Patients who are in renal failure but who are not admitted for intermittent dialysis are coded differently from renal failure patients who are admitted for intermittent dialysis. For the latter group, the principal diagnosis is actually "Admission for Dialysis"; the renal failure becomes a secondary diagnosis.

Introduction

DEFINITION AND TIME FOCUS

Acute renal failure (ARF) is a sudden cessation or decrease in renal function. In ARF, the kidneys cannot maintain fluid and electrolyte balance and cannot filter metabolic waste products. ARF disrupts all body systems and may cause problems in cardiac, respiratory, gastrointestinal, neurologic, musculoskeletal, integumentary, genitourinary, and endocrine-metabolic functions. Mortality can be high depending on the cause, the patient's age, and related physical problems.

ARF patients who recover progress through three stages: oliguria, diuresis, and recovery. The oliguric stage lasts about 2 weeks (a shorter period represents a better prognosis). The diuretic stage may last several weeks. The recovery stage may last up to a year, with initial rapid improvement and a continuing slow return to near-normal function. If the patient does not recover, long-term hemodialysis, peritoneal dialysis, or kidney transplantation is necessary.

This clinical plan focuses on the patient admitted to the critical care unit for ARF treatment, including identification of its cause and support of body systems until the kidneys begin to recover, or evaluation for dialysis or transplantation.

ETIOLOGY AND PRECIPITATING FACTORS

- prerenal problems leading to decreased renal perfusion, such as hemorrhage, all forms of shock, excessive vomiting or diarrhea, heart failure or other causes of decreased cardiac output, burns, excessive diuresis, third-spacing of fluids, hypotension, vasodilation, or obstruction of the aorta or renal arteries
- renal (parenchymal) problems leading to destruction of kidney tissue, such as acute tubular necrosis from ischemia or nephrotoxins, glomerulonephritis, emboli, allergic inflammation, or infections
- postrenal problems leading to obstruction of urine flow, such as calculi, prostate enlargement, tumors, or retroperitoneal fibrosis
- preexisting multisystem problems increase risk of ARF, especially in an older patient

Focused assessment guidelines

NURSING HISTORY (Functional health pattern findings)

Health perception–health management pattern

- may report decreased amount and frequency of urination
- may report headaches, swelling of feet and ankles, and palpitations
- may report a recent high ARF risk episode, such as infection; cardiac, aortic, or biliary surgery; trauma; ingestion of aspirin, antibiotics, or other drugs; exposure to toxins; or an allergic response to food, drugs, or blood transfusions
- may have a history of urinary tract infections, diabetes mellitus, hypertension, kidney disease, or cardiac or liver problems
- may report pain around the flank or costal margin areas

Nutritional-metabolic pattern

- may report loss of appetite, nausea
- may report a weight gain or loss
- may report a "funny" taste in mouth
- may report increased saliva or a dry mouth

Elimination pattern

- may report decreased or absent urination
- may report a change in urine color and smell
- may report abdominal cramps, a feeling of fullness, diarrhea, or constipation
- may report pruritus

Activity-exercise pattern
• may report difficulty in breathing at rest and during exercise
• may report weakness and fatigue
• may report muscle cramps

Sleep-rest pattern
• may report longer sleep periods than usual

Cognitive-perceptual pattern
• may report periods of dizziness
• may report memory loss and inability to concentrate

Role-relationship pattern
• may have job with exposure to nephrotoxic chemicals, such as carbon tetrachloride, dyes, fungicides, pesticides, or heavy metals

Sexuality-reproductive pattern
• may report loss of sexual drive, impotence, or loss of menstruation

Coping–stress tolerance pattern
• may report increased irritability and decreased ability to handle stress

PHYSICAL FINDINGS
Note: Physical findings may vary, depending on the cause, type, and stage of ARF.

Genitourinary
• oliguria (<400 ml/24 hours)
• less commonly, anuria (<50 ml/24 hours) or high urine output (1 to 2 liters/24 hours)
• abnormal urine color, clarity, or smell (such as red or brown color, cloudiness, or foul smell)

Neurologic
• lethargy, apathy
• tremors, convulsions
• memory loss, confusion
• coma

Cardiovascular
• dysrhythmias
• bounding, rapid pulse; normal or high blood pressure; and distended neck veins (with hypervolemia)
• tachycardia, low blood pressure, or orthostatic hypotension (with hypovolemia)
• pericardial-type chest pain (mild to severe pain that may increase with movement or decrease with leaning forward)
• anemia

Pulmonary
• rapid respirations, dyspnea, or crackles (with hypervolemia)
• tachypnea (with hypovolemia)
• Kussmaul's respirations (with acidosis)

Gastrointestinal
• moist tongue and increased saliva (with hypervolemia)
• dry tongue and mucous membranes (with hypovolemia)
• vomiting
• diarrhea
• stomatitis

Musculoskeletal
• muscle spasms (tetany)
• weakness
• asterixis

Integumentary
• moist, warm skin and pitting edema over bony areas (with hypervolemia)
• decreased skin turgor and dry skin (with hypovolemia)
• bruises
• thin, brittle hair and nails
• pallor

DIAGNOSTIC STUDIES
• 24-hour urine output and serum creatinine and blood urea nitrogen (BUN) levels—monitor the kidneys' ability to excrete fluid and waste products. Oliguric ARF is characterized by oliguria and rising BUN and creatinine levels. About 25% of patients may have non-oliguric ARF with a urine output of 1 to 2 liters/24 hours and rising BUN and creatinine levels. The diuretic stage is characterized by increasing urine outputs (2 to 3 liters/24 hours), indicating returning glomerular filtration. BUN and creatinine levels remain high during this stage because the kidneys cannot concentrate the urine effectively. As the kidneys regain concentrating ability during the recovery stage, the BUN and creatinine levels begin to fall and stabilize at normal or near-normal levels depending upon the residual damage to the kidneys.
• serum electrolyte panel—monitors fluid, electrolyte, and acid-base status. Elevated potassium, sodium, and phosphate levels; decreased calcium level; and a decreased pH level indicate poor renal function.
• urinalysis—monitors renal excretion and concentration abilities. Sodium and potassium concentrations may vary, depending on the cause and type of ARF. Casts, crystals, hematuria, and proteinuria may be present. White blood cells (WBCs) may indicate infection. With pre-renal conditions, specific gravity and osmolality may be high; with renal conditions, they may be constant at 1.010 mOsm and approximately 300 respectively.
• creatinine clearance—reflects glomerular filtration rate (GFR) and is an accurate indication of renal function. A decrease indicates a poor GFR. A value of 50 to 84 ml/minute indicates mild failure; 10 to 49 ml/minute, moderate failure; and <10 ml/minute, severe failure.
• urine-plasma creatinine concentration ratios and urine-plasma urea concentration ratios—reflect the kidneys' ability to save water and excrete wastes. Values

vary in degree of abnormality depending upon cause and type of ARF. In prerenal failure, ratios are high, reflecting kidney conservation of sodium and water; in acute tubular insufficiency, the kidneys' inability to perform these functions results in low urine-plasma ratios.
• BUN-to-creatinine ratio—reflects GFR and tubular function. In prerenal failure, the ratio is high (usually >20:1), reflecting increased tubular reabsorption of urea. In acute tubular insufficiency, the ratio remains approximately 10:1, reflecting increased reabsorption of both urea and creatinine by the damaged tubules.
• complete blood count (CBC)—may reveal low red blood cell (RBC) count, hemoglobin, and hematocrit, reflecting anemia. An elevated WBC count may reflect infection.
• coagulation studies—may be abnormal if disseminated intravascular coagulation (DIC) is the cause of ARF.
• Renal concentration tests—may show the kidneys' inability to concentrate solutes in urine.
• EKG—may show dysrhythmias or high, peaked T waves and flattened P waves, and widened QRS complexes associated with high potassium levels.
• kidney-ureter-bladder (KUB) X-rays—show size, structure, and position of kidneys, ureters, and bladder. The kidneys may be normal or enlarged in ARF. Changes in bladder or ureters point to a postrenal cause of ARF.
• computed tomography scan—shows cross-sectional views of renal structures.
• ultrasonic scan—may show abnormalities in kidney size and shape, internally and externally.
• I.V. or retrograde pyelogram—may show obstruction, constriction, or masses.
• renal biopsy—may help differentiate parenchymal kidney diseases.
• renal angiography—may show renal artery abnormalities, cysts, or tumors.
• radionuclide tests (renal scan and renogram)—may show abnormal distributions of radioactive compounds, indicating structural abnormalities or impaired perfusion or uptake.
• cystoscopy—may show urethra and bladder abnormalities.

POTENTIAL COMPLICATIONS

Note: Most complications result from the uremic syndrome—the accumulation of waste products in the blood. Some complications result from the kidneys' inability to maintain the normal hormonal functions of stimulating RBC production, regulating calcium absorption, and controlling the renin-angiotensin system.
• infection (sepsis is the most dangerous complication of ARF)
• stress ulcer
• heart failure
• pericarditis
• pneumonitis
• encephalopathy
• peripheral neuropathy
• coagulation defects
• pathologic fractures from bone demineralization
• gastrointestinal bleeding

Collaborative problem: *Electrolyte imbalance related to decreased electrolyte excretion, excessive intake, or metabolic acidosis*

NURSING PRIORITY: Prevent complications of electrolyte imbalance.

Interventions	Rationales
1. Monitor and document electrolyte levels every 8 to 12 hours and as needed, as ordered, particularly potassium, phosphate, calcium, and magnesium. See the "Fluid and Electrolyte Imbalances" appendix, page 317, for general assessment parameters and interventions for abnormal electrolyte levels.	1. The kidneys' inability to regulate electrolyte excretion and reabsorption may result in high potassium and phosphate levels, a low calcium level, and either a high or a low magnesium level. These levels can change quickly and result in such complications as cardiac dysrhythmias, muscle response changes, mentation changes, skin irritation, and even death. General assessment parameters and interventions are included in the "Fluid and Electrolyte Imbalances" appendix.
2. Continuously monitor the EKG and document. See "Monitoring Standards" appendix, page 314. Note and promptly report peaked, high T waves; prolonged PR interval; or a widened QRS.	2. Electrolyte abnormalities can trigger dysrhythmias and cardiac arrest. "Monitoring Standards" appendix contains general assessments for dysrhythmias. The signs listed indicate hyperkalemia severe enough to be an EKG emergency.
3. If hyperkalemia is present, implement the following measures, as ordered, and document:	3. The kidneys' inability to excrete the potassium released into the serum by normal cellular metabolism results in dangerously high potassium levels.

(continued)

Interventions	Rationales
• I.V. glucose (50%) and insulin solution	• Glucose and insulin may transport potassium into cells temporarily, thus lowering the serum potassium in an emergency situation.
• I.V. calcium chloride or calcium gluconate	• Calcium competes with potassium for entry into heart cells, thus decreasing the dangerous effect of hyperkalemia on cardiac rhythm.
• cation-exchange resins, such as sodium polystyrene sulfonate (Kayexalate), orally or rectally. Give sorbitol with Kayexalate. Do not give with fruit juices.	• Kayexalate removes potassium at the rate of 1 mEq/gram of drug by exchanging it for sodium in the bowel. Sorbitol helps remove the exchanged and bound potassium from the bowel by acting as an osmotic diarrheic. Fruit juices may bind with Kayexalate and decrease its effectiveness.
• I.V. sodium bicarbonate solution.	• ARF causes metabolic acidosis, which may increase the release of potassium from cells in exchange for hydrogen ions. Sodium bicarbonate corrects acidosis by combining with hydrogen ions, allowing potassium to move back into the cells.
4. Limit dietary and drug intake of potassium; for example, avoid juices high in potassium and drugs such as potassium penicillin or potassium-containing antacids.	4. When the kidneys cannot excrete potassium, excess intake can push serum potassium to dangerously high levels.
5. Give aluminum hydroxide antacid with meals and every 4 hours, as ordered. Document.	5. The kidneys cannot excrete the phosphates released from normal cellular metabolism or from dietary phosphate intake. Aluminum hydroxide binds with phosphate in the bowels and prevents absorption into the bloodstream, thus decreasing hyperphosphatemia.
6. Give calcium and vitamin supplements as needed and ordered. Document.	6. The kidneys' inability to stimulate the absorption of calcium in the bowel results in hypocalcemia and bone demineralization. High phosphate levels have an inverse effect on calcium levels, also causing hypocalcemia. Calcium and vitamin D supplements increase the serum calcium levels, helping to prevent bone demineralization and other adverse effects of low calcium.
7. Limit intake of magnesium, as in antacids.	7. The kidneys cannot excrete magnesium.
8. Give sodium chloride I.V., as needed and ordered. Document.	8. Usually, sodium intake is restricted to prevent fluid overload. However, major losses through vomiting, diarrhea, and wound drainage may cause a need for sodium replacement.
9. Additional individualized interventions: ______________________	9. Rationales: ______________________

Target outcome criteria

Within 8 hours after treatment for any hyperkalemic episode, the patient will:
- have a serum potassium level within normal limits
- show no EKG signs of hyperkalemia
- have arterial blood gas (ABG) levels within normal limits.

Within 24 hours of admission and then continuously, the patient will:
- have serum electrolyte levels within expected limits
- have normal sinus rhythm.

Nursing diagnosis: *Fluid volume excess related to sodium and water retention*

NURSING PRIORITIES: (a) Maintain adequate hydration, and (b) prevent fluid overload.

Interventions	Rationales
1. See the "Fluid and Electrolyte Imbalances" appendix, page 317.	1. This appendix contains general information on imbalances that is applicable to any patient. This plan presents additional information specific to ARF.
2. Assess for signs of fluid overload and document findings.	2. Inability to maintain normal fluid homeostasis results in fluid overload during the oliguric stage and potential dehydration during the diuretic stage.
• Assess the following every 1 to 2 hours: vital signs (blood pressure, pulse, respirations), central venous pressure (CVP), pulmonary artery wedge pressure (PAWP), pulmonary artery end-diastolic pressure (PAEDP), mean arterial pressure (MAP), adventitious lung sounds such as crackles or rhonchi, and peripheral edema. Measure cardiac output (CO), as ordered, typically every 12 hours. Assess the following daily: weight and CBC, especially hematocrit.	• Regular assessment of indicated parameters provides the tools for early detection of imbalances.
• Report the following promptly: high blood pressure, rapid pulse, rapid respirations, high hemodynamic parameters (CVP, PAWP, PAEDP, MAP), crackles or rhonchi, peripheral edema, increasing daily weight, or low hematocrit.	• Prompt medical intervention is necessary to resolve imbalances. These signs indicate fluid overload. A low hematocrit may reflect the hemodilution of overhydration.
• Also report the following promptly: low hemodynamic monitoring parameters, rapid pulse, low blood pressure, dry skin and mucous membranes, poor skin turgor, decreased weight, high hematocrit.	• These signs reflect a low circulating fluid volume. The high hematocrit may reflect hemoconcentration.
3. Measure intake and output (I&O) every 2 hours and document.	3. A careful comparison of I&O is necessary to prevent either fluid overload or dehydration.
4. Restrict fluid intake to measured losses plus 400 ml/24 hours, unless fluid or weight losses are excessive. Correlate the I&O record with daily weights. Consult with the doctor about adjusting the fluid replacement amount upward if excessive fluid losses are present or if weight loss is >0.5 kg/day. Document fluid administration.	4. Because the kidneys cannot eliminate excess fluids, intake must be restricted to replacement of lost fluids. The 400 ml represents insensible fluid losses (via lungs, skin, and stool). Although such losses are estimated usually at 400 ml/24 hours, excess losses from high temperatures, wound drainage, diarrhea, or vomiting may require upward adjustment of this amount. Daily weight may help guide fluid replacement because ARF patients usually lose 0.3 to 0.5 kg/day from catabolism. A loss of >0.5 kg/day may indicate a need for additional fluids.
5. Give I.V. infusions through infusion pumps continuously, as ordered.	5. Patients with ARF are susceptible to fluid overload. Infusion pumps prevent accidental boluses of fluid.
6. Provide hard candies, ice chips, and mouth care every 2 hours as needed and ordered. Document.	6. Fluid restrictions cause dry mouth and thirst. These measures aid mouth comfort by stimulating salivation and providing cleanliness during severe fluid-restriction periods.
7. Give diuretics, such as mannitol (Osmitrol), furosemide (Lasix), or ethacrynic acid (Edecrin), as needed and ordered. Document administration and results. Administer vasodilators, as ordered, such as low-dose dopamine (Intropin).	7. Diuretics may be given initially in prerenal conditions to increase fluid volume through the kidneys in an attempt to prevent ARF. However, diuretics may cause ARF with marginally functioning kidneys and are not effective in nonfunctioning kidneys. Vasodilators expand the vascular bed, lessening vascular congestion and the risk of pulmonary edema. Low-dose dopamine causes dopaminergic stimulation of renal blood vessels, thus increasing renal perfusion.

(continued)

Interventions	Rationales
8. Additional individualized interventions: ____________	8. Rationales: ____________

Target outcome criteria

By the time of transfer, the patient will:

- have normal vital signs and hemodynamic monitoring parameters
- have clear lungs
- display minimal or absent peripheral edema
- manifest normal skin turgor
- have moist and clean mucous membranes
- maintain a steady weight.

Nursing diagnosis: *Potential for injury: complications related to uremic syndrome*

NURSING PRIORITIES: (a) Assess for signs and symptoms of uremia, (b) monitor for complications, and (c) prevent injuries.

Interventions	Rationales
1. See the "Acid-Base Imbalances" appendix, page 316.	1. General information on acid-base imbalances is contained in the appendix. This care plan presents additional information specific to ARF.
2. Monitor BUN, creatinine, uric acid, and pH levels once a day (or as needed), as ordered. Monitor ABG measurements once a day or as needed and ordered. Document.	2. Accumulation of the waste products of metabolism and increasing levels of acidosis reflect worsening failure and may indicate a need for dialysis.
3. Assess for signs and symptoms of uremia every 2 to 4 hours and as needed. Note headache, mentation changes, fatigue, confusion, lethargy, pruritus, uremic frost, stomatitis, nausea and vomiting, ammonia breath odor, weight loss, muscle wasting, Kussmaul's respirations, seizures, or coma. Document findings. Report significant findings to the doctor.	3. Uremia affects every system and may cause subtle changes as the condition worsens. Careful assessments are valuable in determining the need for dialysis and gauging its frequency.
4. Give sodium bicarbonate I.V. as needed and ordered, typically if the plasma bicarbonate is 10 to 15 mEq/liter or less. Document.	4. Acidosis is commonly treated by dialysis, but severe cases may be treated with sodium bicarbonate.
5. Assess the hemodialysis access site (shunt or catheter), if present, every 2 hours for patency, warmth, color, thrill, and bruit. Check circulation above and below the access site. Do not use the access site for I.V. infusions or blood drawing. Do not take blood pressures on an arm or leg with an access site. Inject heparinized normal saline solution every 12 hours to maintain patency. Keep alligator clamps attached to the dressings. Document access site status and report abnormalities promptly to the doctor.	5. Access sites must remain patent because of the limited number of large vessels available for dialysis. Early discovery of a clotted shunt or catheter may allow declotting and a salvageable site. Use of the site for purposes other than dialysis increases the risk of infection and loss of the site. Regular heparinization prevents clotting. Alligator clamps should be available to clamp the shunt or catheters in the event of accidental connection.
6. Assess the peritoneal dialysis access catheter site, if present, every 24 hours and as needed for signs and symptoms of infection, including redness, swelling, excess warmth, and drainage. Also assess for general signs and symptoms of infection, including fever, malaise, abdominal pain, and cloudy drainage. Maintain surgical aseptic technique when manipulating the site, changing dressings, or adding medication to the dialysate.	6. Patients undergoing peritoneal dialysis are at a high risk for peritonitis, a life-threatening complication. Early detection of infection permits aggressive intervention and increases the likelihood of its success.

Interventions	**Rationales**
7. Prepare for dialysis every 1 to 3 days as needed and ordered, when potassium, BUN, and creatinine levels, and other uremic parameters indicate a worsening condition.	7. Dialysis, either hemodialysis or peritoneal, removes serum waste products and excess fluids and electrolytes, allowing a more homeostatic metabolic state.
8. Monitor drug administration continually. Assess potential nephrotoxicity, electrolyte content, dosage, and timing with dialysis. Monitor blood levels.	8. Renal dysfunction may decrease drug excretion, resulting in excessive blood levels and varying durations of drug effects. Certain drugs, including antibiotics, may be nephrotoxic and may worsen damage to the kidneys. Drugs containing undesirable electrolytes should be limited to prevent untoward effects. Dialysis may remove some drugs from the blood, so drug administration should be timed with dialysis treatments. Monitoring blood levels provides accurate guidelines for drug therapy.
9. Monitor hematocrit and hemoglobin daily for signs of anemia. Give packed cells, folic acid, and iron supplements as needed and ordered. Document.	9. Erythropoietin, a hormone manufactured by the kidneys, normally stimulates RBC production. Diminished production in ARF results in anemia. Folic acid and iron supplements stimulate RBC production and may correct the anemia. Administering packed cells instead of whole blood provides oxygen-carrying RBCs without exacerbating fluid overload.
10. Assess continually for signs and symptoms of hemorrhage, including changes in vital signs, CBC, and coagulation panel. If present, alert the doctor immediately. Give vitamin K, packed red blood cells, and other blood components as needed and ordered, and document. See the "Gastrointestinal Hemorrhage" care plan, page 191.	10. The uremic syndrome places patients at high risk for stress ulcer development and coagulation problems. General interventions for the patient with gastrointestinal bleeding are included in that care plan.
11. Assess daily for signs and symptoms of pericarditis, including tachycardia, fever, friction rub, and pleuritic pain that is relieved by sitting forward. If indicators are present:	11. About 20% of patients with ARF may develop pericarditis (inflammation of the pericardial sac).
• Report to the doctor. Administer steroids or nonsteroidal anti-inflammatory agents, as ordered. Document.	• Untreated, pericarditis can lead to pericardial effusion and cardiac tamponade. The medications listed relieve inflammation.
• Monitor every 4 hours for indicators of pericardial effusion and a small cardiac tamponade: weak peripheral pulses, pulsus paradoxus >10 mm Hg, or a decreased level of consciousness. If present, alert the doctor immediately.	• Pericardial effusion can range from mild to major. Mild effusion produces a small cardiac tamponade and mildly decreased CO. Mild effusions may be treated with increased dialysis to remove the uremic toxins provoking the effusion.
• Monitor continually for indicators of a large cardiac tamponade: distended neck veins, profound hypotension, and rapid loss of consciousness. Summon immediate medical assistance and prepare for emergency pericardial aspiration.	• A large cardiac tamponade—a medical emergency—compromises cardiac output severely. Immediate removal of pericardial fluid is necessary to allow ventricular filling and prevent cardiac arrest.
12. Additional individualized interventions: ____________	12. Rationales: ____________

Target outcome criteria

Immediately on creation of dialysis access, the patient will:
- have a patent dialysis shunt or catheter
- display no signs of infection
- manifest no signs of hemorrhage.

Within 3 days of admission, the patient will:
- have a normal blood pressure
- display strong, regular peripheral pulses
- show a level of consciousness within normal limits
- manifest a normal temperature.

Within 7 days of admission, the patient will:
- have BUN, creatinine, uric acid, and pH values within expected limits
- display ABG levels within normal limits
- manifest no signs or symptoms of uremia
- maintain therapeutic drug levels
- have a hemoglobin level and hematocrit within expected limits
- display no signs of pericarditis.

Nursing diagnosis: *Potential for infection related to decreased immune response and skin changes secondary to uremia*

NURSING PRIORITIES: (a) Assess for signs of infection, and (b) protect from infection.

Interventions	Rationales
1. Assess continually for signs of infection, such as increased temperature, redness, swelling, warmth, and drainage. Document and report to the doctor.	1. The uremic syndrome suppresses normal cell metabolism and immune response, which results in an increased risk for infection, a major cause of death for ARF patients. Continuous assessment is necessary to identify infection and to begin treatment early to prevent the life-threatening developments of sepsis and septicemia.
2. Continually protect from cross-contamination by using careful medical and surgical aseptic techniques.	2. Careful hand washing and other aseptic techniques with procedures and equipment may prevent infection.
3. Give antibiotics every 4 to 12 hours, as ordered, and document. Follow the guidelines for drug administration in the "Potential for injury" nursing diagnosis above.	3. Antibiotics provide a potent arsenal of weapons against infection; however, many are nephrotoxic. Because the kidneys may be unable to excrete antibiotics normally, lower dosages than usual may be needed. Coordination with dialysis timing is important to minimize drug removal and maintain therapeutic levels.
4. Provide site care and dressing changes to access sites of central and peripheral I.V. lines, catheters, and dialysis shunts every 12 to 48 hours, as indicated by hospital policy. Assess and document condition of skin and puncture sites; document date and type of site care given.	4. Site care may prevent the accumulation of secretions that could serve as growth media for infective organisms, whereas appropriate assessments may allow the early identification of infection. Careful documentation of site care promotes continuity of care.
5. Provide skin care at frequent intervals. Use preventive measures such as position changes, range-of-motion exercises, massage, wrinkle-free beds, and protective pads and mattresses. Document skin condition and nursing care given. See the "Impaired Physical Mobility" care plan, page 33.	5. Skin integrity is compromised in a patient who has ARF and uremia because of altered metabolism and the accumulation of fluid and waste products in the tissues. Frequent skin care may counteract the increased susceptibility to skin breakdown and infection. The "Impaired Physical Mobility" care plan provides further detail on preventing skin breakdown.
6. Avoid continuous invasive procedures, such as Foley catheterization. Catheterize intermittently, as needed and as ordered.	6. Continuous invasive procedures provide reservoirs for infective organisms in a patient already at high risk for infection.
7. Collect urine, blood, and secretion specimens as needed and ordered, for culture and sensitivity laboratory tests. Document.	7. Careful monitoring of body secretions for infection may allow timely and appropriate treatment if needed.

Interventions	Rationales
8. Additional individualized interventions: ____________	8. Rationales: ____________

Target outcome criteria

Within 72 hours of admission and then continuously, the patient will:
- have a normal temperature
- have noncontaminated access sites for lines and catheters
- have negative cultures
- if on antibiotics, have a therapeutic blood level.

Nursing diagnosis: *Potential nutritional deficit related to anorexia, nausea and vomiting, and restricted dietary intake*

NURSING PRIORITIES: (a) Maintain nutritional status, and (b) minimize protein catabolism.

Interventions	Rationales
1. See the "Nutritional Deficit" care plan, page 53.	1. General assessments and interventions for the patient with a nutritional deficit are included in that care plan. This nursing diagnosis focuses on additional information specific to ARF.
2. Medicate for nausea and vomiting as needed and as ordered. Document. Provide frequent meals in small servings. Document dietary intake.	2. Patients with ARF commonly have nausea and vomiting because of the effects of uremia on the gastrointestinal system. Medication and smaller servings enhance tolerance to the diet.
3. Collaborate with the doctor and nutritionist to provide a high-carbohydrate diet that includes limited but high-quality proteins (containing essential amino acids), limited fluids, low potassium and low sodium, and vitamin supplements.	3. A high-carbohydrate diet is required to provide calories for energy while sparing proteins and preventing protein catabolism. Because the kidneys cannot excrete the waste products of protein metabolism, proteins are limited to easily used high-quality proteins. The kidneys cannot regulate water balance, thus fluids are limited. Electrolytes, such as potassium, are limited because they cannot be excreted by the kidneys. Sodium is limited to prevent volume overload. Dialysis may remove vitamins, requiring administration of supplements.
4. Additional individualized interventions: ____________	4. Rationales: ____________

Target outcome criteria

Upon transfer from the critical care unit, the patient will:
- be free of nausea and vomiting
- display only limited weight loss, muscle wasting, or edema
- display a pattern of regular and adequate meals
- verbalize having enough energy for activities of daily living.

Nursing diagnosis: *Knowledge deficit: therapeutic regimen related to complexity and life-threatening nature of ARF and dialysis*

NURSING PRIORITY: Provide information on ARF and dialysis, as appropriate.

Interventions	Rationales
1. See the "Knowledge Deficit" care plan, page 45.	1. General interventions appropriate for any patient with a knowledge deficit are included in the "Knowledge Deficit" care plan.
2. Provide, as appropriate, the following information: • the common stages of ARF • medications • signs and symptoms that should be reported to the nurse, such as dizziness and nausea • procedures, including hemodialysis or peritoneal dialysis • diet • activity	2. Critically ill patients may be too ill for teaching. However, if appropriate, teaching may decrease anxiety and enhance recovery.
3. Additional individualized interventions: ____________	3. Rationales: ____________

Target outcome criteria

According to individual readiness, the patient will be able to relate:
- three stages of ARF
- signs and symptoms of uremia, such as headache, nausea, and vomiting, to be reported to the nurse
- rationale for procedures, including dialysis, diet, and activity.

Transfer planning

NURSING TRANSFER CRITERIA

Upon transfer, documentation shows evidence of:
- stable vital signs and monitoring parameters
- absence of infection, hemorrhage, and major complications in all systems
- stabilized fluid and electrolyte status, including limited edema and appropriate potassium, calcium, sodium, phosphate, and magnesium levels
- stabilized BUN, creatinine, uric acid, and pH levels
- intact and healing dialysis access site
- stable nutritional status including a positive nitrogen balance and minimal weight loss
- therapeutic drug levels.

PATIENT-FAMILY TEACHING CHECKLIST

Document evidence that patient and family demonstrate understanding of:

___ common stages of ARF and patient's current stage
___ fluid and diet regimen including limitations of protein, electrolytes, and fluids
___ rest and activity schedule
___ medications, including action and side effects
___ dialysis treatment if appropriate, including schedule and side effects
___ signs and symptoms, including fever, pain, nausea, vomiting, and dizziness, to be communicated to nurse.

DOCUMENTATION CHECKLIST

Using outcome criteria as a guide, document:

___ clinical status on admission
___ significant changes in status
___ pertinent laboratory and diagnostic test findings, including serum drug levels
___ dialysis access site condition and care
___ urine characteristics and quantity if appropriate
___ intake and output
___ weights
___ diet tolerance
___ activity tolerance
___ mentation status
___ skin status
___ pertinent procedures including dialysis.

ASSOCIATED CARE PLANS

Gastrointestinal Bleeding
Knowledge Deficit
Nutritional Deficit

REFERENCES

Alt, C., Balduf, R., and Thompson, E. "When A Vascular Access Site Complicates Care," *RN* 49(10):36-39, October 1986.

Brunner, L.S., and Suddarth, D.S. *The Lippincott Manual of Nursing Practice*, 4th ed. Philadelphia: J.B. Lippincott Co., 1986.

Carbone, V., and Bonato, J. "Nursing Implications in the Care of the Chronic Hemodialysis Patient in the Critical Care Setting," *Heart Lung* 14(6):570-78, November 1985.

Carpenito, L.J. *Nursing Diagnosis, Application to Clinical Practice,* 2nd ed. Philadelphia: J.B. Lippincott Co., 1987.

"Clinical Highlights; Acute Renal Failure: Classification," *Hospital Medicine* 21(9):51, 54, September 1985.

Coleman, E.A. "When the Kidneys Fail," *RN* 49(7):28-38, July 1986.

Kenner, C.V., Guzzetta, C.E., and Dossey, B.M. *Critical Care Nursing: Body-Mind-Spirit,* 2nd ed. Boston: Little, Brown & Co., 1985.

Lancaster, L. *The Patient with End Stage Renal Disease,* 2nd ed. New York: John Wiley & Sons, 1984.

Lewis, S.M., and Collier, I.C. *Medical-Surgical Nursing, Assessment and Management of Clinical Problems,* 2nd ed. New York: McGraw-Hill Book Co., 1987.

Luckmann, J., and Sorenson, K.C. *Medical-Surgical Nursing, A Psychophysiologic Approach,* 3rd ed. Philadelphia: W.B. Saunders Co., 1987.

Smolens, P. "Acute Renal Failure," *Hospital Medicine* 20(8):95-106, August 1985.

Solomon, J. "Does Renal Failure Mean Sexual Failure?" *RN* 49(8):41-43, August 1986.

Stark, J.L. "Combating Acute Tubular Necrosis," *Nursing Life* 5(4):33-40, July/August 1985.

Swearingen, P.L. *Manual of Nursing Therapeutics, Applying Nursing Diagnosis to Medical Disorders.* Reading, Mass.: Addison-Wesley Publishing Co., 1986.

Acquired Immunodeficiency Syndrome

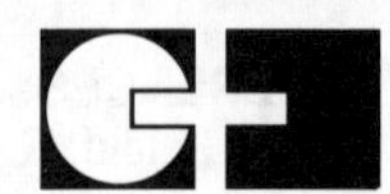

DRG information

DRG 398 Reticuloendothelial and Immunity Disorders. With Complications or Comorbidities (CC).
Mean LOS = 6.4 days
Principal diagnoses include:
- acquired immunodeficiency syndrome
- acquired immunodeficiency syndrome–related complex
- HIV infections (includes those with malignant neoplasm)
- lymphadenitis (acute, chronic, or unspecified)

DRG 399 Reticuloendothelial and Immunity Disorders. Without CC.
Mean LOS = 3.9 days
Principal diagnoses include selected principal diagnoses listed under DRG 398. The distinction is that a patient classified under DRG 399 has no complications or comorbidities.

Additional DRG information: Patients with positive serologic or viral culture findings for HIV are not classified under DRG 398 or 399.

Introduction

DEFINITION AND TIME FOCUS

Acquired immunodeficiency syndrome (AIDS) is a disorder of cell-mediated and humoral immunity. AIDS is caused by the human immunodeficiency virus (HIV), which has previously been called the human T-lymphotropic virus type III (HTLV-III), lymphadenopathy-associated virus (LAV), and other names. The virus, which appears capable of rapid genetic mutation, causes destructive changes in the body's immune system. Specifically, HIV alters the genetic makeup of T_4 helper lymphocytes so that they reproduce HIV instead of themselves. Because B-cell and monocyte function are affected by the activity of these T_4 lymphocytes, further disruption of the immune system follows, and the afflicted person is rendered immunodeficient and susceptible to a wide range of characteristic AIDS-linked disorders. Diagnosis of AIDS is based on clinical findings of opportunistic infection or cancer associated with AIDS, wasting syndrome, or AIDS-related dementia associated with confirmed HIV infection or immunodeficiency not attributable to another cause.

Two disorders seen commonly in AIDS patients (but otherwise uncommon) are *Pneumocystis carinii* pneumonia (PCP) and Kaposi's sarcoma (KS). PCP, the most common opportunistic infection in AIDS patients at the time of diagnosis, is a protozoal pneumonia that frequently has a fulminating course. KS is a malignant neoplasm that begins as reddish or purplish skin lesions in variable distribution and may gradually spread to involve internal organs, lymph nodes, and mucous membranes.

Infections from cytomegalovirus (CMV), *Cryptococcus, Candida, Salmonella,* herpesvirus, and *Mycobacterium avium-intracellulare* are also common.

No cure for AIDS has been discovered, and the prognosis for long-term survival is currently considered very poor, although actual lengths of survival vary significantly depending on the patient's overall health status, the availability of effective and prompt treatment for specific conditions, the patient's response to such treatment, and other factors. More favorable outcomes in acute episodes are associated with early detection.

In the critical care unit, the AIDS patient commonly will be admitted for respiratory support because of PCP or other pulmonary infections, for treatment of early sepsis in cases where the prognosis for recovery is considered good, or for other conditions. AIDS may also be diagnosed initially in the critical care setting when the patient develops overt symptoms or fails to respond appropriately to treatment for another condition that precipitated admission. This care plan focuses on the patient who is admitted with or diagnosed with AIDS in the critical care setting.

ETIOLOGY AND PRECIPITATING FACTORS

Identified risk factors:
- multiple sexual partners, anal intercourse, and other situations contributing to possible sexual transmission of the virus and/or reduction of normal protective barriers
- intravenous (I.V.) drug abuse, multiple blood transfusions, and other conditions that may allow exposure to blood contaminated with the virus.

High-risk groups include male homosexuals or bisexuals, I.V. drug abusers, hemophiliacs, sexual partners of those considered at high risk, and children born to mothers who were HIV-positive during pregnancy.

Focused assessment guidelines

NURSING HISTORY (Functional health pattern findings)

Health perception–health management pattern

- may report weeks to months or sudden recent onset of fatigue, malaise, low-grade fever, night sweats, anorexia, sore throat, cough, shortness of breath, chest discomfort, or congestion
- may describe recurrent infections, amebiasis, or herpes simplex outbreaks
- may have known exposure to AIDS

• may identify self as belonging to one of the high-risk groups, such as male homosexuals or bisexuals, I.V. drug abusers, or hemophiliacs
• may have a history of multiple blood transfusions
• may be the sexual partner of someone in a high-risk group

Nutritional-metabolic pattern
• is likely to report anorexia or dysphagia
• commonly reports weight loss >10 pounds in one month
• commonly reports episodic oral candidiasis (thrush), which may interfere with food intake

Elimination pattern
• commonly reports persistent diarrhea (in many cases despite treatment)
• may report incontinence (from myopathy)

Activity-exercise pattern
• commonly reports severe exertional shortness of breath (with pulmonary involvement)
• may exhibit dry mouth
• is likely to display lack of energy and malaise
• may report leg weakness (from myopathy)

Sleep-rest pattern
• commonly reports drenching night sweats
• may describe erratic sleep patterns because of other symptoms

Cognitive-perceptual pattern
• may exhibit or describe forgetfulness, depression, mental dullness or lability, difficulty concentrating, or other changes in mental status
• may report headache
• may complain of pain from tumor invasion, fever, or neurogenic causes

Role-relationship pattern
• may report close friends or sexual partners who have died of AIDS
• commonly expresses anxiety over potential loss of social contact if diagnosis becomes known to others, or expresses distress over actual losses

Sexuality-reproductive pattern
• may report previous sexual activity with multiple partners
• commonly reports previous infection with other sexually transmitted diseases

Coping–stress tolerance pattern
• typically is a young to middle-aged, previously healthy person who reports little previous experience with illness or death
• may have delayed seeking medical attention until symptoms became severe because of fear, denial, lack of information, or low self-esteem
• commonly expresses extreme anxiety regarding diagnosis, current status, and prognosis
• may exhibit denial ("not me" syndrome) as initial coping behavior
• commonly displays signs of depression
• may express suicidal thoughts

Value-belief pattern
• may express view that illness is retribution for previous behavior

PHYSICAL FINDINGS
General appearance
• wasted, cachectic

Pulmonary
• dyspnea
• dry cough
• crackles

Gastrointestinal
• diarrhea
• hepatomegaly
• splenomegaly
• diffuse abdominal tenderness
• oral candidiasis
• mucosal lesions
• hairy leukoplakia on the tongue

Neurologic
• evidence of decreased intellectual acuity, such as slowed speech, impaired memory, dulled affect
• impaired sense of position or vibration
• tendency not to initiate conversation
• paresthesias
• paralysis
• hyperreflexia
• diffuse retinal hemorrhage or exudates
• positive Babinski's sign
• hypersensitivity to light touch

Integumentary
• drenching night sweats
• red or purple lesions (in KS), varying in size from a few millimeters to a few centimeters in diameter; may be macular or papular, usually appearing first on the head, neck, or mucous membranes
• lymphadenopathy
• dermatitis
• herpes zoster
• herpes simplex lesions on genitalia, oral mucosa, or elsewhere
• anal warts
• diffuse, dry skin
• butterfly rash on nose and cheeks
• tinea
• edema (in advanced KS)

Musculoskeletal
- atrophy
- weakness
- pain
- neck stiffness

DIAGNOSTIC STUDIES
- enzyme-linked immunosorbent assay (ELISA)—identifies HIV antibodies. In the asymptomatic person, the ELISA test is not diagnostic for AIDS; it indicates only development of the antibody to the virus, and it appears that some people may have a positive ELISA test without subsequently developing signs or symptoms of the disease. In addition, the ELISA test may be negative if performed too soon after exposure to the virus, falsely negative, or falsely positive if the person has had recent influenza or other viral illness. A positive ELISA test in a patient who exhibits one of the conditions specifically linked with AIDS is considered diagnostic. Consult current Centers for Disease Control (CDC) guidelines.
- western blot analysis—uses electrophoretically marked proteins to distinguish and differentiate antibodies. This more expensive test is used in combination with the ELISA test to confirm diagnosis.

The following laboratory findings represent characteristic values in patients with AIDS but are not specific or diagnostic AIDS indicators.
- complete blood count (CBC)—reveals leukocytopenia, anemia, and neutropenia.
- total T-cell count—reduced. T_4 cell count is commonly $<400/mm^3$.
- T_4/T_8 ratio (ratio of helper-inducer T cells to cytotoxic-suppressor T cells)—low; decrease depends on patient status but commonly is $<1:2$ (normal T_4/T_8 ratio $= 2:1$).
- immunoglobulin levels—usually elevated, especially IgG and IgA.
- platelet count—reveals thrombocytopenia.
- sedimentation rate—elevated.
- skin test antigen studies—reveal anergy.
- aspartate aminotransferase (AST) level (formerly called serum glutamic-oxaloacetic transaminase)—may be elevated (associated with hepatitis).
- lactic dehydrogenase (LDH) level—may be elevated with PCP.
- serum cholesterol level—may be low.
- serum iron value—may be low.
- hepatitis screen—may demonstrate carrier state or active disease (positive hepatitis B surface antigen).
- stool examination—may reveal parasites, ova, or infections, such as cryptosporidiosis or salmonellosis.
- bronchoscopy—may be done to diagnose PCP or other disorders by transbronchial lung biopsy to examine tissue or by use of bronchoalveolar lavage to obtain specimen containing PCP cysts.
- chest X-ray—may reveal diffuse interstitial infiltrates (associated with PCP); however, it may be nondiagnostic even with active PCP.
- open-lung biopsy—may provide definitive diagnosis of KS-related pulmonary symptoms or evidence of CMV infection.
- lesion cultures—may reveal *Candida* or other organisms.
- lesion biopsy—may demonstrate KS, toxoplasmosis, or other complications.
- gallium scan—may help establish early diagnosis of PCP. This nonspecific test shows radioisotope accumulation in the white blood cells of infected areas.
- blood cultures—may identify pathogens if bacteremia is present.
- lumbar puncture—results vary; they may reveal cryptococcal meningitis; culture of spinal fluid may reveal HIV; results may be inconclusive for CMV infection.
- sputum test for acid-fast bacilli—may indicate *Mycobacterium*.
- computed tomography (CT) scan or magnetic resonance imaging (MRI) testing—may identify lesions for later biopsy; MRI may be the only means of detecting progressive multifocal leukoencephalopathy.
- bone marrow aspiration—may reveal hypoplasia.

POTENTIAL COMPLICATIONS
- Burkitt's lymphoma
- candidal esophagitis
- CMV infection
- cryptococcal meningitis
- cryptosporidiosis
- dementia
- depression
- diffuse organ infection
- disseminated bacterial infection
- encephalopathy
- hemorrhage
- herpes simplex
- multifocal leukoencephalopathy
- *Mycobacterium avium-intracellulare*
- primary lymphoma
- toxoplasmosis
- tuberculosis

Collaborative problem: *Potential hypoxemia related to weakness, ventilation-perfusion imbalance, pneumonia, or other lung pathology*

NURSING PRIORITY: Optimize oxygenation.

Interventions	Rationales
1. Assess respiratory status at least every hour, noting rate and depth of respirations, adequacy of respiratory effort, breath sounds, skin color and temperature, and level of consciousness.	1. Respiratory status in AIDS patients is affected by several factors. The profound weakness experienced by almost all patients during an acute disease episode results in reduced chest expansion. PCP causes the growth of hard cysts in the interstitial lung spaces, which results in alveolar compression, diminished surfactant, and decreased diffusion across the alveolar capillary membrane. KS lesions, nonspecific pneumonitis, and adult respiratory distress syndrome (ARDS) are also common AIDS-linked lung complications that affect adequate oxygenation.
2. Monitor arterial blood gas (ABG) values, as ordered, and report abnormal values or significant changes from previous values.	2. Lung pathology may result in significant impairment of arterial PO_2. A decreasing PO_2 and an increasing PCO_2 indicate hypoventilation and potential respiratory failure. However, arterial PO_2 levels in PCP patients with AIDS tend to be less decreased than PO_2 values in PCP patients without AIDS and are sometimes even within normal values. The reasons for this phenomenon are unclear.
3. Administer oxygen therapy, as ordered.	3. Supplemental oxygen elevates arterial oxygen content and reduces hypoxia.
4. Perform airway clearance measures, as needed:	4. The patient's ability to clear the airway effectively may be impaired from general debilitation and weakness.
• If the patient is able, teach and assist with deep-breathing exercises and encourage use of the incentive spirometer hourly, as ordered. Consult with the doctor about incorporating coughing into the hygiene routine, as indicated.	• Deep breathing helps to expand the lungs fully and prevents areas of atelectasis associated with pneumonia and bed rest. Incentive spirometry also promotes fuller lung expansion. However, caution is warranted in incorporating cough or positive-pressure breathing into the hygiene routine for the PCP patient because alveolar rupture or collapse may occur secondary to decreased surfactant.
• If the patient cannot deep-breathe voluntarily, perform artificial sighing with a manual resuscitation (Ambu) bag hourly.	• Use of the manual resuscitation bag helps promote full lung expansion.
• Suction if needed, as indicated by noisy respirations or rhonchi auscultated over the large airways. Use supplemental oxygen before, during, and after suctioning.	• Even partial obstruction of the airway may result in significant hypoxemia if corrective measures are not instituted promptly. Suctioning may cause marked reductions in arterial PO_2. Supplemental oxygen may be provided during suctioning by using nasal prongs.
5. Evaluate and document the following respiratory parameters at least every 2 hours and as needed: presence or absence of effective cough and airway clearance, sputum color and character, and respiratory effort (including effort with activity, if the patient can engage in voluntary movement). Administer antibiotics, as ordered, documenting and noting effectiveness. Observe for signs of pleural effusion.	5. Careful serial observations of respiratory status are essential to detect subtle changes that may indicate the need for reevaluation of therapy. The PCP patient commonly requires multiple antibiotics as other infections superimpose themselves on the already compromised lungs. Malignant pleural invasion by KS lesions may cause pleural effusion, but diagnosis of KS in the lung is difficult without open-lung biopsy.

(continued)

Interventions	Rationales
6. Immediately report increasing restlessness, anxiety, tachycardia, cyanosis or pallor, increasing or sudden dyspnea, or inadequate respiratory effort. If any of these occur, anticipate immediate endotracheal intubation and mechanical ventilation. See the "Mechanical Ventilation" care plan, page 108, and the "Adult Respiratory Distress Syndrome" care plan, page 101, for further details.	6. The signs and symptoms listed are indicators of hypoxia and may signal impending respiratory failure, a common cause of death in the AIDS patient. Development of adult respiratory distress syndrome is a grave sign and associated with a poor prognosis. If respiratory compromise is present, ventilatory support is indicated until the acute infection resolves or the patient regains sufficient strength to breathe effectively. The "Mechanical Ventilation" and "Adult Respiratory Distress Syndrome" care plans provide further interventions for the care of the patient experiencing respiratory distress.
7. If the patient has undergone bronchoscopy, observe for bleeding, edema, or other complications.	7. Irritation from the bronchoscope may cause bleeding, further threatening airway patency.
8. Watch for signs of respiratory depression following administration of narcotic analgesics, if ordered. Report an excessively slowed respiratory rate, frequent sighing, decreased alertness, or other indications of reduced respiratory effort.	8. Narcotics depress the brain's respiratory center, which can precipitate CO_2 narcosis or respiratory arrest in an AIDS patient with an already precarious oxygenation status.
9. Anticipate activity intolerance and assist with self-care as needed. When the patient begins to resume normal activity, teach energy conservation measures, such as grouping procedures, using large muscles, taking frequent rest periods, sitting during showers, and avoiding activities that involve raising the arms over the head.	9. Because activity increases the body's metabolic rate, it also requires more oxygen; thus, exertion may worsen preexisting hypoxemia or precipitate its development in the susceptible patient. Energy conservation measures help minimize the amount of oxygen needed to perform a given activity. Grouping procedures decreases unnecessary exertion; large muscles are more energy efficient. Sitting requires less energy than standing. Raising the arms over the head causes rapid fatigue and increases cardiac work load.
10. Additional individualized interventions: ____________	10. Rationales: ____________

Target outcome criteria

Within 1 hour of admission, the patient will:
- display decreased dyspnea
- have improved ABG values.

Within 24 hours, if conscious, the patient will:
- participate in airway clearance measures (to extent possible)
- use energy conservation principles.

Collaborative problem: *Immunosuppression related to low number of T_4 cells, or low T_4 / T_8 ratio, or both*

NURSING PRIORITY: Prevent or promptly treat new infections.

Interventions	Rationales
1. Institute precautions recommended by the CDC and your institution for the immunosuppressed patient, including meticulous hand washing before entering the patient's room and after leaving, providing only cooked foods, avoiding standing water in the room (such as in flower vases), screening visitors to prevent those with infections from contact with the patient, and preventing the patient from handling live flowers or plants.	1. The immunosuppressed patient is at risk of infection from any source, even those usually considered benign to healthy persons, such as raw fruits or vegetables. Such precautions minimize the patient's exposure to organisms. Hand washing is the primary infection control measure for any patient. (However, gloves are recommended along with protective gowns and eye wear, as indicated, to protect others from exposure to HIV-contaminated blood or bodily secretions.) Raw produce may be a source of gram-negative bacilli; standing water provides a medium for the growth of microorganisms, particularly *Pseudomonas*. Visitors may transmit organisms to the patient through direct contact or by exposing the patient to airborne bacteria. Plants and soil may harbor fungi.
2. Monitor vital signs, including temperature, at least every 4 hours. Report fever onset or temperature spikes immediately.	2. Fever is produced as the body responds to pyrogens released from invading microorganisms. The increase in metabolic rate is accompanied by a corresponding increase in heart rate and respiratory rate. In the severely immunocompromised patient, however, the body's usual response mechanisms may fail, and the patient may become septic in the absence of fever. For this reason, careful, frequent observation to detect subtle changes in the patient's condition is essential.
3. Monitor CBC daily and report increasing leukopenia or neutropenia.	3. These changes indicate further compromise to the body's ability to resist or fight infection.
4. Monitor potential sites of infection daily. Check I.V. and injection sites, mucous membranes, rectum, vagina, and any wounds or breaks in the skin for changes in color, texture, or sensation, or the development of swelling, pain, induration, purulent drainage, or other abnormalities. If the patient is alert, discuss the importance of ongoing monitoring and early reporting of signs or symptoms of infection.	4. The skin forms one of the body's most important protective barriers against infection, and any break in the skin provides access for the entry of microorganisms. Classic signs and symptoms of infection may be masked or delayed in the immunocompromised patient, so regular, careful observation for changes is essential. Any change may herald an infection. For example, dysphagia may indicate esophagitis, or white patches in the mouth may signal candidiasis (both are common in AIDS patients). Any suspicious area must be investigated promptly, because even relatively benign microorganisms can cause life-threatening illness in the AIDS patient.

(continued)

Interventions	Rationales
5. Be alert for signs and symptoms of neurologic infection, including stiff neck, headache, visual or motor abnormalities, memory impairment, and alterations in level of consciousness. Compare new findings with baseline neurologic or mental status findings, and report new or changed abnormalities to the doctor immediately. Consult with the doctor about possible lumbar puncture or a magnetic resonance imaging (MRI) series.	5. Neurologic abnormalities are common in AIDS patients, with 30% to 40% or more experiencing some neurologic involvement during the course of the disease. About 10% of the patients seek medical attention initially because of neurologic symptoms from the HIV infection or a secondary infection. Encephalitis, the most common complication, may be caused by various microorganisms, including CMV and *Toxoplasma gondii.* Progressive multifocal leukoencephalopathy, another common finding, is usually detectable only by MRI scanning. Early detection and treatment of neurologic symptoms may result in improvement; once such involvement is advanced, however, the prognosis is poor.
6. Monitor for evidence of new pulmonary infections, checking lung sounds at least every 4 hours. Report crackles, decreased breath sounds, or other new abnormal findings promptly.	6. The most common AIDS-linked pulmonary infection is PCP, but other infections—including tuberculosis—may occur. Although current pharmacologic treatment measures for PCP appear to have limited effectiveness, prompt treatment of other infections may be lifesaving for the immunocompromised patient.
7. Obtain cultures, as ordered, from blood, stool, urine, sputum, or wound drainage. Evaluate sensitivity results and verify appropriateness of antibiotic therapy.	7. If new infection is suspected, immediate cultures will identify causative organisms. Sensitivity results provide a guide for antibiotic therapy.
8. Administer antibiotics and anti-infectives, as ordered. The following medications are used commonly in protocols for AIDS-related infections, but others may be used depending on the causative organism.	8. Depending on the organism, antibiotic therapy may be instituted with several drugs at a time. Antibiotics may also be ordered prophylactically for these patients. Effectiveness is variable, particularly in a second episode of PCP, which is associated with a mortality of approximately 75%. If CMV is also involved, mortality is higher still.
• co-trimoxazole (Bactrim, Septra): Observe for and report side effects, such as rash, leukopenia, sore throat, purpura, jaundice, or signs of renal failure. Discontinue use if rash occurs.	• Co-trimoxazole is the antibiotic of choice for PCP treatment. The drug also fights infections caused by *Shigella, Proteus, Klebsiella, Enterobacter,* and other bacteria. Skin rash in a patient on this drug may be an early sign of a severe, even life-threatening, reaction.
• pentamidine isethionate (Pentam): Observe for and report any side effects such as leukopenia, hypotension, hypoglycemia, and formation of sterile abscesses at injection sites. (If the medication is ordered I.V., give over 45 to 90 minutes.)	• Pentamidine is used for PCP and administered I.M., I.V., or by aerosol. Slow I.V. administration lessens the risk of hypotension.
• sulfadoxine and pyrimethamine (Fansidar), or pyrimethamine (Daraprim): Observe for and report leukopenia, rash, purpura, or pruritus. Administer folic acid supplements, as ordered, and observe for glossitis.	• Sulfadoxine and pyrimethamine are indicated for infections caused by toxoplasmosis. Because pyrimethamine is a folic acid inhibitor, folic acid supplementation is recommended. Rash may be an early sign of a severe reaction to the drug. Glossitis may indicate folic acid deficiency.
9. If zidovudine (Retrovir) is ordered, consult current administration guidelines and provide patient teaching, as appropriate to patient's condition, as follows:	9. Zidovudine, an antiviral agent that has shown some promise against the HIV virus in early studies, is made from thymidine, a component of deoxyribonucleic acid (DNA), and appears to block reproduction of HIV, probably by interfering with reverse transcriptase. Early tests also revealed increased T cell counts, restoration of reactivity to skin test antigens, reduction in fever, and improved neurologic status. Although zidovudine may improve a patient's overall status, it does not kill the virus, cure AIDS, or prevent transmission.

Interventions	Rationales
• Avoid concurrent use of acetaminophen (Tylenol), aspirin, indomethacin (Indocin), probenecid (Benemid), cimetidine (Tagamet), lorazepam (Ativan), or ranitidine (Zantac) with zidovudine. Advise the patient to consult the doctor before taking any other medications, including nonprescription medications, while on zidovudine.	• These medications may impair the metabolism of zidovudine or increase the risk of developing toxicity.
• Obtain and monitor laboratory tests, as ordered (usually T-cell count, liver and renal function tests, and CBC initially and serially). Prepare for possible blood transfusions if toxicity develops.	• To qualify for zidovudine, the patient must exhibit evidence of PCP or a T-cell count below established limits (check current CDC recommendations). Because zidovudine use may result in severe neutropenia, anemia, or other blood dyscrasias, ongoing monitoring is essential, and transfusion may become necessary.
• Observe for and report any known side effects, such as headache, abdominal discomfort, anxiety, rash, or itching. Also report any new symptom or worsening of an existing symptom.	• Because no long-term studies of this drug have been completed, the side effects listed are based on results from a small, controlled trial group. Any new symptom, or worsening of an existing symptom, should be promptly investigated.
10. Institute fever control measures, as ordered, including the following, as appropriate: alternating doses of aspirin and acetaminophen, unless the patient is taking zidovudine or exhibits prolonged clotting times; using hypothermia blanket; monitoring for signs of dehydration; and replacing fluid, as needed. See "Fluid and Electrolyte Imbalances" appendix, page 317, for further information regarding such imbalances.	10. Aspirin and acetaminophen act to reduce fever by inhibiting the effects of pyrogens on the thermoregulatory center. Alternating aspirin and acetaminophen is necessary to control fever while avoiding toxicity from too-frequent administration of either drug. However, these drugs may increase the likelihood of toxicity if used with zidovudine. In addition, they decrease platelet adhesion, thus prolonging clotting time. A hypothermia blanket may be necessary if aspirin and acetaminophen are ineffective or contraindicated. Prolonged fever increases the metabolic rate and promotes diaphoresis, contributing to dehydration and electrolyte imbalances.
11. Additional individualized interventions: ____________	11. Rationales: ____________

Target outcome criteria

Throughout the critical care unit stay, the patient will:

• receive continuous protective measures for the immunosuppressed patient
• receive prompt treatment for new infections
• exhibit no unanticipated side effects of medication
• display reduced or controlled fever
• exhibit no signs or symptoms of dehydration.

Nursing diagnosis: *Sensory-perceptual alteration related to neurologic involvement, anxiety, or effects of critical care unit environment*

NURSING PRIORITY: Maximize sensory-perceptual acuity.

Interventions	Rationales
1. Assess the patient's mental and neurologic status on admission and at least daily thereafter, including level of consciousness, orientation, long-term and recent memory, ability to follow directions and think abstractly, speech, pupillary responses, and strength and sensation of arms and legs.	1. Baseline and ongoing assessments of mental and neurologic status allow for early detection of neurologic involvement, a common and ominous finding in many AIDS patients.

(continued)

Interventions	**Rationales**
2. Evaluate the patient's emotional state, considering the effects of depression, anxiety, grieving, or other emotions on mental status findings. Also be alert for possible side effects of medications that may be the cause of confusion, memory impairment, or other unusual findings.	2. Emotional responses or medication side effects may contribute to changes in neurologic or mental status findings.
3. Assess for possible visual impairment by using an eye chart, if possible. If the patient has significant visual impairment, prevent injury by such precautions as placing items within easy reach and ensuring that side rails are always up.	3. CMV infection involving the optic nerve can cause blindness. Precautions, particularly if confusion is a factor, reduce the patient's risk of injury.
4. As much as possible, explain the patient's symptoms to family and friends. Emphasize supportive behaviors, such as changing the subject if repetitive or irrational behavior is exhibited, using humor and providing gentle reminders of appropriate behavior.	4. Both patient and family may find mentation changes difficult to accept. Providing explanations and guidelines for responding to such behavior can reduce distress for all concerned.
5. Institute protective measures and consult with the doctor regarding any paresthesias, numbness, weakness, involuntary arm or leg movements, pain or marked atrophy of arms and legs.	5. Distal symmetrical sensorimotor neuropathy is a common peripheral nerve complication in AIDS patients. Its cause is unknown, and although a relatively benign condition, it may cause the patient significant discomfort. Treatment includes range-of-motion exercises, electrical stimulation, and other measures.
6. See the "Sensory-Perceptual Alteration" care plan, page 60.	6. The "Sensory-Perceptual Alteration" care plan provides additional detailed interventions for the care of the patient experiencing such alterations in the critical care setting.
7. See the "Acute Pain" care plan, page 10.	7. Patients with AIDS may experience pain of varying intensity, duration, and locale, depending on the specific manifestations of the illness.
8. Additional individualized interventions: ______	8. Rationales: ______

Target outcome criteria

Throughout the critical-care unit stay, the patient will experience no injury because of sensory-perceptual alterations.

Nursing diagnosis: *Nutritional deficit related to nausea, vomiting, diarrhea, anorexia, medication side effects, or decreased nutrient absorption secondary to disease process*

NURSING PRIORITY: Promote adequate nutritional intake.

Interventions	Rationales
1. See the "Nutritional Deficit" care plan, page 53, for detailed interventions regarding this common problem of the AIDS patient.	1. The AIDS patient is likely to experience nutritional deficits for several reasons. The immunosuppressed patient has an increased need for nutrients to help repair damaged tissue and decrease muscle wasting. Symptoms of the disease, or side effects of medications, may reduce the patient's appetite or ability to retain ingested nutrients. Severe diarrhea from such infections as cryptosporidiosis or salmonellosis, or intestinal KS lesions, may reduce gastrointestinal absorption of nutrients. Depending on the patient's status, nasogastric feedings or total parenteral nutrition may be indicated. The "Nutritional Deficit" care plan contains detailed interventions for the care of a patient experiencing a nutritional deficit for any reason.
2. Additional individualized interventions: ____________	2. Rationales: ____________

Target outcome criteria
Throughout the critical care unit stay, the patient will:
- tolerate adequate oral intake of food, or tolerate enteral or parenteral feedings without complications
- exhibit no further weight loss.

Nursing diagnosis: *Impaired physical mobility related to weakness, hypoxemia, neuropathy, orthostatic hypotension, and other effects of disease process*

NURSING PRIORITIES: (a) Promote maximum physical mobility, and (b) prevent complications associated with decreased mobility.

Interventions	Rationales
1. Assess for signs and symptoms of activity intolerance, such as tachypnea, tachycardia, increased fatigue, or cyanosis. If present, adjust the patient's activity level to minimize them.	1. The effort required for even minimal activity may overtax the patient's ventilatory capability and reduce the motivation to continue. Fatigue further contributes to hypoxemia. Adjusting the activity level as needed minimizes hypoxemia and may help maintain motivation and a sense of well-being.
2. See the "Impaired Physical Mobility" care plan, page 33, for further information.	2. The "Impaired Physical Mobility" care plan contains detailed interventions for the patient experiencing impairment in normal mobility, including patient assessment and prevention of complications.
3. Additional individualized interventions: ____________	3. Rationales: ____________

Target outcome criteria
Throughout the critical care unit stay, the patient will:
- engage in physical activity as tolerated
- develop no complications from impaired mobility.

Nursing diagnosis: *Potential fluid volume deficit related to chronic, persistent diarrhea and fever associated with opportunistic infection*

NURSING PRIORITY: Maintain optimal fluid status.

Interventions

1. Monitor intake and output scrupulously, collaborating with the doctor to maintain fluid balance. See the "Fluid and Electrolyte Imbalances" appendix, page 317, and the "Acid-Base Imbalances" appendix, page 316.

2. Additional individualized interventions: ____________

Rationales

1. Diarrhea commonly is one of the most problematic symptoms experienced by the AIDS patient. Various microorganisms can contribute to the problem, which may be exacerbated by rectal mucosal lesions, hemorrhoids, or nutritional deficit. Fever contributes further to the potential for dehydration. The appendices listed provide further guidelines for monitoring fluid and electrolyte status and intervening to maintain optimal hydration and metabolic balance.

2. Rationales: ____________

Target outcome criteria
Throughout the critical care unit stay, the patient will maintain normal fluid and electrolyte status, or receive prompt corrective measures if imbalances occur.

Nursing diagnosis: *Social isolation related to communicable disease, associated social stigma, and fear of infection from social contact*

NURSING PRIORITY: Promote social acceptance and integration.

Interventions

1. Assess the patient's family (including significant others and friends) for emotional supportiveness. Ask about recent losses and changes in living situation, job, habits, and attitudes of others toward the patient's illness.

Rationales

1. For many patients with AIDS, the diagnosis and hospitalization represent the continuation of a series of catastrophic life events. In many cases, the patient has recently experienced the loss of a lover or friend to the disease. In addition, the lack of knowledge about AIDS common among persons without previous experience with it and the extreme fear of the disease perpetuate an unwarranted social stigma. The patient, too, may experience self-imposed isolation because of fear of contracting infections from others or giving AIDS to them. Careful assessment of the patient's support systems and recent history guides intervention to promote social contact and reduce the spread of misinformation.

Interventions	Rationales
2. Promote an atmosphere of acceptance. Encourage physical contact, observing and teaching others about recommended precautions, such as wearing gloves and protective attire only when anticipating contact with bodily secretions.	2. An accepting environment contributes to normalizing feelings between the patient and family members; encourages the patient to verbalize his feelings, thus decreasing isolation; and promotes relaxation, thus reducing anxiety. Physical contact provides a direct demonstration of caring and helps reduce the "outcast" feelings so many AIDS patients experience. The nurse can be a good role model for family and friends while teaching and correcting damaging misconceptions about the disease.
3. Teach significant others about ways the virus is *not* transmitted, including contact with toilet seats, swimming pools, food utensils, hugging, social (dry) kissing and other nonsexual gestures of affection, pets (though animals may carry microorganisms that may threaten the patient), and other casual contact. Saliva, tears, and coughing are currently considered unlikely sources of transmission, although the CDC recommends avoiding contact with any body fluid. Provide the family with literature reinforcing these points. See the "Knowledge Deficit" care plan, page 45.	3. The "worried well" (those who are healthy but concerned about catching AIDS themselves) may be torn between their desire to support the patient and their fears of contracting the disease. Specific education may help reduce their conflicts and encourage normal interaction with the patient. The AIDS virus does not survive on inanimate objects and is killed by soap and hot water. Opportunistic infections do represent a potential threat for others, but healthy individuals are at no greater risk than usual. Literature provides a source for future reference and increases the likelihood of retention of information given. The "Knowledge Deficit" care plan contains specific information to help in planning a patient-family teaching program.
4. Provide the patient and family with telephone numbers of available resources for counseling, support, and information, such as those listed below. Also check with the local Public Health Department for resources in your area. • National AIDS Hotline, Atlanta: 800-342-AIDS • CDC information, Atlanta: 800-231-7514 • AIDS Foundation, San Francisco: 415-864-4376 • National Gay Task Force, New York: 800-221-7044	4. Ongoing support is essential for the AIDS patient and the family at all stages of the illness. Support groups offer understanding, practical advice, and the latest information on new developments, which may surpass the necessarily limited support clinicians can provide. In addition, social contacts in such groups may develop into life-enriching relationships that enhance the patient's ability to cope with the disease. Referral to a social services department is essential because most patients cannot afford expensive treatments and need special housing arrangements. Ensure that a social services department referral is made for assistance with financial planning.
5. Additional individualized interventions: ____________	5. Rationales: ____________

Target outcome criteria

Throughout the critical care unit stay, the patient will:
- experience supportive social interaction and physical contact with others
- receive assistance with financial matters, as appropriate.

Nursing diagnosis: *Potential ineffective coping related to diagnosis of life-threatening illness, loss of ability to maintain usual roles, complex decisions regarding treatment options, and anticipatory grieving*

NURSING PRIORITY: Promote coping ability.

Interventions	Rationales
1. See the "Ineffective Coping" care plan, page 26.	1. The "Ineffective Coping" care plan contains detailed interventions helpful in caring for the patient whose coping abilities are threatened by illness, hospitalization, or other circumstances.
2. Be supportive of various patient defense mechanisms, such as allowing the newly diagnosed patient to maintain some level of denial. In the more critically ill patient, encourage hope while facilitating realistic planning.	2. Patients who are permitted to maintain a certain level of denial have been shown to have a more positive prognosis. Maintaining hope promotes general well-being and helps the patient feel less helpless.
3. Anticipate fear, guilt, and anger and accept the expression of these as normal responses. If uncomfortable with discussion of difficult or explicit issues, arrange for another professional to care for the patient. Whenever possible, refer the patient to a mental health professional who can follow the patient on an ongoing basis.	3. The diagnosis of AIDS carries an enormous psychosocial impact that may be overwhelming initially. The patient may have difficulty using usual defense mechanisms; for example, friends or family may abandon the patient once the diagnosis is confirmed. If the disease was contracted through sexual contact, the patient may experience guilt over unresolved issues, anxiety or anger with previous sexual partners, or ambivalence or regret about previous sexual choices. The patient may view the illness as retribution for behaviors that were valued in the past but are now viewed as negative. Unconditional support and consistency in care provide the patient with a resource base from which to begin restructuring his or her future plans.
4. As appropriate, provide the patient and family with information regarding the legal rights of AIDS patients, including privacy, confidentiality of medical records, housing and employment discrimination, preparing wills, and granting power of attorney to trusted persons. The patient also has the right to choose treatment options, resuscitation (code) status, and participation in research studies or surveys. As appropriate, refer the patient, family members, and friends to AIDS support groups and other resources.	4. Because of the widespread fear of AIDS among the general public, the patient may encounter discriminatory practices or pressures. Knowledge of legal rights and options may help avert further losses. Exploring the issue of making a will or arranging legal affairs is important, particularly because such a high percentage of patients with AIDS experience neurologic impairment later in the course of the disease. Support groups can provide the patient or family with more detailed information and "how-to" specifics regarding these problems.
5. See the "Grieving and Dying" care plan, page 15.	5. The care plan on "Grieving and Dying" contains detailed interventions on assisting the patient who is facing the prospect of his or her own death. This plan also provides information regarding the families and friends of the critically ill or dying patient and their special needs.
6. Additional individualized interventions: ________	6. Rationales: ________

Target outcome criteria
Throughout the critical care unit stay, the patient will:
• use positive coping behaviors
• display awareness of legal rights and available support, if appropriate to condition
• have opportunities to address issues of grieving and dying.

Transfer planning

NURSING TRANSFER CRITERIA

Upon transfer, documentation shows evidence of:
• vital signs within normal limits for patient
• spontaneous respirations of 12 to 24 breaths per minute
• balanced intake and output
• weight stable or increased since admission
• ABG values within normal parameters
• fever absent or controlled
• patient-family preferences regarding treatment options, resuscitation (code) status, and confidentiality identified
• mental health referral.

PATIENT-FAMILY TEACHING CHECKLIST

Document evidence that patient and family demonstrate understanding of:
__ disease process and implications
__ treatment options
__ available support groups and resources
__ symptoms to report to health care providers
__ infection prevention measures
__ safety precautions
__ how the virus is (and is not) spread
__ ways to prevent HIV transmission to others
__ legal rights and resources.

DOCUMENTATION CHECKLIST

Using outcome criteria as a guide, document:
__ clinical status on admission
__ significant changes in status
__ pertinent diagnostic test findings
__ occurrence and type of opportunistic infections
__ treatment decisions
__ nutritional program and support
__ intake and output
__ breathing patterns
__ emotional coping
__ support for family and significant others
__ referrals made
__ patient-family teaching
__ transfer planning.

ASSOCIATED CARE PLANS

Acute Pain
Adult Respiratory Distress Syndrome
Grieving and Dying
Impaired Physical Mobility
Ineffective Coping
Knowledge Deficit
Mechanical Ventilation
Nutritional Deficit
Sensory-Perceptual Alteration

REFERENCES

Abbott Diagnostics HTLV-III Education Series Monograph. Irving, Tex.: Abbott Laboratories, 1986.

Abrams, D. "AIDS: In Search of Hope," *California Nurse Review* 9(1):5-40, January 1987.

Abrams, D., et al. "Routine Care and Psychosocial Support of the Patient with Acquired Immunodeficiency Syndrome," *Medical Clinics of North America* 70(3):707-19, May 1986.

Bennett, J. "HTLV-III AIDS Link," *American Journal of Nursing 85:* 1086-89, October 1985.

Bennett, J. "What We Know About AIDS," *American Journal of Nursing 86:* 1016-21, September 1986.

Berger, J. "Neurologic Complications of HIV Infection," *Postgraduate Medicine* 81(1):73-79, 1987.

Boland, M., and Klug, R. "AIDS: The Implications for Home Care," *MCN* 11:404-11, November/December 1986.

Centers for Disease Control. "Morbidity and Mortality Weekly Report: Recommendations for Preventing Transmission of Infection with Human T-lymphotropic Virus Type III/Lymphadenopathy-associated Virus During Invasive Procedures," *Journal of the American Medical Association* 256:1257-58, 1986.

City and County of San Francisco, Department of Public Health Epidemiologic Bulletin. "Human Immunodeficiency Virus Infections in Health-Care Workers Exposed to Blood of Infected Patients," July 1987.

Devita, V.T., et al., eds. *Aids: Etiology, Diagnosis, Treatment, and Prevention.* Philadelphia: J.B. Lippincott Co., 1985.

Donlou, J., et al. "Psychosocial Aspects of AIDS and AIDS-related Complex: A Pilot Study," *Journal of Psychosocial Oncology* 3:2, Summer 1985.

Fischinger, P.J., and Bolognesi, D.P. "Prospects for Diagnostic Tests, Intervention and Vaccine Development in AIDS," in *AIDS: Etiology, Diagnosis, Treatment, and Prevention.* Edited by Devita, V.T., et al. Philadelphia: J.B. Lippincott Co., 1985.

Friedland, G.H., et al. "Lack of Transmission of HTLV-III/LAV Infection to Household Contacts of Patients with AIDS or AIDS Related Complex with Oral Candidiasis," *New England Journal of Medicine* 314:344-49, 1986.

Griffin, J.P. "Nursing Care of the Immunosuppressed Patient in an Intensive Care Unit," *Heart & Lung* 15:179-87, 1986.

Guyton, A. *Textbook of Medical Physiology,* 7th ed. Philadelphia: W.B. Saunders, 1986.

Halliburton, P. "Impaired Immunocompetence," in *Pathophysiological Phenomena in Nursing.* Edited by Carrieri, V., et al. Philadelphia: W.B. Saunders Co., 1986.

Klug, R. "Children with AIDS," *American Journal of Nursing* 86:1125-32, October 1986.

LaCamera, D.J., et al. "The Acquired Immunodeficiency Syndrome," *Nursing Clinics of North America* 20:241-56, 1985.

Lotze, M.T. "Treatment of Immunologic Disorders in AIDS," in *AIDS: Etiology, Diagnosis, Treatment, and Prevention.* Edited by Devita, V.T., et al. Philadelphia: J.B. Lippincott Co., 1985.

Mitsuya, H., et al. "3-Azido-3-deoxythymidine: An Antiviral Agent that Inhibits the Infectivity and Cytopathic Effect of Human T-lymphotropic Virus Type III/Lymphadenopathy-Associated Virus in Vitro," *Proceedings of the National Academy of Sciences* 82:7096-7100, October 1985.

Peabody, B. "Living with AIDS: A Mother's Perspective," *American Journal of Nursing* 86:45-46, 1986.

Porth, C.M. *Pathophysiology Concepts of Altered Health States,* 2nd ed. Philadelphia: J.B. Lippincott Co., 1986.

Price, J.H. "AIDS, the Schools, and Policy Issues," *Journal of School Health* 56(4):137-39, April 1986.

Shaw, G.M., et al. "HTLV-III Infection in Brains of Children and Adults with AIDS Encephalopathy," *Science* 227:177-82, 1985.

Tueller, B., and Malone, R. "Acquired Immune Deficiency Syndrome," in *Medical Surgical Care Plans.* Edited by Holloway, N. Springhouse, Pa.: Springhouse Corp., 1988.

Turner, J., and Williamson, K. "AIDS: A Challenge for Contemporary Nursing," *Focus Critical Care* 13(3):53-61, 1986.

Disseminated Intravascular Coagulation

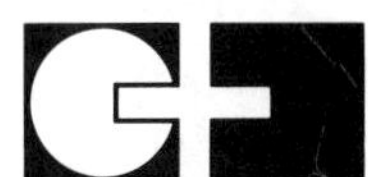

DRG information

DRG 397 Coagulation Disorders.
Mean LOS = 5.5 days
Principal diagnoses include all types of coagulation defects or disorders, including disseminated intravascular coagulation (DIC).

Introduction

DEFINITION AND TIME FOCUS

Disseminated intravascular coagulation (DIC) is a complex, acquired hematologic disorder characterized by a paradoxical blend of coagulation and hemorrhage. One or more procoagulants—such as bacterial toxins, exposure of collagen in damaged blood vessel walls, or tissue fragments—provoke uncontrolled microcirculatory coagulation via the intrinsic clotting pathway, extrinsic clotting pathway, or both.

The explosive production of thrombin precipitates widespread microcirculatory deposition of fibrin and rapid consumption of clotting factors. It also triggers the body's fibrinolytic system, a homeostatic mechanism to limit coagulation. Fibrin split products (FSPs) are produced as a by-product of fibrinolysis and exacerbate bleeding because they function as anticoagulants. Because of the anticoagulants and the scarcity of clotting factors, the patient cannot form stable clots and bleeding occurs at multiple sites throughout the body.

ETIOLOGY AND PRECIPITATING FACTORS

- shock
- sepsis
- severe hypoxia
- transfusion reactions or other hemolytic conditions
- trauma, burns, neoplasms, lengthy cardiopulmonary bypass operations, or other types of tissue injury

Focused assessment guidelines

NURSING HISTORY (Functional health pattern findings)

Health perception–health management pattern

Patient reports are relatively unimportant in diagnosis of this disorder. Patients commonly are too ill from the primary disorder to be aware of or report subjective manifestations. Even if they are able to report symptoms, the widespread manifestations of the disorder may cause symptoms to be variable and nonspecific.

Nutritional-metabolic pattern

- may complain of nausea or vomiting

Activity-exercise pattern

- may report dyspnea
- may report fatigue

Cognitive-perceptual pattern

- may report confusion

PHYSICAL FINDINGS

Physical findings are quite variable, depending on the underlying disorder, degree of organ involvement, and stage of DIC.

Cardiovascular

- blood oozing from multiple sites, such as I.V. insertion sites, incisions, and nasal mucosa around endotracheal or nasogastric tubes
- repeated episodes of minor bleeding
- frank hemorrhage
- hypotension

Integumentary

- acral cyanosis (irregularly shaped, patchy cyanosis of fingers, toes, or ears), considered diagnostic of DIC
- petechiae
- purpura
- ecchymoses
- hematomas

Pulmonary

- tachypnea
- epistaxis

Gastrointestinal

- hematemesis
- melena

Neurologic

- coma
- seizures

Renal

- hematuria

DIAGNOSTIC STUDIES

Note: DIC is a laboratory diagnosis based on a characteristic pattern of abnormal values.

- prothrombin time (PT)—prolonged, indicating dysfunction of the extrinsic clotting pathway.
- partial thromboplastin time (PTT)—prolonged, indicating dysfunction of the intrinsic clotting pathway.
- thrombin time—reveals circulating anticoagulants, such as fibrin split products, if prolonged at 1:1 dilution with normal plasma.

• fibrinogen level—decreased because of fibrinogen consumption.
• platelet count—diminished because of platelet consumption.
• fibrin split products—increased because of fibrinolysis.
• antithrombin III levels—decreased, indicating consumption by excessive thrombin formation.
• peripheral blood smear—reveals large platelets, reflecting rapid platelet usage, and red blood cell fragments, reflecting damage during red blood cell passage through areas of fibrin web formation.

POTENTIAL COMPLICATIONS

• organ necrosis

Collaborative problem: *Potential hemorrhage related to consumption of clotting factors, increased fibrinolysis, and presence of endogenous anticoagulants*

NURSING PRIORITY: Control clotting and bleeding.

Interventions	Rationales
1. Collaborate with the doctor to identify and treat the cause of DIC; for example, administer I.V. fluids to correct hypovolemia or antibiotics to combat sepsis, as ordered.	1. Removing or controlling the underlying cause of DIC is essential to effective treatment.
2. Monitor the presence and degree of hemorrhage. Observe for persistent oozing of blood at multiple sites, petechiae, purpura, ecchymoses, and hemorrhagic gingivitis. Note bleeding from wound sites, drains, and chest tubes. In the female patient, check for vaginal bleeding. Test all drainage for occult blood.	2. The presence and degree of bleeding provides a rough indicator of the severity of DIC.
3. Monitor coagulation panel, as ordered.	3. Coagulation values document the degree of DIC. They may be abnormal even if the patient is not yet showing clinical signs of the disorder.
4. Administer heparin, as ordered, typically as a bolus of 10,000 or more units, followed by continuous I.V. infusion of up to 30,000 units/24 hours *or* intermittent subcutaneous administration of 2,500 to 5,000 units every 4 to 8 hours (low-dose or minidose heparin therapy). Monitor the clotting time, as ordered, and report values exceeding 2½ times normal.	4. Heparin disrupts the vicious cycle of clotting and bleeding that is present in DIC. Although it cannot lyse clots already formed, it can prevent further clot formation. Its complex pharmacologic actions include inhibition of thrombin (therefore limiting platelet aggregation and conversion of fibrinogen to fibrin) and Factor X (therefore blocking both intrinsic and extrinsic pathways that lead to thrombin formation). Monitoring the clotting time allows the doctor to adjust the heparin dose to maintain a therapeutic blood level.
5. Administer transfusion therapy, as ordered, typically fresh whole blood, fresh frozen plasma, platelet concentrate, or factor concentrates.	5. Transfusion therapy replaces depleted clotting factors. Some doctors order it only after initiating heparinization, theorizing that replacing factors before interrupting the clotting cycle is like "adding fuel to the fire" (that is, only potentiating the DIC process).
6. Maintain a normal blood pressure by giving fluid and medications, as ordered.	6. Both hypotension and hypertension are detrimental to the DIC patient. Hypotension is one of the precipitating factors of the disease, whereas hypertension can dislodge precarious blood clots and initiate fresh bleeding.
7. Monitor for fluid overload. Observe for crackles, neck-vein distention, or increased pulmonary artery (PA) and wedge pressures. If present, collaborate with the doctor to reduce fluid volume, such as by administering diuretics.	7. DIC patients usually receive large amounts of fluid and frequent transfusions in an attempt to maintain optimal blood volume and cardiac output. Also, pulmonary capillary fragility makes them prone to develop interstitial edema. Untreated, fluid overload can progress to pulmonary edema.

Interventions	Rationales
8. Additional individualized interventions: ____________	8. Rationales: ____________

Target outcome criteria
Within 72 hours of the onset of bleeding, the patient will have:
- no further episodes of oozing or frank hemorrhage
- vital signs within normal limits for the patient
- coagulation laboratory values within normal limits.

Collaborative problem: *Ischemia related to microcirculatory thrombosis*

NURSING PRIORITY: Restore tissue perfusion.

Interventions	Rationales
1. Assess status of organ systems at least every 4 hours, including: • neurologic function, such as level of consciousness, pupils, and sensorimotor function of the arms and legs • cardiovascular function, such as pulse rate and volume, blood pressure, EKG pattern, and PA and wedge pressures • gastrointestinal function, such as bowel sounds and abdominal girth.	1. Tissue ischemia and necrosis can occur in any body system from the widespread deposition of thrombus in the microcirculation. In addition, hypotension activates the complement system, resulting in increased vascular permeability and blood cell lysis, and the kallikrein system, resulting in increased vascular permeability and vasodilation. The net results are arteriolar vasoconstriction, capillary dilation, and arteriovenous shunting. Stagnant blood accumulates in the dilated, bypassed capillaries and becomes acidotic, further damaging tissue and contributing to the clotting process.
2. Monitor renal function closely. Document hourly urine output, noting and reporting any decreasing trend. Summarize intake and output every 8 hours, noting and reporting any undesirable fluid retention.	2. The renal system is most likely to suffer from thrombosis, resulting in acute tubular necrosis. A trend of decreasing hourly urine outputs or oliguria may reflect this development. Because oliguria may also reflect other factors common in DIC, such as hypotension, cardiac failure, or hypovolemia, it must be interpreted only in the context of the patient's overall condition.
3. As ordered, implement measures (for example, fluid administration) to treat the underlying cause of tissue ischemia.	3. Tissue ischemia is best treated by attacking its causes, such as hypovolemia.
4. Additional individualized interventions: ____________	4. Rationales: ____________

Target outcome criteria
Within 72 hours, the patient will:
- produce hourly urine outputs exceeding 60 ml/hour
- exhibit a balanced fluid intake and output
- display normal vital signs.

Collaborative problem: *Potential hypoxemia related to increased pulmonary shunting, anemia, and acidosis*

NURSING PRIORITY: Optimize oxygenation.

Interventions	Rationales
1. Monitor arterial blood gas (ABG) values, as ordered, for hypoxemia and acidosis.	1. Ischemic damage to the pulmonary parenchyma increases pulmonary shunting, impairing oxygen uptake in the lungs. Red blood cell destruction produces a hemolytic anemia. Both of these factors lessen arterial oxygen content. Also, acidosis and decreased tissue perfusion impair oxygen delivery to the tissues.
2. Assess physical indicators of pulmonary status at least every 4 hours. Note increasing respiratory rate, abnormal respiratory rhythm, and crackles or other abnormal lung sounds. Observe nail beds and buccal mucosa for pallor and central cyanosis.	2. Respiratory rate accelerates to compensate for hypoxemia. Rhythm changes may reflect medullary hypoxemia. Adventitious lung sounds may reflect alveolar accumulation of fluid as the heart fails from ischemia. Pallor and cyanosis reflect arterial oxygen desaturation.
3. Administer supplemental oxygen, positive end-expiratory pressure (PEEP), or mechanical ventilation, as ordered.	3. Supplemental oxygen alone may be insufficient to raise low arterial oxygen content from pulmonary shunting. In that case, PEEP and mechanical ventilation may be necessary to improve functional residual capacity enough to combat hypoxemia.
4. Additional individualized interventions: ______________	4. Rationales: ______________

Target outcome criteria

Within 72 hours, the patient will:

- have ABG values within normal limits for the patient
- display a eupneic respiratory pattern
- have a respiratory rate between 18 and 24 breaths per minute
- display pink nail beds and buccal mucosa.

Nursing diagnosis: *Impaired skin integrity related to capillary fragility*

NURSING PRIORITY: Prevent further bleeding.

Interventions	Rationales
1. Avoid needle punctures, whenever possible. If a needle puncture is essential, use the smallest gauge needle possible and apply pressure to the site for 10 minutes afterward. Whenever possible, administer medications I.V., as ordered.	1. These measures may help reduce the incidence of hematoma formation. In addition, because of poor tissue perfusion, medication deposited I.M. may be absorbed erratically, if at all. Administering medications I.V. provides for more effective absorption and avoids creating a needle puncture site from which the patient may bleed.
2. Handle the patient very gently. Be particularly careful to avoid disturbing healing areas.	2. Gentle handling minimizes skin trauma. Being particularly careful around healing sites minimizes the risk of dislodging unstable clots.
3. Use cushioning and pressure-relieving devices, such as sheepskin. Pad the bed rails.	3. Such action minimizes the risk of hematoma development from extreme capillary fragility.
4. Provide gentle mouth care with swabs and diluted mouthwash.	4. A toothbrush may damage fragile capillaries and result in gingival bleeding.

Target outcome criteria
Within 72 hours of onset of DIC, the patient will have no new hematoma formation.

Nursing diagnosis: *Pain related to tissue ischemia, hematomas, or bleeding into organ or joint capsules*

NURSING PRIORITY: Relieve pain.

Interventions	Rationales
1. Assess for pain frequently. Use various pain-relieving measures, such as ice packs for hematomas or soothing music. Promote rest and provide emotional support. Consult the "Acute Pain" care plan, page 10, for details.	1. The "Acute Pain" care plan contains details applicable to any patient in pain. This care plan contains interventions specific to DIC. Soothing music is useful for relieving tension and lessening pain perception.
2. Administer pain medications I.V.	2. DIC may cause erratic absorption of I.M. medications.
3. Additional individualized interventions: ____________	3. Rationales: ____________

Target outcome criteria
Within 1 hour of pain onset, the patient will:
• have a relaxed facial expression and body posture
• if able to communicate, indicate that pain is relieved.

Transfer planning

NURSING TRANSFER CRITERIA
Upon transfer, documentation shows evidence of:
• stable vital signs
• laboratory coagulation panel within normal limits for the patient
• no bleeding episodes for at least 24 hours.

PATIENT-FAMILY TEACHING CHECKLIST
Document evidence that patient and family demonstrate understanding of:
__ basic pathophysiology and implications of DIC
__ rationale for therapy
__ pain relief measures.

DOCUMENTATION CHECKLIST
Using outcome criteria as a guide, document:
__ clinical status on admission
__ significant changes in status
__ pertinent diagnostic test findings
__ bleeding episodes
__ transfusion and fluid replacement therapy
__ pain relief measures
__ patient-family teaching
__ transfer planning.

ASSOCIATED CARE PLANS
Acute Heart Failure
Acute Pain
Adult Respiratory Distress Syndrome
Cardiac Surgery
Impaired Physical Mobility
Ineffective Coping
Liver Failure
Major Burns
Mechanical Ventilation
Multiple Trauma
Nutritional Deficit
Renal Failure
Shock

REFERENCES
Griffin, J. "The Bleeding Patient," *Nursing86* 34-42, June 1986.
Holloway, N. *Nursing the Critically Ill Adult,* 3rd ed. Menlo Park, Calif.: Addison-Wesley Publishing Company, in press.
Ives, J. "Disseminated Intravascular Coagulation (DIC)," in *Critical Care Nursing,* 4th ed. Edited by Hudak, C., et al. Philadelphia: J.B. Lippincott Co., 1986.

SUBSTANCE ABUSE

Drug Overdose

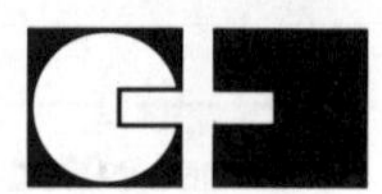

DRG information

DRG 449 Poisoning and Toxic Effects of Drugs.
Age >17. With Complications or Comorbidities (CC).
Mean LOS = 6.1 days
Principal diagnoses include:
• poisoning by drugs of all varieties, affecting multiple body systems
• toxic effects of alcohol.

DRG 450 Poisoning and Toxic Effects of Drugs.
Age >17. Without CC.
Mean LOS = 4.1 days
Principal diagnoses include selected principal diagnoses listed under DRG 449. The distinction is that DRG 450 excludes complications or comorbidities.

DRG 451 Poisoning and Toxic Effects of Drugs.
Age 0 to 17.
Mean LOS = 4.4 days
Principal diagnoses include selected principal diagnoses listed under DRG 449. The distinction is that DRG 451 excludes patients >17 years.

Introduction

DEFINITION AND TIME FOCUS

The patient admitted to the critical care unit (CCU) following a drug overdose (OD) presents a particular challenge. In many cases, the patient is comatose, withdrawn, agitated, somnolent, or otherwise unable to provide clear historical data. The type of drug involved may be unknown, or evidence may suggest multiple drug ingestion. If illegal substances are involved, family members may be reluctant to provide a full history because they fear possible criminal prosecution, even if assured of medical confidentiality.

Even when the patient or family clearly identifies a specific drug that was taken, the possibility of multiple drug ingestion or potential interaction of other medications with the drug involved must always be considered. For the purposes of this care plan, overdose will be defined as an intentional act in which the patient ingests, injects, sniffs, inhales, or otherwise self-administers a dosage that proves to be toxic.

Using this definition, the care plan omits discussion of overdoses from accidental poisoning, toxic reactions to prescribed medications taken at recommended doses, and industrial or agricultural exposure to toxic substances. This care plan focuses on the patient who is admitted to the CCU for treatment of an intentional overdose, commonly associated with a suicide gesture or attempt.

ETIOLOGY AND PRECIPITATING FACTORS

For each patient, different factors precipitate the overdose event, but usually one or more of the following are involved:
• drug or alcohol abuse or addiction
• unhealthy coping patterns
• unusually stressful life event or circumstances
• despair, depression, anger, or the desire for revenge

Focused assessment guidelines

NURSING HISTORY (Functional health pattern findings)

Health perception–health management pattern

• may reveal history of short- or long-term drug or alcohol abuse or addiction
• may reveal intent to commit suicide
• may admit previous suicide attempt

Sleep-rest pattern

• may give history of insomnia or early morning awakening (associated with depression)

Cognitive-perceptual pattern

• may show poor concentration or memory impairment
• may experience difficulty making decisions

Self-perception–self-concept pattern

• expresses helpless or hopeless self-perception commonly
• may make self-deprecating statements

Role-relationship pattern

• may lack a significant other
• may describe recent conflict or breakup with significant other
• may reveal recent or chronic job difficulties
• may have experienced the death of a loved one recently

Coping–stress tolerance pattern

• may use unhealthful coping behavior habitually, such as drug abuse

Value-belief pattern

• may express surprise or disbelief about seriousness of overdose

PHYSICAL FINDINGS

Because physical findings vary so widely in patients with drug overdoses, depending on the specific drug taken, this section is omitted. See the *Nurse's Guide to Common Drug Overdoses* or consult pharmacologic references for findings associated with specific drug overdoses.

DIAGNOSTIC STUDIES

Appropriate laboratory tests vary widely, depending on the specific drug taken. The following are commonly performed for toxicity screening and evaluation.

• serum electrolyte levels—may be abnormal; several drugs commonly seen in overdose cases, including salicylates and alcohol, may cause electrolyte abnormalities.

• arterial blood gas (ABG) values—essential for monitoring the adequacy of respiratory efforts; salicylates and other drugs cause acid-base abnormalities.

• liver enzymes—may reveal liver damage; many medications can cause liver damage at toxic levels, most notably acetaminophen and alcohol.

• blood alcohol level—an important screening test in any overdose because many drug effects are potentiated by alcohol, thus increasing central nervous system depression.

• toxicology screening assay—checks for various substances, depending on the laboratory, but usually includes barbiturates, narcotics, amphetamines, salicylates, and acetaminophen, among others.

• serum salicylate level—may reveal toxicity; time-elapsed nomograms are obtained in acute overdosage to assess toxicity level. Because salicylates have a prolonged half-life, the sample should be obtained at least 6 hours after ingestion. Toxic range is >150 mcg/ml.

• urine narcotic levels—determine narcotic presence and concentration; most narcotics are excreted in urine within 48 hours of administration. Toxic levels vary depending on specific narcotic.

• serum barbiturate levels—determine the concentration of barbiturates in the blood. Salicylates may interfere with the test; alcohol ingestion may increase barbiturate levels. Toxic levels vary depending on the barbiturate taken.

• serum antidepressant levels—identify drug presence and concentration. Toxic levels vary, depending on the specific antidepressant; for most tricyclic antidepressants, toxic range is >1,000 ng/ml.

• abdominal X-rays—can reveal a mass of pills in the stomach.

• gastroscopy—may be performed to remove substances if X-rays reveal a coalesced mass of material that cannot be removed by lavage.

POTENTIAL COMPLICATIONS

See *Nurse's Guide to Common Drug Overdoses.*

NURSE'S GUIDE TO COMMON DRUG OVERDOSES

Drug	Effects	Signs and symptoms	Treatment	Complications
acetaminophen	Fever reduction by hypothalamic impairment; raised pain threshold; exact mechanisms unclear; metabolized in liver	• Anorexia • Nausea and vomiting • Diaphoresis • Right upper quadrant abdominal pain • Jaundice • Hypotension • Altered level of consciousness	• Emesis or lavage • Cathartics • Acetylcysteine (Mucomyst), if >7.5 g ingested; ingested within 24 hours; and serum level in toxic range 4 hours after ingestion	• Hepatic failure • Coagulation defects • Renal failure • Hepatic encephalopathy • Shock
alcohol (ethanol)	Central nervous system (CNS) depression; peripheral vasodilatation; direct destruction of brain cells by acetaldehyde; potentiation with many other drugs	• Ataxia • Reduced comprehension • Vomiting • Respiratory depression • Hypotension • Seizures • Flushing • Coma	• Emesis or lavage, if ingestion within 4 hours • I.V. fluids • Thiamine, dextrose, or multivitamins • Ventilatory support, especially in multiple drug overdose • Observation for withdrawal, including anxiety, tremor, diaphoresis, tachycardia, hypertension (usually occurs 24 to 48 hours after last alcohol intake) • If withdrawal symptoms are noted, sedation	• Massive respiratory depression • Aspiration • Liver failure • GI tract bleeding

(continued)

NURSE'S GUIDE TO COMMON DRUG OVERDOSES *(continued)*

Drug	Effects	Signs and symptoms	Treatment	Complications
barbiturates	CNS depression	• Cardiopulmonary depression • Hypotension • Sluggish pupil response • Nystagmus • Bullae • Hypothermia • Coma	• Ventilatory support • Emesis or lavage • Activated charcoal • Cathartics • I.V. fluids • Observation for withdrawal, including tremors, vomiting, weakness, hallucinations • Dialysis possible for large doses of long-acting barbiturates	• Dysrhythmias • Respiratory arrest • Shock • Seizures • Pulmonary edema
benzodiazepines	CNS depression	• Lethargy • Hypotension • Tachycardia • Respiratory depression • Confusion • Coma	• Ventilatory support • Emesis or lavage • Activated charcoal • Cathartics • Physostigmine salicylate (Antilirium), if severe CNS depression • I.V. fluids • Hemodialysis or forced diuresis: not effective	• Taken alone, no fatalities, but possible potentiating effects in multiple-drug overdoses
cocaine	CNS stimulation	• Hyperexcitability • Anxiety • Hypertension or hypotension • Fever • Tachypnea • Tachycardia • Confusion • Hallucinations • Dilated pupils • Diaphoresis • Convulsions • Coma	• Anticonvulsants • Cardiac monitoring • Emesis or lavage, if ingested • Activated charcoal, if ingested • Cathartic, if ingested • Fever control measures	• Myocardial infarction • Cerebral hemorrhage • Respiratory arrest • Status epilepticus
narcotics	CNS depression	• Respiratory depression • Constricted pupils • Reduced level of consciousness • Hypothermia • Hypotension • Bradycardia	• Ventilatory support • Naloxone (Narcan) I.M. or I.V. in repeated doses • Close monitoring, because respiratory depression may recur • Cardiac monitoring • Emesis or lavage, if ingested	• Respiratory arrest • Shock • Dysrhythmias
salicylates	Direct respiratory stimulation; interference with normal clotting; increased gastric motility	• Nausea and vomiting • Hyperthermia • Electrolyte imbalances • Acid-base imbalances (usually respiratory alkalosis and metabolic acidosis) • Hyperglycemia (in children, hypoglycemia) • Hyperpnea • Hyperventilation • Oliguria • Tinnitus • Confusion • Convulsions • Petechiae	• Ventilatory support • Cardiac monitoring • I.V. fluids • Cooling measures • Correction of electrolyte and acid-base abnormalities • Emesis or lavage • Activated charcoal • Cathartics • Alkalinization of urine with sodium bicarbonate and potassium chloride (a urine pH between 7.5 and 8.5 promotes increased renal excretion)	• Respiratory failure • Dysrhythmias or other life-threatening conditions caused by electrolyte or acid-base abnormalities • Renal tubular necrosis • GI bleeding • Hepatotoxicity • Pulmonary edema • Shock

NURSE'S GUIDE TO COMMON DRUG OVERDOSES *(continued)*

Drug	Effects	Signs and symptoms	Treatment	Complications
tricyclic antidepressants	Central and peripheral anticholinergic effects; myocardial depression; rapid absorption rate	• Lethargy • Dry mouth • Dilated pupils • Confusion • Tremors • Urinary retention • Tachycardia • Hypotension • Respiratory depression • Cardiac conduction delay • Hypothermia • Convulsions • Coma	• Ventilatory support • Cardiac monitoring • Emesis or lavage • Activated charcoal • Cathartics • I.V. fluids • Sodium physostigmine 1 to 3 mg I.V., if large amount ingested • Cardiac pacing, if complete heart block • Anticonvulsants • Alkalinization with sodium bicarbonate • Temperature regulation measures • Dialysis: ineffective	• Dysrhythmias • Complete heart block • Congestive heart failure • Shock • Paralytic ileus

Nursing diagnosis: *Potential ineffective airway clearance related to reduced alertness, decreased or absent gag reflex, obstruction by tongue, vomiting, or lavage procedures*

NURSING PRIORITY: Maintain a clear airway.

Interventions	Rationales
1. Assess the patient's airway status continually by noting the adequacy of spontaneous respiratory effort, chest excursion, breath sounds, gag reflex, skin color, and level of consciousness.	1. Initial and ongoing airway evaluation is essential in the patient who has taken a drug overdose because many medications cause central nervous system (CNS) depression. If several medications were taken, their combining or potentiating effects may further reduce the patient's ability to clear the airway.
2. Position the patient on his side. Ensure that suction equipment is at the bedside, ready for use.	2. The side-lying position facilitates drainage from the mouth and reduces the possibility of aspiration. Suctioning may be needed if the patient vomits.
3. If lavage is initiated, ensure airway protection by placing the patient in a head-down position or assisting with placement of a cuffed endotracheal tube if the patient is obtunded.	3. Aspiration of gastric contents predisposes the patient to aspiration pneumonitis, a complication associated with increased morbidity and mortality.
4. If the patient's gag reflex is reduced or absent or if respirations are <12 or >24/minute, shallow, or labored, anticipate and assist with endotracheal intubation and mechanical ventilation. See the "Mechanical Ventilation" care plan, page 108, for details.	4. Toxic CNS effects may interfere with vital functions. Unless promptly corrected, respiratory impairment results in permanent damage to the brain and other organs.
5. Monitor ABG levels, as ordered. See the "Acid-base Imbalances" appendix, page 316.	5. Changes in ABG levels may provide early warning of impaired ventilatory status even before clinical evidence is apparent. Also, toxic levels of many medications cause acid-base abnormalities; ABG studies serve as a guide for corrective intervention.
6. Additional individualized interventions: ______	6. Rationales: ______

Target outcome criteria
Throughout the CCU stay, the patient will:
• maintain a clear airway
• maintain spontaneous respiratory rate of 12 to 24 breaths per minute or receive mechanical ventilatory assistance.

Collaborative problem: *Potential multi-organ dysfunction related to systemic toxic effects of drug(s)*

NURSING PRIORITIES: (a) Support and monitor vital organ functions, and (b) identify and counteract effects of drugs.

Interventions

1. Collect as much historical data as possible about the overdose by questioning the patient, family, friends, and other caregivers. Determine the following, if at all possible:
• what was taken
• how much was taken
• when it was taken
• how it was taken (for example, ingested or injected)
• concomitant alcohol use
• underlying health problems
• other medications taken
• what has been done for the patient so far.

2. Monitor vital signs, hemodynamic pressures, and EKG findings according to the "Monitoring Standards" appendix, page 314, or unit protocol.

3. Collaborate with the doctor and the regional poison control center personnel in selecting and initiating measures to reverse or eliminate the drug(s) from the body (some of the measures may have already been implemented in the emergency department). Initiate one or more of the following, as appropriate:

• Induced emesis with ipecac syrup, 30 ml orally with fluids. Observe for onset of vomiting within 15 to 30 minutes. If no emesis, the dose may be repeated once. If still no emesis, consult the doctor and prepare for gastric lavage. Never administer ipecac if the patient has an absent gag reflex, signs of decreasing alertness, or seizures or if he has ingested corrosives. Consult with the poison center before administering ipecac in patients with hydrocarbon ingestion.

Rationales

1. Thorough history-taking may be difficult, but it provides vital clues for effective intervention and ongoing monitoring.

2. At toxic levels, many drugs can interfere with the vasomotor center's control of cardiac function and blood vessel constriction. Baseline and ongoing assessment of these parameters provides early warning of cardiovascular dysfunction.

3. Since the institution of regional poison control centers, with their "hot line" consultative services, the mortality from poisonings has fallen significantly. The poison control center provides expert advice on treating all types of drug overdoses.

• Ipecac syrup is thought to act both centrally and locally on the gastrointestinal tract to stimulate vomiting. Fluids are given with ipecac because, without adequate gastric volume, esophageal injury may occur from forceful retching. Doses >60 ml may have cardiotoxic effects. Ipecac administration is contraindicated in the circumstances noted because vomiting under such conditions may result in aspiration. Also, vomiting of corrosives may cause or increase damage to esophageal and oropharyngeal mucosal surfaces. Treating hydrocarbon ingestion depends on the specific substance ingested. Ipecac may not be effective if the patient has taken an overdose of antiemetic medication, such as phenothiazine.

Interventions	Rationales
• Gastric lavage, using a large-bore Ewald tube and the irrigant that the doctor prefers, usually normal saline solution. Lavage with 100 to 200 ml fluid boluses and avoid overdistending the stomach with fluid. Lavage until return is clear, unless otherwise ordered, usually 1,000 to 1,500 ml total. Monitor inflow and outflow volumes and report discrepancies. Save aspirated fluid for analysis, as needed. Monitor serum electrolyte levels in conjunction with large-volume or prolonged lavage.	• Gastric lavage is used when vomiting is contraindicated (for example, if the patient has a reduced or absent gag reflex). It effectively removes ingested substances from the stomach, but is thought to be somewhat less effective than induced emesis. The choice of fluid is controversial and may depend on the specific drug ingested. Fluid boluses larger than 200 ml are thought to wash the toxin into the small bowel. A discrepancy between the amounts of instilled irrigant and returned fluid may indicate a need to reposition the patient to promote drainage or may indicate fluid reabsorption and risk of fluid overload. The aspirate may be examined for diagnostic clues. Electrolyte imbalances, and their cardiovascular sequelae, may result from prolonged or large-volume lavage.
• Dilution, usually with milk or water, unless the patient is obtunded.	• Dilution is used primarily to treat ingestion of corrosives or other substances that preclude emesis. Distending the abdomen with fluid, if the patient is obtunded, may increase the risk of aspiration.
• Gut lavage, using a peristaltic pump to deliver warmed electrolyte solution to the stomach.	• This relatively new therapy may be used to aid clearance of certain herbicides from the bowel.
• Activated charcoal, usually 25 to 50 g in a slurry, administered orally or via gastric tube after the emesis or lavage is completed. Do not give charcoal with ipecac syrup.	• Activated charcoal is an inert substance that adsorbs toxins. It should not be given at the same time as ipecac syrup because it will inactivate the ipecac and prevent emesis. Clinicians' opinions vary on whether the charcoal should be removed after a given time or allowed to pass through the gut.
• Cathartics, as ordered, usually mixed with charcoal. Cathartics ordered include magnesium sulfate and magnesium citrate.	• Saline cathartics stimulate peristaltic activity by drawing fluid into the bowel through osmotic effects, thus hastening drug excretion and reducing absorption in the gut.
• Specific antidotes-antagonists, as ordered. See the *Nurse's Guide to Common Drug Overdoses*, page 259, for further details.	• A few drugs, notably narcotics and acetaminophen, are effectively treated with antidote-antagonist substances; however, multiple drug ingestion is always a possibility, so the clinician must remain vigilant even if these measures are employed.
• Other measures, as recommended by the doctor or poison control center, such as forced diuresis, peritoneal dialysis, hemodialysis, exchange transfusion, or gastroscopy.	• Forced diuresis may be used if the drug involved is excreted primarily through the urinary tract. Dialysis may help remove certain substances, but its effectiveness depends on the drug's pharmacologic properties and its distribution within body tissues. Exchange transfusion may be used for certain drugs if the dosage is massive and recent enough that absorption by tissues has not yet taken place. Gastroscopy may be performed if abdominal X-rays reveal a coalesced mass of pills in the stomach.
4. Perform meticulous serial evaluations of level of consciousness, mental status, and protective reflex status (gag and corneal) every 1 to 2 hours during the first 24 hours or until the patient's condition stabilizes.	4. Decreasing alertness and diminished or absent protective reflexes indicate CNS impairment and impending need for airway management or ventilatory support. Serial evaluations allow early detection of subtle changes.
5. Monitor intake and output and report dropping urinary output (<60 ml/hour) promptly to the doctor.	5. Because many medications are detoxified or excreted through the renal system, the possibility of renal failure from toxic effects must always be considered. Also, a dropping urine output is a clue to the early development of shock, another potential complication of drug toxicity.

(continued)

Interventions	Rationales
6. Assess and monitor initial or serial laboratory test findings, as ordered, for specific overdose substance(s). See the *Nurse's Guide to Common Drug Overdoses*, page 259, for further details.	6. Specific initial and serial urine or serum studies provide information about the amount of drug(s) taken and the rate of absorption, guiding therapeutic treatment.
7. Additional individualized interventions: ________	7. Rationales: ________

Target outcome criteria

Within 1 hour of admission to the hospital, the patient will receive initial treatment for specific drugs taken.

Throughout the unit stay, the patient will maintain vital organ functions.

Nursing diagnosis: *Hopelessness related to low self-esteem, emotional disorganization, or sense of having inadequate resources to cope with life*

NURSING PRIORITIES: (a) Promote a sense of hope, and (b) foster self-esteem.

Interventions	Rationales
1. Examine your own attitudes toward suicide and drug abuse. Assume a concerned but nonjudgmental attitude and avoid vindictive or "punishing" behavior when providing care. Seek peer support or consult with a psychiatric liaison nurse if negative attitudes affect patient care.	1. Many health professionals have difficulty caring for suicidal or self-abusive patients. Frustration and anger are common when the patient seems to be undermining the efforts of health care providers. "Punishing" attitudes, however, tend to further decrease the patient's already fragile self-esteem and reduce coping ability. The patient is likely to interpret such behavior as "just one more sign I'm no good for anything," further adding to self-directed anger and hopelessness. Peer or psychiatric liaison support can help professionals address and resolve issues raised by abusive or noncompliant responses to care.
2. Foster communication.	2. Commonly, the patient who has overdosed perceives himself to be without resources or cannot communicate feelings because of emotional disorganization. Opening communication is the first step in identifying more positive responses to the problems that may have resulted in the overdose.
• Use touch, as appropriate.	• Touch can convey profound messages of acceptance and caring and may, for some patients, be less threatening than verbal interaction as a way to initiate the therapeutic relationship.
• Use active listening skills.	• Active listening involves an attentive attitude, feedback, and rephrasing or reflection to help the patient clarify feelings and ideas. This reassures the patient that his feelings are worthy of attention and that he is important.
• Note and acknowledge nonverbal cues (body posture and gestures, facial expression, tone of voice, silences).	• Acknowledging nonverbal communication may help verify expressed feelings or open discussion of unexpressed feelings.
• Make eye contact.	• Making eye contact in a nonthreatening manner is a simple way to express interest and the intent to communicate.

Interventions	Rationales
3. Encourage the patient to participate in care-related decisions, as soon as his condition permits.	3. Consideration of the patient's stated wishes may, in many cases, be secondary to saving the patient's life. However, as the patient's condition stabilizes, a return to participation in self-care helps bolster self-respect and reduces feelings of powerlessness.
4. Arrange referral to psychiatric resources (such as a psychiatric nurse specialist, psychiatrist, or other mental health professional). Place the patient on suicide precautions, if appropriate.	4. Any patient admitted with an intentional overdose warrants psychiatric evaluation and counseling as part of the treatment plan. Careful evaluation of suicide potential is essential. If continuing suicidal ideation is present, suicide precautions are warranted to avoid a repeated suicide attempt during hospitalization.
5. See the "Ineffective Coping" care plan, page 26, and the "Grieving and Dying" care plan, page 15.	5. The "Ineffective Coping" care plan contains interventions for patients struggling with emotional adjustments. The "Grieving and Dying" care plan addresses issues that may relate to the care of the patient who has attempted suicide.
6. Ensure appropriate follow-up care arrangements before discharge from the unit, including continuation of suicide precautions, if appropriate.	6. The patient who has been severely depressed may attempt suicide again once physical energy has been restored and he begins to appear "better." Careful follow-up, both on the unit to which the patient is transferred and after discharge from the hospital, is vital in assisting the patient's transition back to everyday life.
7. Additional individualized interventions: ____________ ____________	7. Rationales: ____________ ____________

Target outcome criteria
Before transfer from the unit, the patient will:
- discuss reasons for the overdose and identify precipitating factors
- participate, to the extent possible, in self-care and care planning
- begin to display coping behaviors that are health-promoting
- make contact with follow-up care providers.

Transfer planning

NURSING TRANSFER CRITERIA

Upon transfer, documentation shows evidence of:
- spontaneous respirations and airway clearance
- stable vital signs for at least 12 hours
- completion of specific measures to remove or reverse drugs consumed
- drug levels (if applicable) declining since admission
- urinary output >60 ml/hour
- ABG values within normal limits
- initial psychiatric evaluation and follow-up arrangements made
- implementation of suicide precautions, if appropriate.

PATIENT-FAMILY TEACHING CHECKLIST

Document evidence that patient and family demonstrate understanding of:
__ toxic effects of drugs and possible later complications
__ treatment measures undertaken
__ signs and symptoms of complications, if any anticipated
__ health-promoting coping behaviors
__ resources available for help.

DOCUMENTATION CHECKLIST

Using outcome criteria as a guide, document:
__ clinical status on admission
__ significant changes in status
__ pertinent laboratory and diagnostic test findings
__ effectiveness of measures to promote elimination or reversal of drugs
__ mental health measures
__ suicide precautions, if used
__ follow-up plans
__ patient-family teaching
__ transfer planning.

ASSOCIATED CARE PLANS

Acute Renal Failure
Grieving and Dying

Ineffective Coping
Impaired Physical Mobility
Mechanical Ventilation
Sensory-Perceptual Alteration
Shock

REFERENCES

Acee, A., and Smith, D. "Crack," *American Journal of Nursing* 87(5):614-17, May 1987.

Alspach, J., and Williams, S. *Core Curriculum for Critical Care Nursing,* 3rd ed. Philadelphia: W.B. Saunders Co., 1985.

Diagnostics. Nurse's Reference Library series. Springhouse, Pa.: Springhouse Corp., 1983.

Emergencies. Nurse's Reference Library series. Springhouse, Pa.: Springhouse Corp., 1985.

Lasater, M. "Nursing Care of the Patient with a Tricyclic Antidepressant Overdose," *Critical Care Nurse* 4(4):28-30, 1984.

Leoni, M.P. "Management of Acetaminophen Overdose," *Critical Care Nurse* 5(4):44-57.

Moisan, D. "Poison and Drug Overdose," in *Critical Care Nursing: A Holistic Approach,* 4th ed. Edited by Hudak, C., et al. Philadelphia: J. B. Lippincott Co., 1986.

Strasen, L. "Acute Alcohol Withdrawal Syndrome in the Critical Care Unit," *Critical Care Nurse* 2(12):24-31, November/December 1982.

Thurkauf, G. "Acetaminophen Overdose," *Critical Care Nurse* 7(1):20-30, 1987.

Major Burns

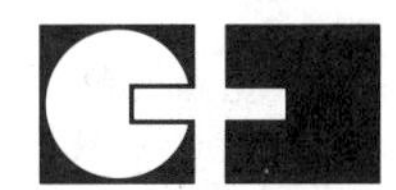

DRG information

DRGs involving burns are assigned based on specific sites, percent of body surface burned, percent of third-degree burns, and operative procedures

DRG 456 Burns Transferred to Another Acute Care Facility.
Mean LOS = 4.6 days

DRG 457 Extensive Burns, Without Operating Room Procedures.
Mean LOS = 4.1 days
Principal diagnoses include, in general, burns involving 20% to 90% or more of body surface, with 10% to 90% or more third-degree burns.

DRG 458 Non-Extensive Burns With Skin Grafts.
Mean LOS = 16.1 days
Principal diagnoses include first-, second-, or third-degree burns of face, scalp, head, or neck (with or without loss of body part). Usually, burns involving 10% to 49% of body surface, with 10% to 19% third-degree burns.
Additional DRG information: One or more of these diagnoses must be accompanied by one or more of the following principal procedures:
- graft (free skin, full-thickness, or split-thickness) to breast, hand, or other site
- heterograft or homograft to skin.

DRG 459 Non-Extensive Burns With Wound Debridement and Other Operating Room Procedures.
Mean LOS = 10.0 days
Principal diagnoses include selected principal diagnoses listed under DRG 458.
Additional DRG information: One or more of these diagnoses must be accompanied by one or more of the following selected principal procedures:
- debridement of infection or burn
- amputation of upper or lower limb, or penis
- revision of amputation stump
- closure of oral, bronchial, tracheal, thoracic, or gastric fistula
- reconstruction, repair, or plastic operations and reattachments of body parts or organs.

DRG 460 Non-Extensive Burns Without Operating Room Procedures.
Mean LOS = 6.4 days
Principal diagnoses include selected principal diagnoses listed under DRG 458.

DRG 472 Extensive Burns With Operating Room Procedure.
Mean LOS = 17.1 days
Principal diagnoses include selected principal diagnoses listed under DRG 457, accompanied by a principal procedure listed under DRG 458 or DRG 459.

Introduction

DEFINITION AND TIME FOCUS

A burn is an integumentary injury caused by an exposure to a thermal, chemical, or electrical source of trauma. The severity of the burn depends on the depth of the tissue burned and the amount of body surface area affected. Partial-thickness burns can be superficial (first-degree), involving only the epidermis, or deep (second-degree), involving the epidermal and dermal layers of the skin. Some epithelial tissue remains uninjured, particularly the hair follicles, and can regenerate new skin. Full-thickness burns (third- and fourth-degree) involve the epidermis, dermis, subcutaneous tissues, and, sometimes, underlying muscle, tendon, and bone. Full-thickness burns require skin grafting for healing.

The total body surface area (TBSA) burned is estimated using the Rule of Nines or the Lund and Browder chart. Both the depth and the area of the burn are used as criteria to determine the initial treatment and the necessity for admission to a burn unit. Patients with more than 25% partial-thickness TBSA; more than 10% full-thickness TBSA; burn injuries complicated by trauma, chronic illness, or inhalation or electrical injuries; or burns affecting special areas such as the face, eyes, ears, hands, feet, or the perineum should be treated in burn units. This also applies to children under age 2 or adults over age 60.

Patients with moderate burns without complications can be treated in a general critical care unit (CCU). Minor burns can be treated in the emergency department or in the doctor's office. This clinical plan focuses on the patient who is admitted to the CCU for treatment of superficial and deep partial-thickness burns involving more than 25% of the body.

ETIOLOGY AND PRECIPITATING FACTORS

- occupational sources of burn injuries, such as fuels, chemicals, electricity, or hot substances
- home sources of burn injuries, such as cooking, electricity, heaters, chemicals, matches, or cigarettes

- outdoor sources of burn injuries, such as sunburn, lightning, barbecues, or flammable liquids
- high-risk populations, such as young children, elderly persons, drug or alcohol abusers, chronically ill or debilitated patients, or those working in high-risk jobs

Focused assessment guidelines

NURSING HISTORY (Functional health pattern findings)

Health perception–health management pattern
- may report a high-risk job for burn injuries
- may report a high-risk activity that caused the burn
- may report chronic illness or debilitation

Nutritional-metabolic pattern
- may report thirst
- may report nausea, vomiting, and loss of appetite
- may report feelings of fullness in abdomen

Elimination pattern
- may report decreased or absent urination

Activity-exercise pattern
- may report pain and stiffness when moving involved area
- may report difficulty in breathing at rest and during movement

Cognitive-perceptual pattern
- may report pain
- may repeatedly verbalize the circumstances of the burn injury, or may report confusion and loss of memory about burn incident

Self-perception–self-concept pattern
- may express fear of loss of body part or disfigurement
- may express fear of dying

Role-relationship pattern
- may express concern about whereabouts and condition of others involved in the burn incident
- may express fear about maintaining role in family and in relationships
- may express concern over effects of injury on family
- may express fear about not being able to work again

Sexuality-reproductive pattern
- may express fear about not being able to perform sexually in the future
- may express fear about lack of sexual attractiveness because of injury

Coping–stress tolerance pattern
- initially may express lack of concern about burn injury
- may express fear and anxiety
- may express being overwhelmed by burn injury

Value-belief pattern
- may express need to see member of clergy

PHYSICAL FINDINGS

Note: Physical findings may vary depending on the type, depth, surface area involved, and location of the burn injuries.

Pulmonary
- apnea
- tachypnea, dyspnea, shortness of breath on exertion
- if an inhalation injury, soot in nostrils or sputum
- stridor
- wheezing
- hoarse voice
- diminished breath sounds
- mucosal edema, vesicles, redness

Cardiovascular
- tachycardia
- hypotension
- dysrhythmias
- pale, clammy, diaphoretic, or cool skin
- if an electrical injury, cardiac arrest with ventricular fibrillation; chest pain; or cardiac irritability

Neurologic
- agitation
- memory loss
- confusion
- headache
- mentation changes

Gastrointestinal
- decreased or absent bowel sounds
- distention
- vomiting
- dry mouth and mucous membranes

Genitourinary
- oliguria to anuria
- cloudy or tea-colored urine

Musculoskeletal
- pain and stiffness on movement of affected areas
- if electrical injury is involved, tetany and bone fractures caused by tetany or fall

Integumentary
- if a superficial partial-thickness burn is involved, bright red to pink color, glistening blisters, blanching on pressure, and pain
- if a deep partial-thickness burn is involved, pink to white color, blanching, pain, sensitive to pressure, and blisters
- if a full-thickness burn is involved, white, gray, brown, or black skin color; eschar (coagulated and necrotic burned tissue) formation; no pain or pressure sensations; no blanching; dry, easily pulled out hair

- massive edema
- hypothermia
- shivering

DIAGNOSTIC STUDIES

- complete blood count—determines red blood cell count and hemoglobin and hematocrit levels, reflecting any blood loss or destruction and indicating the oxygen-carrying ability of the blood. The white blood cell (WBC) count reflects the adequacy of the WBCs to respond to the inflammatory process. Baseline data and serial evaluations may reflect the seriousness of the fluid shifts and cellular destruction accompanying major burns.
- serum electrolyte level—monitors fluid, electrolyte, and acid-base status. Hyperkalemia occurs initially because of the release of potassium into the serum during cell destruction and the hemoconcentration caused by the fluid shifts into the interstitium. Hypokalemia may occur during the second postburn day as electrolytes are excreted into the urine. Other electrolytes may be low during the initial period after injury because of the massive fluid and electrolyte shifts into the interstitium.
- blood glucose level—monitors the effect of the catabolic burn state on sugar metabolism and insulin production.
- blood urea nitrogen and creatinine levels—monitor the adequacy of kidney function; acute tubular necrosis is a common complication after major tissue destruction.
- clotting time (prothrombin time and partial thromboplastin time)—may reflect coagulation problems associated with major tissue destruction.
- serum proteins (albumin and globulin) and serum osmolality—may reflect movement of intravascular colloids in and out of the interstitium.
- arterial blood gas (ABG) values—monitor oxygenation, ventilation, and acid-base status, especially with a suspected inhalation injury. Initially, they reveal respiratory alkalosis, reflecting hyperventilation; later, metabolic acidosis, reflecting hypoxemia and shock.
- carboxyhemoglobin level—may be elevated, confirming carbon monoxide poisoning and smoke inhalation.
- urinalysis, specific gravity, urine electrolytes, and urine myoglobin levels—monitor kidney status. Total urine output monitors adequacy of hydration.
- blood and tissue cultures—provide baseline data and monitor infections.
- chest X-ray—usually normal at first; in 1 to 2 days, it may reveal atelectasis or pulmonary edema.
- electrocardiogram—may reveal dysrhythmias.
- ventilation-perfusion pulmonary scan—may reveal areas of nonventilation and nonperfusion.
- bronchoscopy—may reveal abnormalities of the bronchial tree such as redness, blistering, edema, or soot.
- tissue biopsies and cultures—may reveal excessive wound contamination.

POTENTIAL COMPLICATIONS

- hypovolemic shock
- cardiac dysrhythmias
- cardiac arrest
- respiratory arrest
- atelectasis, pneumonia
- pulmonary edema
- infection, sepsis, septic shock
- acute tubular necrosis
- acute renal failure
- conversion of partial-thickness burns to full-thickness burns
- contractures
- loss of mobility and function
- scarring
- social and emotional isolation
- hematologic disorders

Nursing diagnosis: *Potential for injury: continuing tissue injury related to continued exposure to heat or chemicals*

NURSING PRIORITY: Stop the burning process.

Interventions	Rationales
1. Remove any jewelry, belts, coins, or other metal objects. Flush the burned area with cool water for 10 to 15 minutes immediately after the burn injury. Document.	1. Metal items retain heat and permit continued thermal burning. Immediate flushing with cool water will cool the tissue and may limit the damage. Prolonged flushing or the use of ice water may cause complications such as dysrhythmias, hypothermia, or shock.

(continued)

Interventions	Rationales
2. If a chemical burn is present, quickly remove the patient's clothes, brush off dry chemicals, and flush the burns with large amounts of water. Observe the site for chemical residues. After flushing, use a neutralizer, if appropriate, to neutralize any remaining chemical; consult a burn center or poison control center to determine appropriate neutralizing agents. Assess the site hourly and as needed for continuing damage, such as spreading redness, blistering, or loss of sensation. Document.	2. Clothes may contain chemical residues and should be removed to prevent further injury. Copious flushing with water will remove most chemicals. Neutralization may be helpful for some chemicals, but time should not be spent initially finding an appropriate neutralizer. Some chemicals, such as alkalies, may cause continuous damage even when neutralized, making continual assessments necessary.
3. Temporarily cover the flushed burn area with a clean or sterile dressing or sheet while stabilization of status continues.	3. Covering the burn area may limit contamination and decrease pain from air exposure. Further burn wound care, such as debridement and application of local skin antibiotics, has a low priority in the emergent care period as compared with stabilization of airway, breathing, and circulation.
4. Additional individualized interventions: ____________	4. Rationales: ____________

Target outcome criteria

Within the first hour of admission, the patient will:

- display minimal or absent continuing tissue damage, such as additional areas of redness, blistering, or sensation loss
- manifest no signs of chemical residue on skin.

Collaborative problem: *Potential hypoxemia related to airway burns and carbon monoxide inhalation*

NURSING PRIORITY: Promote ventilation and gas exchange.

Interventions	Rationales
1. Maintain a patent airway. Anticipate the need for endotracheal intubation and mechanical ventilation.	1. Airway burns or inhalation of hot air can cause laryngospasms, progressive edema, and rapid airway occlusion up to 8 hours after the burn. Intubation is commonly performed for the patient with an inhalation injury before progressive edema occludes the airway.
2. Assess respiratory status initially, then every 15 minutes until stable, then every 1 to 2 hours. Monitor respiratory rate; chest movements; use of accessory muscles; signs of anxiety or restlessness; color; breath sounds; adventitious sounds such as crackles, rhonchi, or wheezes; the presence of hoarseness when speaking; and the presence of soot around the nares. Notify doctor and document findings. Be prepared to assist with chest wall escharotomy, if necessary.	2. Abnormal findings, including hoarseness, crackles, wheezes, rhonchi, signs of hypoxemia, restlessness, and soot around the nostrils, may indicate an inhalation injury and impending respiratory failure. Circumferential chest burns can restrict chest wall expansion and require escharotomy to allow ventilation.
3. Monitor ABG values initially and then every shift and as needed for suspected changes in respiratory status. Monitor initial and serial carboxyhemoglobin levels. Notify doctor of abnormalities and document.	3. ABG values reflect general oxygenation and acid-base levels. Low oxygen and high carbon dioxide levels may indicate a need for oxygen therapy or mechanical ventilation. Carbon monoxide inhalation interferes with oxygen transport because of its strong affinity for hemoglobin. Carboxyhemoglobin levels reflect the amount of abnormal hemoglobin present.

Interventions	Rationales
4. Provide 100% humidified oxygen therapy, as needed and ordered, especially for smoke inhalation or respiratory distress. Document.	4. Oxygen therapy may be required during the initial postinjury period to maintain desirable ABG levels, help eliminate carbon monoxide, and assist burn wound healing.
5. Obtain initial and serial chest X-rays, as ordered.	5. Pulmonary involvement may not appear on X-ray for up to 24 hours.
6. Encourage deep breathing and coughing every hour and as needed. Assist with the use of an incentive spirometer. Document.	6. Regular deep breathing and coughing promotes expansion of the lungs, mobilizes secretions, and prevents atelectasis. Spirometers encourage deep inspiratory efforts that more effectively expand the alveoli than forceful expiratory efforts.
7. Administer bronchodilators every 4 to 8 hours, if ordered. Document.	7. Bronchodilators may interrupt bronchospasms and counteract the airway-narrowing effect of the airway edema.
8. Assess amount, color, and consistency of sputum, including soot, every shift. Notify doctor and document.	8. Soot in the sputum may confirm an inhalation injury. Excessive sputum may indicate an infection.
9. Assist with bronchoscopy.	9. Bronchoscopy is used diagnostically to determine soot in smaller airways, airway burns, and pulmonary inflammation. It also is used therapeutically to remove excess soot and secretions to minimize the risk of later infection and atelectasis.
10. After stabilization, assist with intermittent positive-pressure breathing (IPPB) every 4 hours, if ordered. Document.	10. IPPB promotes lung expansion by the deep delivery of bronchodilators and positive-pressure breaths.
11. Additional individualized interventions: ____________	11. Rationales: ____________

Target outcome criteria

Within 24 hours of admission, the patient will:

- display no signs of respiratory distress
- display improving breath sounds
- have moist mucous membranes.

Collaborative problem: *Hypovolemia related to movement of vascular fluids to the interstitium and water evaporation from burned areas*

NURSING PRIORITY: Maintain vascular fluid volume.

Interventions	Rationales
1. On admission, place one or two large-bore I.V. lines in large veins in the arms, using aseptic technique. Document.	1. Large I.V. access lines are needed to give the large amounts of fluids required during the fluid resuscitation period.
2. Collaborate with the doctor about fluid replacement therapy. Administer fluids, as ordered, and document, typically:	2. Appropriate fluid therapy is critical to the patient's survival.

(continued)

Interventions	Rationales
• On admission, assess the fluid therapy needed. Use the Rule of Nines or the Lund and Browder chart for the TBSA, and a fluid replacement formula, preferably the Parkland formula (4 ml Ringer's lactate × kg body weight × % TBSA for the volume needed) in the first 24 hours after injury.	• The TBSA calculations and fluid replacement formulas estimate the total fluid replacements needed every 24 hours. Numerous fluid replacement formulas are available. The American College of Surgeons and the American Burn Association recommend the Parkland formula.
• Give crystalloid fluid replacements during the first 24 hours after the burn injury. According to the Parkland formula, administer half the volume in the first 8 hours, a quarter in the next 8 hours, and a quarter in the last 8 hours post burn.	• Large amounts of crystalloid fluids are needed to replace the massive amounts of vascular fluids that leak into the interstitium during the first 24 hours, a time of inflammation and increased capillary permeability.
• After 24 to 48 hours, add colloids and dextrose in water solutions.	• After the capillary membranes stabilize, colloids such as plasma can be added to replace colloid losses. Dextrose in water solutions are also added to replace evaporation loss and as a maintenance solution.
3. Assess adequacy of fluid replacement every 1 to 2 hours and as needed, including vital signs, urine output, specific gravity, mentation, weight, serum electrolytes and osmolality, and hematocrit. Document.	3. Vital signs within a normal range, a urine output of 50 to 100 ml/hour, a normal range of specific gravity and osmolality, absence of mentation changes, normal serum electrolyte levels, and normal hematocrit all reflect adequate fluid replacement. Diuresis commonly begins on the third postinjury day. A weight loss of <2% a day during this time reflects adequate fluid replacement.
4. Assess serum electrolyte levels, as ordered. Replace as ordered. Document. See the "Fluid and Electrolyte Imbalances" appendix, page 317, for general assessments and interventions for electrolyte imbalances.	4. During the first 24 to 48 hours, electrolytes follow the fluid shifts into the interstitial areas, reducing the amounts available in the intravascular areas. Electrolytes may need replacing at this time, the exception being potassium, which is increased in the serum because of cellular destruction during the immediate postburn period. Careful monitoring guides electrolyte replacement. The "Fluid and Electrolyte Imbalances" appendix includes general assessments and interventions for electrolyte imbalances.
5. After completion of fluid resuscitation and the return of gastrointestinal function, begin enteral feedings and remove the I.V. lines. Document.	5. Enteral feedings should be instituted as soon as possible to decrease the risk of infection at insertion sites of I.V. lines.
6. Additional individualized interventions: ____________	6. Rationales: ____________

Target outcome criteria

Within 24 hours of admission, the patient will:
- manifest normal vital signs
- have urine output of 50 to 100 ml/hour
- stay within normal ranges for specific gravity, serum electrolytes, osmolality, and hematocrit
- have no observable changes in mentation.

Within 48 to 72 hours of admission, the patient will manifest a weight loss of no more than 2% a day.

Collaborative problem: *Potential peripheral ischemia related to circumferential eschar formation on arms and legs, compartmental syndrome, or vascular disruption*

NURSING PRIORITY: Maintain adequate tissue perfusion.

Interventions	Rationales
1. When possible, elevate burned areas, but not above the level of the heart.	1. Elevation may decrease edema formation by using gravity to optimize venous return.
2. Assess tissue perfusion distal to the burn site every 1 to 2 hours, noting color, temperature, capillary refill, pulses, sensation, function, and pain. If abnormalities are present, notify the doctor and document.	2. As an eschar hardens, it may constrict circulation, particularly if it is circumferential. The patient with arm or leg burns also is at great risk for compartmental syndrome, in which edema increases pressure in a fascial compartment and compresses nerves, blood vessels, and muscle. Early recognition of impaired circulation allows early intervention and minimizes the risk of permanent damage.
3. Assist the doctor in performing an escharotomy, if necessary. Assess the escharotomy site for bleeding and circulation return. Apply dressings to the site. Document.	3. Incisions across areas of eschar formation release tissue tension and allow circulation to return to constricted areas. Assessments provide for early identification and correction of complications.
4. If ordered, apply proteolytic enzymes, such as sutilains (Travase), to eschar areas. Assess effect and document.	4. Proteolytic enzymes selectively digest necrotic tissue. By softening the eschar, they decrease its constricting effects.
5. Additional individualized interventions: ____________	5. Rationales: ____________

Target outcome criteria

Within 1 to 2 days of admission, the patient will:

- display signs of adequate tissue perfusion distal to the burned area, such as pink color, good capillary refill, warmth, sensation, function, and minimal pain
- display minimal bleeding or other complications at eschar site.

Nursing diagnosis: *Potential for infection of burn wound(s) related to loss of protective integument, exposure to contamination, decreased perfusion, and impaired immunologic response*

NURSING PRIORITIES: (a) Protect burn wound(s), and (b) prevent or minimize infection.

Interventions	Rationales
1. Explain the purpose and methods of wound care to the patient and family.	1. Understanding the purpose of wound care helps the patient establish a perspective that may be helpful in coping with the inevitable pain the care causes, whereas understanding the general methods may decrease fear of the unknown. Involving family members in teaching and care, when appropriate, acknowledges their learning needs and the importance of their emotional support to the patient.

(continued)

Interventions	Rationales
2. Use strict aseptic technique including cap, mask, gown, and sterile gloves during all wound care. Wash the burned area once or twice daily with a mild soap or normal saline solution. A hydrotherapy tub, shower stretcher, or basins at the bedside may be used. Use a gentle circular scrubbing motion. Debride with scissors if necessary. Shave hair over involved areas, with the exception of eyebrows. Rinse with water. Document.	2. Strict aseptic technique to prevent sepsis must be used when the burn wounds are uncovered. Regular washing and debridement removes dead tissue and stimulates the development of granulation tissue, which serves as the base for skin grafting. Shaving excess hair removes a growth medium for bacteria. Eyebrows are not shaved because they may not grow back, leaving the patient with an odd facial appearance.
3. During the washing and debridement procedure, assess the wound area for color, drainage, size, odor, elevations or depressions, and pain. Document.	3. Regular assessments may identify early signs of infection and allow timely treatment before sepsis occurs.
4. Apply topical antibiotics, if ordered, after washing and debridement, typically silver nitrate, mafenide acetate (Sulfamylon), silver sulfadiazine (Silvadene), or povidone-iodine. Use aseptic technique including masks, caps, gowns, and sterile gloves. Cover the wound with gauze or stretch bandages after applying antibiotics. Monitor for medication-related complications such as pain, leukopenia, tissue damage, or electrolyte depletion. If signs of medication-related complications occur, notify the doctor and document.	4. Topical antibiotics are commonly used to prevent massive bacterial colonization of burn wounds from the patient's own skin flora or contaminants. Strict aseptic technique should always be used when the burn wounds are uncovered. Side effects or complications of antibiotic therapy should be monitored to avoid further compromise of patient's status.
5. Leave partial-thickness burns open to air, if ordered. Document scab formation and condition of wound.	5. Partial-thickness burns may heal in a week without complications when left open to air.
6. Monitor temporary wound covers, such as biologic, biosynthetic, or synthetic dressings, if used. Change as needed, observing for infection and excessive exudate. Remove excess liquid, as necessary. Document.	6. Early temporary wound coverage prevents infection and evaporative losses and promotes development of granulation tissue. The dressings are left in place for varying amounts of time. Usually, excessive exudate should be removed to enhance the dressing's adherence.
7. Maintain patient warmth during washing, debridement, and dressing changes. Limit procedures to 30 minutes or less. Document the procedure and the patient's tolerance.	7. Water loss by evaporation during procedures may increase the risks of volume deficit, electrolyte loss, and shock.
8. Assist in obtaining needle biopsy cultures from burn wounds, as ordered. Document.	8. Needle biopsy cultures are more accurate monitors of potential wound infection than surface cultures. Early detection of wound infection allows timely treatment and may prevent sepsis.
9. Assess for signs of sepsis, including increased pulse rate, respiratory rate and temperature, decreased blood pressure, decreased urine output, and mentation changes, every 2 to 4 hours and as needed. Notify doctor about abnormal findings and document.	9. Loss of the skin barrier, frequent manipulation of the burn wounds, and the general catabolic state place the burn patient at high risk for sepsis. Early recognition and treatment may prevent irreversible sepsis and septic shock, a major cause of death in burn patients.
10. Administer tetanus toxoid on admission, as ordered. Administer tetanus immunoglobulin in another site, if tetanus toxoid has not been given during the preceding 10 years. Document.	10. Burn wounds are at high risk for anaerobic infections, including tetanus. Tetanus toxoid stimulates antibody production. Tetanus immunoglobulin provides protection until the tetanus antibodies are developed. Different sites should be used to prevent inactivation of the immunoglobulin.
11. Give I.V. antibiotics, as ordered, if major wound sepsis occurs. Observe for secondary infections of the mouth, GI tract, and the genitalia. Monitor for resistance to topical and systemic antibiotics. Document.	11. I.V. antibiotics usually are given only for major wound sepsis because eschar areas have poor circulation and are better treated with topical antibiotics. Secondary infections may result from overgrowth of normally suppressed pathogens. Development of resistant strains of microorganisms is common because of the long-term use of topical antibiotics.

Interventions	Rationales
12. Additional individualized interventions: ________	12. Rationales: ________

Target outcome criteria
Within 1 week of admission, the patient will:
- display clean and healing superficial burn wounds including scab formation
- display development of red granulation tissue over deeper partial-thickness wounds that are also free of odor, purulent drainage, and elevations or depressions
- display no topical antibiotic complications, such as pain, leukopenia, tissue damage, electrolyte or fluid loss, or secondary infections
- display intact wound covers
- manifest normal range of vital signs, WBC, urine output, and mentation.

Nursing diagnosis: *Pain related to tissue destruction and exposure of nerves in partially destroyed tissue*

NURSING PRIORITY: Relieve pain.

Interventions	Rationales
1. See the "Acute Pain" care plan, page 10, for general assessments and interventions for a patient with pain.	1. The "Acute Pain" care plan includes general assessments and interventions for a patient with pain. This plan contains additional information specific to the burn patient.
2. Administer I.V. analgesics 10 to 20 minutes before wound cleansing, debridement, and dressing application. Medicate frequently and liberally within the ordered parameters. Document administration and degree of pain relief achieved.	2. The wound care procedures are excruciatingly painful and may need to be repeated several times in 24 hours. Patient anticipation increases the perceived pain. Frequent and liberal medication may decrease the pain experience by not allowing the pain to reach intolerable levels. Pain medication addiction is rare in burn patients. The I.V. route should be used because medication absorption is poor through the subcutaneous and intramuscular routes because of the massive edema and inflammatory response.
3. Decrease anxiety and fear by explaining procedures and treatments thoroughly. Document teaching. Refer to the "Knowledge Deficit" care plan, page 45, and "Ineffective Coping" care plan, page 26.	3. Pain may be increased by fear of the unknown, helplessness, and powerlessness. Burn care is complex and long term. Thorough teaching and emotional support may allay fear of the unknown and provide some sense of control concerning the treatment, which may lessen the pain experience. The "Knowledge Deficit" and the "Ineffective Coping" care plans contain general assessments and interventions applicable to any patient.
4. Additional individualized interventions: ________	4. Rationales: ________

Target outcome criteria
Within 1 to 2 days of admission, the patient will experience minimal pain during the wound care procedure.

Nursing diagnosis: *Impaired skin integrity related to potential nonadherence of graft and impaired donor site healing*

NURSING PRIORITY: Optimize wound healing process.

Interventions	Rationales
1. Apply homografts or heterografts in single sheets to freshly cleaned wound sites, as ordered, using aseptic technique. Trim to prevent overlapping. Smooth the graft, removing wrinkles and air. Apply thin gauze with or without antibiotic ointment over the graft, as ordered. Apply a dressing over the gauze. Protect the site from movement or trauma. Document.	1. Homografts or heterografts are used as temporary biological dressings to protect wound sites and stimulate formation of granulation tissue until autografts can be applied. Application without air pockets promotes adherence. Gauze and dressings protect the graft. Freshly grafted sites must be protected from accidental dislodgment until circulation has been established with underlying tissue.
2. After surgery for autografting, immobilize the graft and protect from injury for at least 48 to 72 hours. Keep the large, bulky dressings in place. Use a bed cradle. Prevent prolonged pressure over the graft. Elevate the graft site to the highest position possible. Use splints and elastic bandages over graft sites, particularly when the patient is walking. Discontinue activities, such as hydrotherapy or active physical therapy, for several days after grafting. Document.	2. The graft must be immobilized and protected from trauma and movement for several days to prevent dislodgment and promote circulation until adherence occurs. Large dressings provide protective padding. A bed cradle prevents pressure from bed linens. Elevation limits edema. Splints and elastic bandages provide support, maintain the placement of the dressings, prevent excessive movements of the graft site, and allow some activity. Excessive moisture or exercise may dislodge the graft in the initial days after grafting.
3. Protect the donor site from infection or trauma. If outer dressings are used, keep them in place by using splints and limiting exercise for several days. Leave the inner gauze dressing in place until it falls off in 2 to 3 weeks. Use a heat lamp or hair dryer to dry the site for 15 to 20 minutes four times a day or as ordered. If ordered, leave the site open to air. Document treatments and condition of the site every shift.	3. The donor site must be protected to prevent the potential conversion of the site from a partial-thickness wound to a deeper-thickness wound. Dressings, splints, and limited exercise may protect the site and promote tissue regeneration. The inner gauze is left in place to stabilize and cover the site while tissue regeneration occurs. Early removal could traumatize the new tissue. Heat increases circulation and promotes healing. Air exposure promotes drying and scab formation.
4. Observe the homograft, heterograft, autograft, or donor sites for adherence and signs of infection. Report immediately any redness, exudate, blood under the graft, swelling, separation, drainage, foul odor, increased temperature, pulse rate, or respirations. Document.	4. Regular assessments may reveal the complications of graft rejection or wound sepsis.
5. Apply moist warm compresses to the donor site, if ordered, for 20 to 30 minutes four times a day. Document.	5. Warmth and moisture may increase circulation and promote epithelization.
6. Apply topical antibiotics to the burn and donor site and administer systemic antibiotics intravenously, if ordered. Document.	6. As previously described, topical antibiotics are commonly used to prevent wound sepsis from the patient's own skin flora. Systemic antibiotics are used when major wound sepsis occurs.
7. Additional individualized interventions: ____________	7. Rationales: ____________

Target outcome criteria

Within 2 to 5 days after grafting, the patient will:
- display an intact and healing graft without redness, swelling, exudate formation, bleeding, or foul odor
- display a dry and healed donor site
- manifest normal vital signs
- display no signs of wound sepsis
- maintain activity limitations.

Nursing diagnosis: *Nutritional deficit related to increased metabolic needs of burn wound healing*

NURSING PRIORITY: Provide adequate nutrition to promote wound healing.

Interventions	Rationales
1. Refer to the "Nutritional Deficit" care plan, page 53.	1. The "Nutritional Deficit" care plan contains general assessments and interventions for a patient with a nutritional deficit. This diagnosis provides additional information pertinent to the burn patient.
2. During the immediate postburn period, insert a nasogastric tube and withhold food and fluids until bowel sounds return. Provide I.V. fluids and total parenteral nutrition continuously, as ordered. Assess patient tolerance, including weights; intake and output; edema; and blood glucose, electrolyte, and protein levels. Document.	2. A burn injury commonly causes paralytic ileus, which prevents oral intake for 2 to 4 days after the burn injury. Requirements are met using the I.V. route. Regular assessments monitor the adequacy of fluid and nutrient intake.
3. After bowel function returns, provide a high-calorie and high-protein diet with vitamin supplements, as ordered. Provide high-calorie liquids, such as milk shakes or prepared liquid diet supplements, instead of water. Document daily intake.	3. A high-calorie and high-protein diet, between 5,000 to 6,000 calories a day, may be required to meet the increased needs for tissue healing. All intake must count toward meeting these increased needs, so milk shakes are preferable to water, especially because the patient commonly loses his appetite and needs to be encouraged to take anything. Extra vitamins are needed to meet tissue-healing needs.
4. Additional individualized interventions: ____________	4. Rationales: ____________

Target outcome criteria
Within 1 week of admission, the patient will:
- display minimal or no signs of nutritional deficit
- manifest expected wound healing
- display no more than a 10% weight loss.

Nursing diagnosis: *Impaired physical mobility related to prescribed position and movement limitations*

NURSING PRIORITY: Maintain mobility within range of limitations.

Interventions	Rationales
1. Implement measures in the "Impaired Physical Mobility" care plan, page 33, as appropriate.	1. The "Impaired Physical Mobility" care plan covers general information about this problem. This plan provides additional information pertinent to burns.
2. Provide active and passive range-of-motion (ROM) exercises to arms and legs with healing graft every 2 hours and as needed. Document patient tolerance.	2. ROM exercises prevent contractures and promote circulation, healing, and a sense of well-being.
3. Promote self-care within the range of limitations.	3. Self-care increases active exercise and promotes a sense of well-being and control over the environment.
4. Provide protective devices, such as splints and dressings during exercise, as ordered. Document.	4. Protective devices allow mobility while maintaining the integrity of the graft site.

(continued)

Interventions	Rationales
5. Position body parts in anatomic and functional alignment. Document.	5. Anatomic and functional alignment prevents contracture formation and promotes eventual return of normal activities.
6. Provide pain medication, as needed and ordered. Document.	6. Relief from pain encourages movement and activity.
7. Additional individualized interventions: ____________	7. Rationales: ____________

Target outcome criteria

Within 2 weeks of admission, the patient will:
- have no contractures
- manifest anatomic and functional positions of arms and legs
- perform ROM and other exercises
- experience minimal pain during activities.

Nursing diagnosis: *Disturbed body image related to extensive burn wounds and potential scarring*

NURSING PRIORITY: Promote adjustments to body changes.

Interventions	Rationales
1. Refer to the "Ineffective Coping" care plan, page 26, and the "Grieving and Dying" care plan, page 15.	1. The extensive emotional adjustments necessary to recover from the burn trauma may severely tax the patient's and family's coping abilities. Grieving for the lost appearance or function of body parts is a necessary first step in emotional recovery. The plans listed provide multiple interventions helpful in facilitating the recovery process.
2. Encourage verbalizations of feelings about burn injury, potential scarring, and loss of function. Document concerns.	2. Verbalization of concerns decreases anxiety and fear and encourages self-appraisals of realistic future goals.
3. Provide information about procedures and expected results. Document teaching and patient's response.	3. Knowledge of procedures and expected results decreases fear of the unknown and encourages patient participation and cooperation during the recovery process.
4. Encourage realistic goal setting.	4. Focusing on realistic goals, such as small, obtainable daily goals, may prevent disappointment and despair during recovery.
5. Additional individualized interventions: ____________	5. Rationales: ____________

Target outcome criteria
Throughout the recovery period, the patient will:
- express fears and concerns openly
- set small, realistic goals for recovery
- participate in the recovery process.

Transfer planning

NURSING TRANSFER CRITERIA

Upon transfer, documentation shows evidence of:
- stable vital signs and monitoring parameters
- healing graft and donor sites
- absence of wound or systemic sepsis
- stable fluid and electrolyte status
- renal status within normal limits
- adequate nutrition and fluid intake
- ability to perform ROM and other exercises
- anatomic and functional positions of arms and legs
- absence of such complications as shock, cardiac dysrhythmias, renal failure, contractures, or bleeding
- minimal edema.

PATIENT-FAMILY TEACHING CHECKLIST

Document evidence that patient and family demonstrate understanding of:

___ grafting and wound care procedures, including expected course of healing
___ signs and symptoms of such complications as shock, bleeding, infection, and graft rejection
___ importance of ROM and anatomic and functional positioning of affected arms and legs
___ nutritional intake needs
___ comfort measures for pain
___ protective measures such as splints and dressings for wounds
___ long-term recovery goals.

DOCUMENTATION CHECKLIST

Using outcome criteria as a guide, document:

___ clinical status on admission
___ significant changes in status
___ pertinent diagnostic test findings
___ status of graft and donor sites
___ complications, such as shock, dysrhythmias, sepsis, renal failure, or contractures
___ oxygen therapy
___ ROM and other exercises
___ tolerance of tubbing, debridement, and wound care
___ pain and effect of medication
___ mental and emotional status
___ patient-family teaching
___ transfer planning.

ASSOCIATED CARE PLANS

Acute Pain
Impaired Physical Mobility
Ineffective Individual Coping
Knowledge Deficit
Nutritional Deficit

REFERENCES

American Burn Association: Specific Optimal Criteria for Hospital Resources for Care of Patients with Burn Injury. The Association, 1976.

Bayley, E., and Smith, G. "The Three Degrees of Burn Care," *Nursing87* 17(3):34-41, March 1987.

Brodt, D. *Medical-Surgical Nursing and the Nursing Process.* Boston: Little, Brown & Co., 1986.

Carpenito, L. *Nursing Diagnosis: Application to Clinical Practice,* 2nd ed. Philadelphia: J.B. Lippincott Co., 1987.

Cooke, S. "Major Thermal Injury—The First 48 Hours," *Critical Care Nurse* 6(1):55-63, 1986.

Cuzzell, J. "The Crucial First Days," *American Journal of Nursing* 86:29-50, January 1986.

Freeman, J. "Nursing Care of the Patient With a Burn Injury," *Critical Care Nurse* 4(6):52-68, 1984.

Jacobs, M., ed. *Signs and Symptoms in Nursing.* Philadelphia: J.B. Lippincott Co., 1984.

Jacoby, F. "Care of the Massive Burn Wound," *Critical Care Quarterly* 7(3):44-53, 1984.

Kenner, C., et al. *Critical Care Nursing: Body-Mind-Spirit.* Boston: Little, Brown & Co., 1985.

Kibbee, E. "Burn Pain Management," *Critical Care Quarterly* 7(3):54-62.

Lewis, S., and Collier, I. *Medical-Surgical Nursing: Assessment and Management of Clinical Problems,* 2nd ed. New York: McGraw-Hill Book Co., 1987.

The Lippincott Manual of Nursing Practice. Philadelphia: J.B. Lippincott Co., 1986.

Long, B., and Phipps, W. *Essentials of Medical-Surgical Nursing.* St. Louis: C.V. Mosby Co., 1985.

Luckman, J., and Sorensen, K. *Medical-Surgical Nursing: A Psychophysiological Approach,* 3rd ed. Philadelphia: W.B. Saunders Co., 1987.

Swearingen, P. *Manual of Nursing Therapeutics: Applying Nursing Diagnosis to Medical Disorders.* Reading, Mass.: Addison-Wesley Publishing Co., 1986.

Multiple Trauma

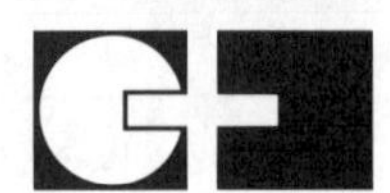

DRG information

DRG 444 Multiple Trauma. Age >17. With Complications or Comorbidities (CC).
Mean LOS = 5.3 days
Principal diagnoses include:
- traumatic amputation of extremities
- crushing injuries of various sites (external)
- injuries to blood vessels of various sites (internal)
- open wounds complicated by delayed treatment, delayed healing, or primary infection.

DRG 445 Multiple Trauma. Age 0 to 17. Without CC.
Mean LOS = 3.7 days
Principal diagnoses include selected principal diagnoses listed under DRG 444. The distinction is that DRG 445 excludes complications or comorbidities.

DRG 446 Multiple Trauma. Age 0 to 17.
Mean LOS = 2.4 days
Principal diagnoses include selected principal diagnoses listed under DRG 444. The distinction is that DRG 446 excludes patients >17 years.

Additional DRG information: Specific details of injuries sustained and treatment received for those injuries must be known before a DRG can be assigned. Usually, coding guidelines suggest listing the most severe injury or the injury requiring surgical treatment as the principal diagnosis. Therefore, the DRG classification could be based on the most severe injury's diagnosis code or the principal procedure code.

For example, for a patient with multiple open and closed fractures, none requiring surgical treatment, the open fracture would be considered the principal diagnosis. If, however, one of the fractures required an open reduction and internal fixation, the surgical code would determine the DRG grouping. A laceration involving fascia and muscle would be coded higher than a superficial laceration. Consequently, a laceration requiring extensive surgical repair would be coded higher than an open wound not requiring repair. Predicting DRG classification without specific details is even more difficult for multiple fractures requiring multiple surgeries.

Introduction

DEFINITION AND TIME FOCUS

Multiple trauma results from accidental or intentional injury to more than one body part, organ, or system. Trauma usually can be described as either blunt or penetrating, depending on whether the skin is broken.

This care plan focuses on the first few days after trauma—the acute-care phase in the critical care unit. It assumes that the patient has been moved from the field to the emergency department for stabilization, to surgery where essential repairs have been accomplished by the time of unit admission, and then to the critical care unit. If stabilization has not been accomplished already, plan and implement appropriate cardiopulmonary support and cervical spine protection as well as provide preoperative care based on institution policies. Although every possible complication cannot be included, the care plan reviews major complications in detail and provides cross-references to other care plans in this book where appropriate. Long-term rehabilitation is not covered here, but prevention of long-term disability—the focus of the critical care nurse—is discussed. The plan refers to special equipment used to care for the trauma patient, but the author implies no endorsement of a specific product or manufacturer.

ETIOLOGY AND PRECIPITATING FACTORS

- chemical impairment of mentation and judgment, such as by alcohol, narcotics, cocaine, or other street drugs
- suicide attempts
- assaults
- falls
- industrial accidents
- motor vehicle accidents
- pedestrian-vehicle collisions
- sports injuries
- underlying physical problems, such as acute myocardial infarction or cerebrovascular accident
- major psychiatric disorders
- recent personal stress

Focused assessment guidelines

NURSING HISTORY (Functional health pattern findings)

Health perception–health management pattern

- likely to be a male age 15 to 35; about 75% of trauma patients are male

Nutritional-metabolic pattern

- usually well-nourished

Activity-exercise pattern

- may have a history of athletic competition

Cognitive-perceptual pattern

- complains of pain, if conscious
- is likely to report or display confusion, anxiety, or amnesia, if conscious

Coping–stress tolerance pattern
• may be undergoing a situational or maturational life crisis
• may have a history of psychiatric problems

PHYSICAL FINDINGS
Note: Alcohol, drugs, anxiety, restlessness, decreased level of consciousness (LOC), or altered sensory function commonly interfere with accurate assessment. Serial observations and analysis of trends in findings are critical. Physical findings vary with the particular types of trauma present.

Cardiovascular
• hypotension and tachycardia (if shock is present)
• hypertension and tachycardia (if shock is absent)
• diminished or absent pulse (if trauma is to an extremity)
• dysrhythmias
• jugular venous distention (if cardiac tamponade is present)
• muffled heart sounds (if cardiac tamponade is present)
• capillary refill time >3 seconds (if shock or vascular disruption is present)

Pulmonary
• tachypnea
• shallow respirations
• paradoxical chest movement (if flail chest is present)
• crepitus and ecchymoses (if chest trauma is present)

Gastrointestinal
• Cullen's sign (ecchymoses around umbilicus) and Turner's sign (ecchymoses in flanks) if intra-abdominal or retroperitoneal bleeding present—a late sign

Neurologic
• decreased LOC
• rhinorrhea or otorrhea (if cerebrospinal fluid leak is present)
• pupillary changes
• sensory or motor impairment (if the trauma is to the head, the spinal cord, or an extremity)

Integumentary
• abrasions
• lacerations
• ecchymoses
• road burns
• Battle's sign (ecchymosis over mastoid area) and raccoon's eyes (periorbital ecchymosis) (if basilar skull fracture or facial fracture is present)
• pallor, mottling, or cyanosis
• cool, cold, or clammy skin

Musculoskeletal
• fractures
• amputations

DIAGNOSTIC STUDIES
• complete blood count—commonly reveals decreased hemoglobin and hematocrit levels secondary to hemorrhage; white blood cell count may be elevated.
• serum electrolytes—used to monitor fluid and electrolyte status.
• blood urea nitrogen and serum creatinine levels—may be elevated secondary to decreased renal perfusion in shock.
• lactate levels—may be elevated, reflecting anaerobic metabolism in shock; high initial levels are associated with low probability of survival.
• serum bilirubin—used to assess hepatic damage.
• cardiac isoenzymes—used to determine acute myocardial infarction, a common precipitator of trauma, or cardiac injury
• arterial blood gas (ABG) levels—vary, depending on cardiopulmonary status; usually, respiratory alkalosis occurs if tachypnea is present; respiratory acidosis occurs if respiratory depression is present; metabolic acidosis occurs if shock is present.
• coagulation panel—used to monitor for disseminated intravascular coagulation.
• aspartate transaminase, alanine transaminase, and lactic dehydrogenase—used to monitor for liver damage.
• anteroposterior, odontoid, and lateral cervical spine (C-spine) radiography—an essential procedure to visualize C1 to C7; can detect spinal injury or "clear" the C-spine of fractures.
• the 12-lead EKG—can help evaluate myocardial infarction or contusion, dysrhythmias, electrolyte imbalance, or antidysrhythmic agent effects.
• chest X-ray—can detect fractured ribs, widened mediastinum, pneumothorax, hemothorax, or other life-threatening chest injuries; a chest X-ray can also confirm placement of an endotracheal tube and central lines and monitor for adult respiratory distress syndrome, pneumonia, and other complications.
• anteroposterior pelvic X-ray, including both hips—can detect pelvic ring disruption or hip dislocation.
• diagnostic peritoneal lavage—may reveal blood, feces, bile, or amylase, indicating abdominal injury.
• excretory urogram, cystogram, or ureterogram—used to identify the size, location, and filling of the renal pelvis, ureters, and urethra.
• computed tomography (CT) scan—can visualize injuries to the head, neck, spine, abdomen, and kidneys.
• arteriography—determines vessel integrity.
• radionuclide scanning and sonography—assists in the identification of organ structure and function; especially useful in suspected chest, abdominal, or pelvic injuries.

POTENTIAL COMPLICATIONS
• infection or sepsis
• pulmonary embolism
• atelectasis or pneumonia
• adult respiratory distress syndrome

- disseminated intravascular coagulation
- renal failure
- cardiac failure
- liver failure
- increased intracranial pressure
- paralysis
- fat embolism
- compartmental syndrome
- malnutrition
- multisystem organ failure
- post-traumatic stress disorder

Collaborative problem: *Potential hypoxemia related to pulmonary injury, head injury, shock, or other factors*

NURSING PRIORITY: Maintain optimal airway, ventilation, and oxygenation.

Interventions	Rationales
1. Maintain a patent airway. Maintain cervical spine precautions until radiologic or tomographic findings have ruled out ligamentous injury or fracture.	1. Although airway patency will have been evaluated before unit admission, trauma to the head, face, neck, or torso can compromise a previously patent airway at any time. Although cervical spine clearance usually is done before unit admission, general precautions may still be required while awaiting the official radiologic reading. In many cases, the C6 and C7 vertebrae are difficult to clear in patients with large shoulders, and CT scan may be required.
2. Monitor ventilatory status. Observe respiratory rate, rhythm, effort of breathing, and tidal volume. Monitor trends in ABG values. Prepare for intubation and mechanical ventilation, as ordered, particularly if the patient has flail chest, pulmonary contusion, or shock. Refer to the "Mechanical Ventilation" care plan on page 108.	2. If the patient's condition deteriorates, ventilatory status may change abruptly. Deterioration also may be insidious (for example, if the patient tires), so close monitoring is essential. The "Mechanical Ventilation" care plan presents comprehensive information on indications for, types of, and nursing care for mechanical ventilation.
3. Provide supplemental oxygen, as ordered.	3. All multiple trauma patients need supplemental oxygenation. Hypoxemia is multifactorial and may result from pulmonary injury, depressed LOC, decreased cardiac output, ischemia, acidosis, and other factors. Supplemental oxygen elevates arterial oxygen tension, ensuring that the blood reaching the tissues provides the maximum amount of oxygen possible.
4. Obtain serial chest X-rays at least daily, as ordered.	4. Serial chest X-rays can detect complications in time for corrective action.
5. Additional individualized interventions: ____________	5. Rationales: ____________

Target outcome criteria

According to individual readiness, the patient will:
- display ABG levels within normal limits
- have clear breath sounds bilaterally
- have clear lung fields on chest X-ray.

Collaborative problem: *Potential shock related to hypovolemia, cardiac injury, spinal cord injury, or sepsis*

NURSING PRIORITIES: (a) Monitor for shock, and (b) restore circulating blood volume and tissue perfusion if shock occurs.

Interventions	Rationales
1. Implement measures in the "Shock" care plan on page 173, as appropriate, such as monitoring LOC, vital signs, urinary output, EKG pattern, hemodynamic measurements, and laboratory values; maintaining patency of two large-bore I.V. lines; and administering fluids and positive inotropic agents, as ordered.	1. The "Shock" care plan covers assessment and interventions for this potential problem in detail. This plan provides additional information specific to trauma patients.
2. Implement autotransfusion, when possible. Follow the manufacturer's directions for citration, if used, and reinfusion.	2. The patient's own blood, when captured in drainage, is an ideal source of blood replacement because it decreases the possibility of transfusion reactions and infection. Citration may be used to prevent the retrieved blood from coagulating in the autotransfusor.
3. Monitor continually for new or ongoing bleeding.	3. Commonly, restoration of adequate blood pressure reverses peripheral vasoconstriction and dislodges fragile clots, so additional bleeding becomes apparent.
4. Collaborate with the doctor to adjust blood replacement needs according to the sites of suspected or obvious bleeding and estimated amount lost.	4. Rough guidelines exist for the amount of blood loss to expect with particular types of injuries, for example, with the following closed orthopedic injuries: humerus, 1 to 2 units; ulna-radius, ½ to 1 unit; pelvis, 2 to 12 units; tibia-fibula, ½ to 4 units; and ankle, ½ to 2 units. With open injuries, an estimated 1 to 3 additional units may be lost per site. Such guidelines, when used with the clinical picture, help determine appropriate blood replacement.
5. Warm I.V. fluids before administration.	5. The volume of fluid required in a major trauma resuscitation is so massive that infusing room temperature solutions and cold blood products may precipitate hypothermia and shivering. Shivering requires an extraordinary energy expenditure the patient can ill afford.
6. Additional individualized interventions: ____________	6. Rationales: ____________

Target outcome criteria

Within 24 hours of the onset of therapy, the patient will:

- have an adequate circulating volume, as manifested by normal vital signs; warm, dry skin; urinary output within normal limits; and strong, bilaterally equal, peripheral pulses
- have a core temperature within normal limits.

Collaborative problem: *Potential undetected injury related to mechanism of injury*

NURSING PRIORITIES: (a) Correlate the mechanism of injury with the patient's clinical presentation, and (b) remain alert for new signs of injury.

Interventions	Rationales
BLUNT HEAD TRAUMA	
1. Implement measures in the "Increased Intracranial Pressure" care plan on page 82, as appropriate.	1. Brain damage may not reflect velocity and duration of the injuring force because a contracoup injury may be worse than the coup injury to the head. Preadmission health status, the specific type of injury, and immediate detection of and treatment of increased intracranial pressure are critical to survival. The "Increased Intracranial Pressure" care plan discusses these problems in detail.
2. Monitor LOC, pupillary reactions, motor function, and sensory function. Alert the doctor immediately to any signs of neurologic deterioration.	2. Brain damage may not be apparent until days or weeks after injury. Signs of acute subdural hematoma usually appear within 24 hours of injury. An epidural hematoma, usually from arterial bleeding secondary to blows to the temple that tear the middle meningeal artery, is life-threatening and requires immediate surgical evacuation. Signs of concussion usually reverse within 24 hours, whereas those from contusion may persist for several days. Failure to recover within the expected time may indicate ongoing pathology or previously undetected injury and requires medical evaluation.
3. Additional individualized interventions: ____________	3. Rationales: ____________
BLUNT CHEST TRAUMA	
1. Notify the doctor promptly of the onset of subcutaneous emphysema in the chest or neck, gastric contents in tracheal secretions, severe chest pain, deteriorating ABG values, or dyspnea.	1. These signs may indicate tracheal disruption or esophageal or bronchial tears. The trachea, esophagus, and bronchi are attached to other body structures by "stalks" that are prone to tear from direct impact, deceleration, and shearing or rotary forces associated with blunt trauma.
2. Monitor for indicators of cardiac tamponade, such as rising central venous pressure, falling blood pressure, neck-vein distention, or muffled heart sounds. Notify the doctor immediately and prepare for pericardiocentesis.	2. When the chest strikes the steering wheel in a motor vehicle accident, for example, the heart is compressed between the sternum and vertebrae. The abrupt increase in intracardiac pressure may cause cardiac rupture. Damage may also occur to great vessels, especially to the vena cava and pulmonary veins, which are thought to have different deceleration rates than the atria. Cardiac damage may occur even without thoracic injury, if a lap belt compresses the abdomen and knees strike the dashboard. A "hydraulic ram" effect occurs because of abdominal and leg compression, which displaces abdominal viscera and blood upward, increasing intracardiac pressure and causing cardiac damage.

Interventions	Rationales
3. Monitor for signs of cardiac contusion, including tachycardia, chest pain, dysrhythmias, elevated pulmonary capillary wedge pressure, and indicators of heart failure. Obtain serial EKGs, cardiac enzymes, and a Doppler echocardiogram during the diagnostic phase, as ordered. Provide care, as ordered, depending on the contusion's effect on the particular patient.	3. Cardiac contusion may result from horizontal or vertical deceleration, compression, or shock wave damage in a gunshot wound to the chest or abdomen. Some controversy exists over management of cardiac contusion. Recent studies show little risk for most patients. If an EKG and Doppler echocardiogram do not reveal electrical or mechanical dysfunction, this disorder need not be treated in a critical care unit. If function is impaired or dysrhythmias threaten cardiac output, however, treatment should be similar to that for acute myocardial infarction.
4. Monitor for signs of pulmonary contusion, such as dyspnea, increasing pulmonary secretions (usually bloody), increasing inspiratory pressure while on a volume ventilator, and hypoxemia. Follow serial ABG measurements and chest X-ray results.	4. Pulmonary insufficiency from contusions increases within the first several hours after injury. Contusion creates swelling, a natural inflammatory process, and a capillary leak, which is worsened by the aggressive fluid resuscitation necessary for the multiple trauma patient.
5. Additional individualized interventions: ________	5. Rationales: ________
BLUNT ABDOMINAL TRAUMA	
1. Report changes in abdominal pain, tenderness, rebound tenderness, absent bowel sounds, and increased abdominal distention.	1. Lap belt restraints may produce intraperitoneal, retroperitoneal, or pelvic disruption, resulting in life-threatening hemorrhage. These acceleration-deceleration injuries may not appear immediately after injury but hours or even days later.
2. Maintain placement and patency of gastric and urinary catheters, as ordered. Avoid nasogastric tube placement if facial fractures or cribriform plate injury is suspected. Avoid urinary catheter insertion if blood is present at the urinary meatus; notify the doctor.	2. A gastric catheter decompresses the stomach and aids in detection of gastric bleeding, whereas a urinary catheter does the same for the bladder. Attempts to insert a nasogastric tube when facial fractures or cribriform plate injury is present may result in catheter placement into the brain. Bleeding at the urinary meatus may indicate urethral transection and requires medical evaluation.
3. Additional individualized interventions: ________	3. Rationales: ________
BLUNT SPINAL CORD INJURY	
1. Perform and document a motor and sensory examination every shift.	1. Mechanisms of spinal cord injury include horizontal loading, vertical loading, and acceleration or deceleration. Horizontal loading is lateral cord motion, such as when the patient hits the ground after being ejected from an automobile. Vertical loading results in cord compression, such as with a vertical fall or diving injury. Acceleration or deceleration injuries are common in falls.
2. Additional individualized interventions: ________	2. Rationales: ________
PENETRATING WOUNDS	
1. With bullet wounds, observe the wound edge for necrosis and distal tissue for perfusion. Also inspect carefully for other wounds.	1. Bullet wounds usually are explored surgically, because of the erratic path the bullet may take as it moves through tissue and because its kinetic energy (which depends on its mass and velocity) creates a much larger internal wound than the surface may indicate.

(continued)

Interventions	Rationales
2. With stab wounds, observe distal vascular supply and tissue integrity, and signs of underlying organ function. Assume underlying vessel, tissue, and organ damage until proven otherwise.	2. Depending on the length of the weapon and the direction of penetration, body areas other than that of the surface wound may be entered. For example, an abdominal stab wound may penetrate the diaphragm and involve the chest cavity, or a buttock stab wound may enter the abdomen. A high index of suspicion is critical.
3. Additional individualized interventions: ___________	3. Rationales: ___________
ALL TYPES OF INJURY	
1. Assess and report to the doctor if the apparent mechanism of injury and observed injuries are dissonant.	1. Dissonance between the apparent mechanism of injury and pattern of observed injuries may indicate previously undetected mechanisms of injury or abuse.
2. Additional individualized interventions: ___________	2. Rationales: ___________

Target outcome criteria
Throughout the unit stay, the patient will have previously unapparent injuries detected and treated promptly.

Nursing diagnosis: *Impaired physical mobility related to orthopedic injury*

NURSING PRIORITIES: (a) Restore maximum mobility, (b) strengthen muscle groups involved in weight bearing and range of motion, and (c) prevent orthopedic complications.

Interventions	Rationales
1. Implement measures in the "Impaired Physical Mobility" care plan, page 33, as appropriate.	1. The "Impaired Physical Mobility" care plan presents comprehensive information on the hazards of immobility and their prevention. This plan provides additional information pertinent to trauma patients.
2. Elevate extremities in casts. Check neurovascular function every 1 to 2 hours. Report to the doctor altered sensation, increased pain, decreased ability to move fingers or toes, and capillary refill time >3 seconds.	2. Extremities in casts commonly swell from tissue edema; elevation decreases the amount of swelling. Altered sensation, increased pain, limited movement, and prolonged capillary refill time indicate that the swelling is causing neurovascular compromise. Unrecognized damage can threaten limb survival or function.
3. Observe uncasted extremities for crepitus, deformity, swelling, discoloration, pain, paralysis, pulse loss, and muscle spasms. If present, splint the extremity and notify the doctor.	3. Occasionally, injuries may be missed during resuscitation, especially if other life-threatening injuries require immediate surgical intervention.
4. If reimplantation is planned, maintain the severed body part in a sealed plastic bag on ice; do not soak, wrap, or pack in ice. Prepare the patient for reimplantation surgery.	4. Several hours may elapse before reimplantation. Maintaining the body part as described preserves viability.
5. Maintain traction and immobilization of all cervical spinal injuries and all other unstable spinal fractures. Besides halo traction, methods include using Gardner-Wells, Barton-Cone, or Crutchfield tongs.	5. Maintaining traction prevents further injury to the spinal cord. Although cervical spinal injuries require immediate treatment along with other life-threatening injuries, treatment of thoracolumbar injuries can be deferred until the patient is stable.

Interventions

6. Prevent skin breakdown and other hazards of immobility by obtaining turning orders and restrictions, as appropriate, instituting a program of diligent side-to-side turning, at least every 2 hours as ordered, or using trauma beds. The different kinds of trauma beds include:

Rationales

6. Skin breakdown, thromboembolism, and other complications of immobility may threaten life or markedly prolong recovery. Preventive methods depend on the type of injury and degree of activity allowed.

• Roto Rest bed

• A Roto Rest bed cycles automatically through several lateral positions and has been used for all types of patients, including those with cervical spine fractures. Ventilator patients can be cared for easily on this bed.

• Air bag beds (Avoid these for patients in spinal traction.)

• Various air bag beds are available. Benefits include side-to-side turning, bacterial filtration, prevention of skin breakdown, and smaller unit space requirements than the Roto Rest bed. Because of the potential for air bag deflation, a Roto Rest bed is better suited for spinal traction patients.

• Stryker or CircOlectric frames

• Although these beds facilitate turning, they do not automatically change the patient's position and thus require more nursing supervision.

7. Apply, monitor, and maintain continuous passive range-of-motion or sequential compression devices, if ordered.

7. These devices are designed to maintain leg range of motion and prevent deep venous stasis and thromboembolism.

8. Additional individualized interventions: ____________

8. Rationales: ____________

Target outcome criteria
By the third post-trauma day, the patient will have no evidence of skin breakdown or other complications of immobility.

Nursing diagnosis: *Potential post-trauma response related to overwhelming psychological assault from sudden, unexpected injury*

NURSING PRIORITY: Facilitate effective coping.

Interventions

1. Refer to "Ineffective Coping" care plan on page 26 and "Grieving and Dying" care plan on page 15.

Rationales

1. Both plans contain helpful interventions for any trauma patient and the family. This plan provides additional information specifically for trauma patients and their families.

2. Observe for indications of reexperiencing of the traumatic incident, such as flashbacks, intrusive thoughts, nightmares, guilt over survival, and excessive talking about the event. Also observe for indications of psychic numbing, such as confusion, amnesia, limited affect, misinterpretation of reality, and poor impulse control.

2. These signs and symptoms characterize the post-traumatic response that may follow a sudden event over which the victim felt powerless, for example, a motor vehicle accident, natural disaster, or act of violence.

3. Encourage the patient to discuss feelings and reach out to others for help in coping with them. Explicitly acknowledge the intense feelings involved and the difficulty in coping with them.

3. Retelling the incident and verbalizing feelings are important steps toward psychic integration of the experience. Reaching out to others provides comfort and reestablishes psychological security. Explicit recognition of the powerful feelings involved and acknowledgment of the difficulty in coping with the experience conveys respect for the patient and helps establish rapport and trust.

(continued)

Interventions	Rationales
4. Reassure the patient about being safe now. Give praise for behaviors contributing to survival, if appropriate.	4. The post-traumatic syndrome can be so intense that the patient becomes absorbed in reexperiencing the terrifying incident. Reassurance helps reorient the patient to reality and brings closure to the terrifying incident. Praise for survival behaviors helps restore a sense of control.
5. Support the patient's family and assist them in understanding his or her response.	5. Distress at observing the patient's upset feelings may cause the family to shut off verbalizations, crying, and other expressions of feeling. Although well intentioned, such blocking may ultimately interfere with the patient's ability to integrate the experience.
6. With the patient's and family's consent, call in counseling professionals, such as a spiritual advisor, social worker, or trauma stress specialist. Refer the patient and family to a trauma support group, if available.	6. Counseling professionals may provide special skills that facilitate coping. Calling them in without consent, however, may reinforce the powerless feeling experienced during the traumatic incident.
7. Additional individualized interventions: ____________	7. Rationales: ____________

Target outcome criteria

According to individual readiness, the patient will:
- discuss feelings about the traumatic incident
- learn to cope with flashbacks and other signs of the post-traumatic response.

Nursing diagnosis: *Potential for injury: complications related to impaired immunologic defenses, hypermetabolic state, stress, and other factors.*

NURSING PRIORITY: Prevent or minimize complications.

Interventions	Rationales
1. Identify and minimize potential sources of infection. For example, use strict aseptic technique when opening invasive lines; provide care at the insertion site of skeletal pins, wires, and tongs, as ordered; administer antibiotics, as ordered. If a cerebrospinal fluid leak is present, avoid suctioning or blowing of the nose and packing the nose or ears. Ideally, remove and replace I.V. lines and urinary catheters within 24 hours of insertion in the prehospital environment or emergency department.	1. Breach of the skin barrier, ischemia and necrotic tissue, inadequate inflammatory response, chronic disease, large numbers of invasive procedures, malnutrition, and pharmacologic agents contribute to the high risk of infection for trauma patients. The measures listed prevent or treat infection. Lines and catheters hurriedly placed tend to become contaminated and serve as a wick for infection. Early replacement minimizes the infection risk.
2. Verify that tetanus prophylaxis was administered, if needed.	2. Although tetanus prophylaxis usually is accomplished in the emergency department, it may have been overlooked if life-threatening injuries required immediate surgical intervention.

Interventions	Rationales
3. Provide adequate nutrition within 24 hours of admission, as ordered. Refer to the "Nutritional Deficit" care plan on page 53 for details.	3. Adequate nutrition is critically important to recovery, as trauma induces a hypermetabolic response. Commonly, paralytic ileus or facial, airway, esophageal, chest, or abdominal injuries preclude oral nutrition. Ideally, if these injuries are substantial, a jejunostomy tube to facilitate feeding is placed during the initial chest or abdominal surgery. If the enteral route is unavailable, parenteral nutrition should be started. The goals include achieving positive nitrogen balance and preventing complications from inadequate nutrition, such as sepsis, delayed wound healing, and multiple organ failure. The "Nutritional Deficit" care plan discusses this potential complication in detail.
4. Prevent stress ulcers by administering antacids, titrated to gastric pH, and histamine antagonists or anticholinergic agents, as ordered. Monitor gastric drainage for occult blood.	4. Trauma patients are at increased risk for stress ulcers. Prevention is the best therapy. The medications indicated reduce the secretion and acidity of gastric fluids, and gastric drainage monitoring can detect incipient stress ulcers.
5. Monitor for signs and symptoms of compartmental syndrome, such as unrelievable pain, muscle tension, and neurovascular compromise. If any of these signs and symptoms are present, alert the doctor and assist with measurement of compartmental pressure or transfer to surgery for fasciotomy.	5. Compartmental syndrome, also called low-velocity crush syndrome, results from excessive pressure within a fascial compartment as a result of swollen tissue or blood confined within the compartment. Soft tissue injury, burns, use of an pneumatic antishock garment, and tight casts or dressings increase the risk of compartmental syndrome. Neurovascular compromise results, and if the pressure is not relieved by fasciotomy, the end result may be nerve damage or paralysis.
6. Monitor for signs and symptoms of myoglobinuric renal failure, such as decreased urinary output and elevated specific gravity. Notify the doctor and obtain plasma creatine phosphokinase (CPK) and urine myoglobin levels, as ordered. If myoglobinuria is present, administer volume and mannitol, as ordered.	6. Myoglobinuria reflects myoglobin release from muscle damage associated with crush injury or compartmental syndrome. When circulation is restored to the damaged tissue, a flood of myoglobin is released into the central circulation. Myoglobinuria peaks about 3 hours after circulation is restored and may persist for as long as 12 hours after the ischemic event. If myoglobin precipitates in the renal tubules, it may cause acute renal failure. Elevated plasma CPK and urine myoglobin levels confirm the diagnosis. Volume administration and osmotic diuresis maintain renal tubular flow and lessen the risk of myoglobin clogging the renal tubules.
7. If musculoskeletal, soft tissue, burn, arterial, or multisystem trauma is present, observe for signs of fat embolism, such as sudden onset of respiratory distress, tachypnea, tachycardia, decreased LOC, and personality changes. If any of these signs or symptoms are present, alert the doctor.	7. Fat embolism is caused by mobilization of fat globules (for example, fat escaping from a fractured bone) or altered fat metabolism. The signs and symptoms from fat globules lodging in the lungs, brain, and kidneys usually occur 24 to 48 hours after injury. The early signs listed may be followed by petechiae (which appear on the second to fourth days), retinal changes, and hematuria. Untreated, fat embolism may result in adult respiratory distress syndrome. Treatment is controversial but usually includes mechanical ventilation with positive end-expiratory pressure and possibly corticosteroids.
8. If death is imminent, consult with the doctor, family, and organ transplant team about possible organ donation. See "Organ Donation," page 319, for details.	8. Because trauma commonly involves young, previously healthy people, many patients may be suitable organ donors. Although contemplating the end of a loved one's life is naturally distressing, donating organs may bring meaning and comfort to an otherwise senseless experience for the family.

(continued)

Interventions	**Rationales**
9. Additional individualized interventions: __________	9. Rationales: __________

Target outcome criteria

Throughout the critical care stay, the patient will:

• receive care designed to prevent complications

• receive prompt treatments of complications that do occur.

If death is imminent and the patient is a suitable donor, the family will be approached about organ donation.

Transfer planning

NURSING TRANSFER CRITERIA

Upon transfer, documentation shows evidence of:

• stable vital signs

• stable laboratory values

• absence of major complications, such as sepsis, renal failure, and increased intracranial pressure.

Note: Transfer is dependent upon the type of unit available. If a "step down" unit with experienced critical care or ventilator-skilled nurses is available, the patient may be transferred while still on the ventilator. If "step down" trauma care is not available, the patient must be independent of the ventilator before transfer.

PATIENT-FAMILY TEACHING CHECKLIST

Document evidence that patient and family demonstrate understanding of:

__ extent of injuries

__ prognosis

__ treatments

__ pain management

__ post-trauma response

__ coping resources

__ organ donation process, if appropriate.

DOCUMENTATION CHECKLIST

Using outcome criteria as a guide, document:

__ clinical status on admission

__ significant changes in status

__ pertinent laboratory and diagnostic test findings

__ airway and ventilation support

__ volume administration

__ medication administration

__ nutritional support

__ emotional support

__ measures to prevent or treat complications

__ patient-family teaching

__ transfer planning.

ASSOCIATED CARE PLANS

Acute Pain
Acute Renal Failure
Adult Respiratory Distress Syndrome
Disseminated Intravascular Coagulation
Grieving and Dying
Impaired Physical Mobility
Increased Intracranial Pressure
Ineffective Coping
Knowledge Deficit
Mechanical Ventilation
Nutritional Deficit
Sensory-Perceptual Alteration
Shock

REFERENCES

Cardona, V. *Trauma Reference Manual.* Bowie, Md.: Robert J. Brady Co., 1985.

Carrieri, V. *Pathophysiological Phenomena in Nursing.* Philadelphia: W.B. Saunders Co., 1986.

Healy, F. "Fat Embolism Syndrome," *Trauma* 2(4):35-39, February 1986.

Johanson, B. *Standards for Critical Care.* St. Louis: C.V. Mosby Co., 1985.

Knezevich, B. *Trauma Nursing: Principles and Practice.* East Norwalk, Conn.: Appleton & Lange, 1986.

Loser, W. "Nutritional Support of the Traumatized Patient," *Trauma* 2(4):51-56, February 1986.

McLane, A., ed. *Classification of Nursing Diagnoses: Proceedings of the Seventh Conference.* St. Louis: C.V. Mosby Co., 1986.

Rea, R., ed. *Trauma Nursing Core Course Instructor Manual.* Chicago: Emergency Nurses Association, 1987.

Richardson, D., et al. *Trauma Clinical Care and Pathophysiology.* Chicago: Yearbook Medical Pubs., 1987.

Sommers, M. "Cardiac Tamponade after Nonpenetrating Cardiac Trauma," *Dimensions of Critical Care Nursing* 5(4):206-15, July/August 1986.

"Standards and Guidelines for Cardiopulmonary Resuscitation (CPR) and Emergency Cardiac Care (ECC)," *Journal of the American Medical Association* 255(21): 2979-84, June 6, 1986.

Strange, J. *Shock Trauma Care Plans.* Springhouse, Pa.: Springhouse Corp., 1987.

Trunkey, D., and Lewis, F. *Current Therapy of Trauma.* Philadelphia: B.C. Decker, 1986.

Section III

Selected condensed care plans, arranged alphabetically, provide a quick review of nursing diagnoses, collaborative problems, interventions, teaching, and documentation.

Acquired Immunodeficiency Syndrome

COLLABORATIVE PROBLEM: *Potential hypoxemia related to weakness, ventilation/perfusion imbalance, pneumonia, or other lung pathology*

Interventions

1. Assess respiratory status at least every hour.
2. Monitor arterial blood gas levels, as ordered.
3. Administer oxygen therapy, as ordered.
4. Perform airway clearance measures, as needed:
• deep-breathing exercises and incentive spirometer (consult with the doctor about incorporating coughing)
• artificial sighing with a hand-held resuscitator
• suctioning.
5. Evaluate respiratory parameters at least every 2 hours and as needed.
6. Immediately report indicators of hypoxemia and impending respiratory failure. If any occur, anticipate immediate endotracheal intubation and mechanical ventilation.
7. If the patient has undergone bronchoscopy, observe for complications.
8. Watch for signs of respiratory depression following administration of narcotic analgesics, if ordered.
9. Anticipate activity intolerance and assist with self-care as needed. Teach energy conservation measures.
10. Additional individualized interventions: ____________

____

COLLABORATIVE PROBLEM: *Immunosuppression related to low number of T_4 cells, low T_4/T_8 ratio, or both*

Interventions

1. Institute protective precautions for immunosuppressed patients, including meticulous hand washing; providing only cooked foods; avoiding standing water; screening visitors; and preventing the patient from handling live flowers or plants.
2. Monitor vital signs at least every 4 hours. Report fever onset or temperature spikes immediately.
3. Monitor daily complete blood count and report increasing leukopenia or neutropenia.
4. Monitor potential sites of infection daily.
5. Be alert for signs and symptoms of neurologic infection. Compare new findings with baseline findings; report new or changed abnormalities to the doctor immediately.
6. Monitor for evidence of new pulmonary infections, checking lung sounds at least every 4 hours.
7. Obtain cultures, as ordered.
8. Administer antibiotics, as ordered, commonly:
• co-trimoxazole (Bactrim, Septra)
• pentamidine isethionate (Pentam)
• sulfadoxine and pyrimethamine (Fansidar), or pyrimethamine (Daraprim).
9. If zidovudine (Retrovir) is ordered, consult current administration guidelines and provide patient teaching, as appropriate.
10. Institute fever control measures.
11. Additional individualized interventions: ____________

____

NURSING DIAGNOSIS: *Sensory-perceptual alteration related to neurologic involvement, anxiety, or effects of unit environment*

Interventions

1. Assess the patient's mental and neurologic status on admission and at least daily thereafter.
2. Evaluate the patient's emotional state.
3. If the patient is able to read an eye chart, assess for possible visual impairment. Institute precautions to prevent injury if a significant visual deficit is present.
4. Explain the patient's symptoms to family and friends. Emphasize supportive behaviors.
5. Institute protective measures and consult with the doctor regarding any paresthesias, numbness, weakness, involuntary limb movements, pain, or marked atrophy of extremities.
6. See the "Sensory-Perceptual Alteration" care plan, page 60.
7. See the "Acute Pain" care plan, page 10.
8. Additional individualized interventions: ____________

____

NURSING DIAGNOSIS: *Nutritional deficit related to nausea, vomiting, diarrhea, anorexia, medication side effects, or decreased nutrient absorption secondary to disease process*

Interventions

1. See the "Nutritional Deficit" care plan, page 53.
2. Additional individualized interventions: ____________

____

NURSING DIAGNOSIS: *Impaired physical mobility related to weakness, hypoxemia, neuropathy, orthostatic hypotension, and other effects of disease process*

Interventions

1. Assess for signs of activity intolerance. If present, adjust activity level.
2. See the "Impaired Physical Mobility" care plan, page 33.
3. Additional individualized interventions: ____________

____

NURSING DIAGNOSIS: *Potential fluid volume deficit related to chronic, persistent diarrhea and fever associated with opportunistic infection*

Interventions

1. Monitor intake and output, collaborating with doctor to maintain fluid balance. See the "Fluid and Electrolyte" and "Acid-Base Imbalance" appendices, pages 317 and 316, respectively.
2. Additional individualized interventions: ____________

____

NURSING DIAGNOSIS: *Social isolation related to communicable disease, associated social stigma, and fear of infection from social contact*

Interventions

1. Assess the patient's family and friends for emotional supportiveness.
2. Promote an atmosphere of acceptance. Encourage physical contact, teaching others about recommended precautions.

3. Teach family and friends about ways the virus is not transmitted.
4. Provide the patient and family with telephone numbers of available resources for counseling, support, and information.
5. Additional individualized interventions: ____________

____

NURSING DIAGNOSIS: *Potential ineffective coping related to diagnosis of life-threatening illness, loss of ability to maintain usual roles, complex decisions regarding treatment options, and anticipatory grieving*

Interventions

1. See the "Ineffective Coping" care plan, page 26.
2. Support defenses. Encourage hope while facilitating realistic planning.
3. Anticipate fear, guilt, and anger. Whenever possible, link the patient with a mental health professional who will be able to follow the patient on an ongoing basis.
4. Provide the patient and family with information regarding the legal rights of acquired immunodeficiency syndrome patients, as appropriate.
5. See the "Grieving and Dying" care plan, page 15.
6. Additional individualized interventions: ____________

____

PATIENT-FAMILY TEACHING CHECKLIST

__ disease process and implications
__ treatment options
__ available support groups and resources
__ symptoms to report to health care providers
__ infection prevention measures
__ safety precautions
__ how the virus is and is not spread
__ ways to prevent transmission of the virus to others
__ legal rights and resources

DOCUMENTATION CHECKLIST

__ clinical status on admission
__ significant changes in status
__ pertinent laboratory and diagnostic test findings
__ occurrence and type of opportunistic infections
__ treatment decisions
__ nutritional program and support
__ intake and output measurements
__ breathing patterns
__ emotional coping
__ support of family and friends
__ referrals
__ patient-family teaching
__ transfer planning

ASSOCIATED CARE PLANS

Acute Pain
Adult Respiratory Distress Syndrome
Grieving and Dying
Impaired Physical Mobility
Ineffective Coping
Knowledge Deficit
Mechanical Ventilation
Nutritional Deficit
Sensory-Perceptual Alteration

Acute Heart Failure

COLLABORATIVE PROBLEM: *Potential hypoxemia related to pulmonary congestion, decreased systemic perfusion, or both*

Interventions

1. Monitor pulmonary status as needed, typically every 15 minutes until stable, and then every 2 hours.
2. Monitor arterial blood gas levels, as ordered, typically every 4 hours until stable. Obtain chest X-rays, as ordered.
3. Assist the patient to semi-Fowler's or high-Fowler's position.
4. Administer supplemental oxygen, as ordered.
5. Suction as needed.
6. Administer narcotics, sedatives, or tranquilizers, as ordered, only if the patient's respiration rate is >12 breaths/minute.
7. Alert the doctor immediately if the patient has severe dyspnea, pink frothy sputum, marked neck-vein distention, or describes a feeling of impending doom.
8. Additional individualized interventions: ____________

____

COLLABORATIVE PROBLEM: *Inadequate cardiac output related to heart rate abnormalities and/or diminished contractility*

Interventions

1. Observe for signs and symptoms of decreased CO.
2. Monitor the patient's EKG continuously.
3. Assist with inserting a pulmonary artery catheter, as ordered.
4. Monitor cardiac index (CI) and pulmonary capillary wedge pressure (PCWP) every hour, as ordered. Note isolated values and the trend of values.
5. Classify the patient according to the following Forrester subsets:
   - Subset I: PCWP <18 mm Hg and CI >2.2 liters/minute/m (no failure)
   - Subset II: PCWP >18 mm Hg and CI >2.2 liters/minute/m^2 (pulmonary congestion)
   - Subset III: PCWP <18 mm Hg and CI <2.2 liters/minute/m^2 (peripheral hypoperfusion)
   - Subset IV: PCWP >18 mm Hg and CI <2.2 liters/minute/m^2 (pulmonary congestion and peripheral hypoperfusion).
6. Anticipate medical therapy consistent with Forrester subsets. Administer therapy as ordered.
   - For patients with no signs of failure (Subset I), observe for possible development of failure.
   - For patients with pulmonary congestion only (Subset II), see the "Hypervolemia" problem in this care plan.
   - For patients with hypoperfusion but no pulmonary congestion (Subset III):
     - □ For elevated heart rate, administer volume.
     - □ For depressed heart rate, assist with pacemaker insertion.
   - For patients with pulmonary congestion and hypoperfusion (Subset IV), see the "Hypervolemia" problem in this care plan.
7. Additional individualized interventions: ____________

____

COLLABORATIVE PROBLEM: *Hypervolemia related to sodium and water retention from compensatory release of antidiuretic hormone and aldosterone interventions*

Interventions

1. Monitor for signs and symptoms of fluid volume excess.
2. Monitor hourly intake and output levels and 24-hour fluid balance; weigh the patient daily.
3. Administer I.V. solutions, as ordered. Avoid saline solutions.
4. If the patient is placed on fluid restrictions:
• Explain the rationale to the patient and family.
• Establish a fluid intake schedule.
• Teach the patient how to record oral fluid intake.
• Control I.V. intake by using microdrip tubing or an infusion pump.
5. For patients with pulmonary congestion (Subset II), administer pharmacologic therapy, as ordered:
• If blood pressure is normal, administer diuretics.
• If blood pressure is elevated, administer vasodilators—typically, venodilators, such as nitroglycerin or morphine, or arteriolar dilators, such as sodium nitroprusside (Nipride).
6. For patients with pulmonary congestion and peripheral hypoperfusion (Subset IV), administer pharmacologic therapy, as ordered.
• If blood pressure is depressed, administer positive inotropes—typically, digitalis preparations, dopamine hydrochloride (Inotropin), dobutamine hydrochloride (Dobutrex); or combined vasodilator and positive inotrope therapy, such as sodium nitroprusside and dopamine, or amrinone (Inocor).
• If blood pressure is normal, administer vasodilators.
7. Additional individualized interventions: ___________

____

NURSING DIAGNOSIS: *Activity intolerance related to hypoxemia, weakness, or diminished cardiovascular reserve*

Interventions

1. Assess for signs and symptoms of activity intolerance.
2. During periods of physiologic instability, place the patient on complete bed rest or chair rest.
3. Space nursing care to promote rest.
4. When stable, increase activity gradually, as ordered.
5. Additional individualized interventions: ___________

____

NURSING DIAGNOSIS: *Knowledge deficit related to disease process and complex therapeutic regimen*

Interventions

1. Implement the following measures only as the patient's condition allows. See the "Knowledge Deficit" care plan, page 45, for details.
2. Briefly explain the pathophysiology of heart failure.
3. Emphasize the patient's role in controlling the disease and the importance of medical follow-up.
4. In collaboration with the dietitian, review the prescribed diet with the patient and family—typically, low sodium, low fat, low cholesterol, and, if the patient is overweight, low calorie. Refer the patient to a smoking-cessation program, if appropriate. Stress the value of family support.
5. Instruct the patient and family about discharge medications.
6. Emphasize signs and symptoms requiring immediate medical attention after discharge, such as shortness of breath, rapid weight gain, increasing fatigue, or increasing edema.
7. Additional individualized interventions: ___________

____

PATIENT-FAMILY TEACHING CHECKLIST

__ cause and implications of acute heart failure
__ purpose of medications
__ activity restrictions
__ rationales for other therapeutic interventions
__ need for life-style modifications

DOCUMENTATION CHECKLIST

__ clinical status on admission
__ significant changes in status
__ pertinent laboratory and diagnostic test findings
__ hemodynamic measurements
__ oxygen therapy
__ fluid therapy or restrictions
__ response to inotropes, vasodilators, or other pharmacologic agents
__ dietary modifications
__ activity restrictions
__ patient-family teaching
__ transfer planning

ASSOCIATED CARE PLANS

Acute Myocardial Infarction
Impaired Physical Mobility
Knowledge Deficit
Shock

Acute Myocardial Infarction

COLLABORATIVE PROBLEM: *Potential cardiogenic shock related to dysrhythmias, impaired contractility, and/or thrombosis*

Interventions

1. Institute constant EKG monitoring on admission.
2. Record and analyze rhythm strips every 4 hours and as needed for significant variations.
3. Obtain serial 12-lead EKGs on admission, daily for 3 days, and as needed for chest pain.
4. Evaluate hourly, or as needed, level of consciousness, pulse, blood pressure, heart sounds, breath sounds, urinary output, skin color and temperature, and capillary refill time.
5. Establish and maintain a patent I.V. line. Document hourly and cumulative intake and output.
6. Administer heparin or warfarin sodium (Coumadin), or both, as ordered.
7. Prepare the patient for aggressive treatment measures, as ordered, for example:
• emergency coronary arteriography
• streptokinase infusion
• tissue plasminogen activator (tPA) infusion
• percutaneous transluminal coronary angioplasty
• coronary artery bypass surgery.
8. Additional individualized interventions: ___________

____

COLLABORATIVE PROBLEM: *Hypoxemia related to ventilation/perfusion imbalance*

Interventions

1. Observe for signs and symptoms of hypoxemia. Monitor arterial blood gas values, as ordered.
2. Administer oxygen therapy according to medical protocol and nursing judgment.
3. If blood pressure is stable within normal limits, assist the patient to semi-Fowler's position.
4. During the acute instability period, place the patient on bed rest or chair rest. Once stabilized, progress activity as tolerated.
5. Provide adequate rest.
6. Additional individualized interventions: ______

______

COLLABORATIVE PROBLEM: *Chest pain related to myocardial ischemia*

Interventions

1. On admission, teach the patient to report immediately any chest pain, chest tightness, heaviness, or burning.
2. Monitor continually for chest pain complaints.
3. Document pain episodes.
4. Medicate promptly at onset of pain.
5. During the initial cardiovascular instability period, titrate morphine I.V. (if ordered) according to pain level and vital signs.
6. Remain with the patient until pain is relieved.
7. Position the patient comfortably. Use noninvasive pain relief measures as well as medications, as appropriate.
8. Additional individualized interventions: ______

______

NURSING DIAGNOSIS: *Potential ineffective coping related to fear of death, anxiety, denial, or depression*

Interventions

1. Implement measures in the "Ineffective Coping" care plan, page 26, as appropriate.
2. Administer tranquilizers, as ordered, typically diazepam (Valium).
3. Additional individualized interventions: ______

______

NURSING DIAGNOSIS: *Constipation related to diet, bed rest, immobility, or medications*

Interventions

1. Encourage compliance with the prescribed diet, typically low in caloric, salt, and fat content. Limit caffeine intake.
2. Supply a bedside commode when the patient's condition allows.
3. Administer stool softeners and laxatives judiciously, as ordered.
4. Provide privacy while the patient defecates.
5. Additional individualized interventions: ______

______

NURSING DIAGNOSIS: *Potential for injury: complications related to myocardial ischemia, injury, necrosis, inflammation, or dysrhythmias*

Interventions

1. Monitor constantly for general complications of acute myocardial infarction (AMI), including:

DYSRHYTHMIAS
- Observe for ventricular dysrhythmias.
- Observe for supraventricular dysrhythmias.
- Administer antidysrhythmic agents, as ordered:
  - □ class Ia, such as procainamide hydrochloride (Pronestyl)
  - □ class Ib, such as lidocaine hydrochloride
  - □ class II, such as propranolol (Inderal)
  - □ class III, such as hydrochloride bretylium tosylate (Bretylol)
  - □ class IV, such as verapamil hydrochloride (Calan).
- Implement emergency measures as needed.

ACUTE HEART FAILURE
- Implement measures in the "Acute Heart Failure" and "Shock" care plans, pages 140 and 173, respectively, as appropriate.

INFARCT EXTENSION
- Monitor for new, increased, or persistent chest pain. Obtain a 12-lead EKG and administer pain medication, as ordered.
- Notify the doctor about pain as well as any indicators of new infarction reflected by 12-lead EKG.

PERICARDITIS
- Observe for pericardial chest pain, fever, tachycardia, or pericardial friction rub.
- Administer anti-inflammatory agents, as ordered.
- Monitor for pericardial effusion indicators.
- Monitor for cardiac tamponade signs. If present, summon immediate medical assistance and prepare for emergency pericardial aspiration.

VENTRICULAR ANEURYSM
- Observe for ventricular aneurysm signs, which include those of congestive heart failure, thromboembolism, or persistent ectopy.
- Alert the doctor and prepare the patient for surgery, as ordered.

RUPTURE
- Monitor for papillary muscle rupture. Assist with cardiogenic shock treatment or prepare the patient for surgery, as ordered.
- Observe for potential septal rupture. Initiate cardiopulmonary resuscitation, if necessary, and obtain immediate medical assistance. Implement measures to treat cardiogenic shock or prepare the patient for surgery, as ordered.
- Be alert for signs of impending myocardial rupture. Notify the doctor immediately. Assist with emergency pericardiocentesis and cardiogenic shock treatment, as ordered.

2. Monitor constantly for specific complications of particular types of AMI, including:
ANTERIOR, ANTEROSEPTAL, OR ANTEROLATERAL INFARCT
• Monitor for signs of bundle branch block (BBB).
• Alert the doctor if you detect:
  □ Right BBB
  □ Left BBB
  □ Left anterior hemiblock or left posterior hemiblock.
• Observe closely for Mobitz II block or complete heart block. Prepare for prophylactic pacemaker insertion, as ordered.

INFERIOR INFARCT
• Monitor for sinus bradycardia and atrioventricular block.
• Observe for indicators of right ventricular (RV) infarct.
• If the patient has fluid volume depletion on admission, watch for signs of RV infarction after I.V. hydration.
• When recording 12-lead EKGs of patients who have suspected inferior or posterior infarction, routinely record right ventricular leads.
• If infarction indicators appear, alert the doctor.
• If an RV infarction is confirmed, collaborate with the doctor to implement therapy.
  □ Avoid administering diuretics. Administer fluid boluses, as ordered.
  □ Administer inotropes and vasodilators judiciously, as ordered.
• Closely monitor hemodynamic parameters and clinical indicators of therapeutic effectiveness.
3. Additional individualized interventions: ___________

____

NURSING DIAGNOSIS: *Knowledge deficit related to diagnostic procedures, therapeutic interventions, and long-range implications for life-style changes*
Interventions
1. Implement measures in the "Knowledge Deficit" care plan, page 45, as appropriate.
2. Defer participation in a formal rehabilitation and education program until patient attains physiologic stability. In the meantime:
• Establish rapport.
• Assess immediate learning needs.
• As appropriate, provide brief information.
• Note and document long-range learning needs.
3. Additional individualized interventions: ___________

____

PATIENT-FAMILY TEACHING CHECKLIST
__ the extent of infarction
__ activity restrictions
__ recommended dietary modifications
__ smoking cessation program as needed
__ common emotional changes after AMI
__ community resources for life-style–modification support and cardiac rehabilitation

DOCUMENTATION CHECKLIST
__ clinical status on admission
__ significant changes in status
__ pertinent laboratory and diagnostic test findings
__ chest pain episodes
__ pain relief measures
__ rhythm strip analyses
__ emergency protocols
__ hemodynamic and other trend data
__ I.V. line patency
__ oxygen therapy
__ other therapies
__ nutritional intake
__ patient-family teaching
__ transfer planning

ASSOCIATED CARE PLANS
Acute Pain
Grieving and Dying
Acute Heart Failure
Impaired Physical Mobility
Ineffective Coping
Knowledge Deficit
Shock

Acute Renal Failure

COLLABORATIVE PROBLEM: *Electrolyte imbalance related to decreased electrolyte excretion, excessive intake, or metabolic acidosis*
Interventions
1. Monitor and document electrolyte levels every 8 to 12 hours and as needed, as ordered.
2. Continuously monitor EKG.
3. With hyperkalemia, implement the following measures, as ordered:
• I.V. glucose (50%) and insulin
• I.V. calcium chloride or calcium gluconate
• cation-exchange resins
• I.V. sodium bicarbonate.
4. Limit dietary and drug intake of potassium.
5. Give aluminum hydroxide antacid with meals and every 4 hours, as ordered.
6. Give calcium and vitamin supplements as needed and ordered.
7. Limit magnesium intake, such as in antacids.
8. Give sodium chloride I.V., as needed and ordered.
9. Additional individualized interventions: ___________

____

NURSING DIAGNOSIS: *Fluid volume excess related to sodium and water retention*
Interventions
1. See the Appendix C, Fluid-Electrolyte Imbalances.
2. Assess for signs of fluid overload.
• Assess every 1 to 2 hours: vital signs (blood pressure, pulse, respirations), central venous pressure (CVP), pulmonary artery wedge pressure (PAWP), pulmonary artery end-diastolic pressure (PAEDP), mean arterial pressure (MAP), adventitious lung sounds such as crackles or rhonchi, and peripheral edema. Measure cardiac output, as ordered, typically every 12 hours.
• Assess daily: weight and complete blood count, especially hematocrit.

• Report promptly:
 □ high blood pressure (BP), rapid pulse rate, rapid respirations, high hemodynamic parameters (CVP, PAWP, PAEDP, MAP), crackles or rhonchi, peripheral edema, and increasing body weight
 □ low hemodynamic parameters, rapid pulse rate, low BP, dry skin and mucous membranes, poor skin turgor, decreased body weight, and a high hematocrit.

3. Measure intake and output levels every 2 hours.
4. Restrict fluid intake to measured losses plus 400 ml/24 hours, unless fluid or weight losses are excessive. Consult with the doctor about increasing the fluid replacement amount if excessive fluid losses occur or if weight loss exceeds 0.5 kg/day.
5. Give I.V. infusions through infusion pumps continuously, as ordered.
6. Provide hard candies, ice chips, and mouth care every 2 hours and as needed.
7. Give diuretics, such as mannitol, furosemide (Lasix), or ethacrynic acid (Edecrin), as needed and as ordered. Administer vasodilators, as ordered.
8. Additional individualized interventions: ____________

____

NURSING DIAGNOSIS: *Potential for injury: complications related to uremic syndrome*
Interventions
1. See Appendix B, Acid-Base Imbalances, page 316.
2. Monitor blood urea nitrogen, creatinine, uric acid, and pH levels once daily or as needed and ordered. Monitor arterial blood gas values once daily or as needed and ordered.
3. Assess for signs and symptoms of uremia every 2 to 4 hours and as needed.
4. Give sodium bicarbonate I.V., as needed and ordered.
5. Assess the hemodialysis access site (shunt or catheters), if present, every 2 hours for patency, warmth, color, thrill, and bruit. Do not use the access site for I.V. infusions or blood withdrawal. Do not measure BPs on an extremity containing an access site. Keep alligator clamps attached to the dressings.
6. Assess the peritoneal dialysis access catheter site, if present, every 24 hours and as needed for signs and symptoms of infection.
7. Prepare for dialysis every 1 to 3 days, as ordered.
8. Monitor drug administration continually.
9. Monitor hematocrit and hemoglobin values daily for signs of anemia.
10. Assess continually for signs and symptoms of hemorrhage.
11. Assess daily for signs and symptoms of pericarditis. If indicators exist:
• Report to the doctor, and administer steroids or nonsteroidal anti-inflammatory agents, as ordered.
• Monitor every 4 hours for indicators of pericardial effusion and a small cardiac tamponade: weak peripheral pulses, pulsus paradoxus over 10 mm Hg, or a decreased level of consciousness. If present, alert the doctor immediately.
• Monitor continually for indicators of a large cardiac tamponade: distended neck veins, profound hypotension, and rapid loss of consciousness. If present, summon immediate medical assistance and prepare for emergency pericardial aspiration.

12. Additional individualized interventions: ____________

____

NURSING DIAGNOSIS: *Potential for infection related to decreased immune response and skin changes secondary to uremia*
Interventions
1. Assess continually for signs of infection.
2. Continually protect patient from cross-contamination.
3. Give antibiotics every 4 to 12 hours, as ordered.
4. Provide care and dressing changes to central and peripheral I.V. access sites, catheters, and dialysis shunts every 12 to 48 hours.
5. Provide skin care at frequent intervals.
6. Avoid continuously invasive procedures.
7. Collect urine, blood, and secretion specimens as needed and ordered, for culture and sensitivity laboratory tests.
8. Additional individualized interventions: ____________

____

NURSING DIAGNOSIS: *Potential nutritional deficit related to anorexia, nausea and vomiting, and restricted dietary intake*
Interventions
1. See the "Nutritional Deficit" care plan, page 53.
2. Medicate for nausea and vomiting as needed and ordered.
3. Collaborate with the doctor and dietitian to provide a diet reflecting the following:
• high-carbohydrate content
• limited but high-quality protein content
• limited fluids
• low-potassium and low-sodium content
• vitamin supplements.

4. Additional individualized interventions: ____________

____

NURSING DIAGNOSIS: *Knowledge deficit: therapeutic regimen related to complexity and life-threatening nature of ARF and dialysis*
Interventions
1. See the "Knowledge Deficit" care plan, page 45.
2. Provide, as appropriate, information about the following:
• the common stages of acute renal failure (ARF)
• medications
• signs and symptoms, such as dizziness and nausea, to report to the nurse
• procedures, including hemodialysis or peritoneal dialysis
• diet
• activity.

3. Additional individualized interventions: ____________

____

PATIENT-FAMILY TEACHING CHECKLIST
__ common stages of ARF and patient's current stage
__ fluid-diet regimen, including protein, electrolyte, and fluid limits
__ medications, including actions and side effects

___ dialysis treatment if appropriate, including schedule and side effects
___ signs and symptoms to report to nurse, including fever, pain, nausea and vomiting, and dizziness

DOCUMENTATION CHECKLIST
___ clinical status on admission
___ significant changes in status
___ pertinent laboratory and diagnostic test findings, including serum drug levels
___ care and condition of the dialysis access site
___ urine characteristics and quantity, if appropriate
___ intake and output levels
___ body weight
___ diet tolerance
___ activity tolerance
___ mentation status
___ skin status
___ pertinent procedures including dialysis

ASSOCIATED CARE PLANS
Gastrointestinal Hemorrhage
Knowledge Deficit
Nutritional Deficit

Adult Respiratory Distress Syndrome

COLLABORATIVE PROBLEM: *Hypoxemia related to pulmonary shunt, interstitial edema, and/or alveolar edema*
Interventions
1. Monitor clinical signs and symptoms:
• tachypnea
• progressive dyspnea
• abnormal breath sounds
• deteriorating level of consciousness
2. Obtain chest X-ray daily, as ordered.
3. Obtain arterial blood gas values at least every 4 hours, as ordered. Note degree of hypoxemia and acid-base imbalance.
4. Continuously monitor gas exchange status, as ordered, with an ear oximeter or SVO_2 catheter.
5. Prepare for endotracheal intubation, if necessary.
6. Implement mechanical ventilation, as ordered.
7. Implement positive end-expiratory pressure (PEEP), as ordered.
8. Monitor compliance.
9. Administer medications, as ordered:
• corticosteroids
• antibiotics.
10. Additional individualized interventions: ___________

____

NURSING DIAGNOSIS: *Potential for injury: complications related to additional lung insults stemming from dysfunction of other organ systems*
Interventions
1. Maintain adequate cardiac output. Monitor pulmonary artery pressures, vital signs, EKG, and urinary output.
2. Administer packed red blood cells, as ordered.
3. Administer crystalloid or colloid I.V. fluids, as ordered.
4. Obtain an order to institute gastric drainage.
5. Provide nutritional support, as ordered. See the "Nutritional Deficit" care plan, page 53.
6. Monitor for signs and symptoms of infection. Institute aggressive treatment measures, as ordered.
7. Observe for signs of single or multiple organ failure.
8. Implement measures to prevent the complications of immobility. See the "Impaired Physical Mobility" care plan, page 33.
9. Additional individualized interventions: ___________

____

NURSING DIAGNOSIS: *Potential ineffective coping related to abrupt onset of life-threatening illness*
Interventions
1. Implement the measures outlined in the "Ineffective Coping" care plan, page 26.
2. Additional individualized interventions: ___________

____

PATIENT-FAMILY TEACHING CHECKLIST
___ definition and pathophysiology of adult respiratory distress syndrome
___ probable precipitator(s) for this patient
___ prognosis
___ rationale for mechanical ventilation, PEEP, and other therapies

DOCUMENTATION CHECKLIST
___ clinical status on admission
___ significant changes in status
___ pertinent laboratory and diagnostic test findings
___ airway care
___ tolerance of ventilator and PEEP
___ response to medications
___ fluid therapy
___ nutritional support
___ nursing care to combat effects of immobility
___ psychological coping
___ patient-family teaching
___ transfer planning

ASSOCIATED CARE PLANS
Disseminated Intravascular Coagulation
Grieving and Dying
Impaired Physical Mobility
Ineffective Coping
Mechanical Ventilation
Multiple Trauma
Nutritional Deficit
Sensory-Perceptual Alteration

Diabetic Ketoacidosis

COLLABORATIVE PROBLEM: *Hypovolemia related to osmotic diuresis, vomiting, or both*
Interventions
1. Monitor for signs and symptoms of dehydration and shock. Continuously monitor blood pressure and cardiac rate and rhythm.

2. Observe for signs and symptoms of electrolyte imbalances:
• hyperkalemia in the first 1 to 4 hours of treatment
• hypokalemia after 1 to 4 hours of treatment
• hyponatremia early in treatment
• hypernatremia later.
3. Monitor serum osmolality and electrolyte values, as ordered.
4. Establish and maintain one or more I.V. lines in large peripheral veins.
5. Insert an indwelling urinary catheter, as ordered. Monitor intake, output, and urine specific gravity. Weigh the patient daily.
6. Administer I.V. solutions, as ordered, typically:
• normal saline solution (0.9% sodium chloride), 1 to 2 liters in the first 2 hours
• plasma volume expanders if dehydration is severe
• ½ normal saline solution (0.45% sodium chloride) after the first few hours, or 0.45% sodium chloride with dextrose 5% in water when blood glucose level reaches 250 mg/dl or urinary glucose level is <1%.
7. Administer therapy for electrolyte imbalances, as ordered.
8. For at least 24 hours after rapid fluid repletion, observe for signs and symptoms of pulmonary edema. If present, alert the doctor immediately.
9. Additional individualized interventions: ____________

____

COLLABORATIVE PROBLEM: *Hyperglycemia related to decreased cellular glucose uptake and utilization*
Interventions
1. Assess blood glucose levels as ordered. Perform bedside fingerstick to monitor blood glucose level every hour until level reaches normal, then every 6 hours or as ordered.
2. Assess blood ketone level, as ordered. Perform bedside urine ketone monitoring every hour until level stabilizes, then every 6 hours.
3. Administer insulin, as ordered.
4. Alert the doctor when the blood glucose level reaches 250 mg/dl or urinary glucose level is <1%.
5. Observe for signs and symptoms of medication-induced hypoglycemia.
6. Additional individualized interventions: ____________

____

NURSING DIAGNOSIS: *Sensory-perceptual alteration related to cerebral dehydration, decreased perfusion, hypoxemia, or acidosis*
Interventions
1. Implement standard safety precautions.
2. Observe level of consciousness (LOC) continuously.
3. Additional individualized interventions: ____________

____

COLLABORATIVE PROBLEM: *Acidosis related to altered LOC, ketosis, and decreased tissue perfusion*
Interventions
1. Maintain a patent airway.
2. Monitor respiratory status hourly.
3. Anticipate intubation and mechanical ventilation if increasing respiratory distress occurs.
4. Administer oxygen, as ordered.
5. Monitor arterial blood gas values, as ordered.
6. Administer I.V. sodium bicarbonate, as ordered.
7. While the patient is acutely ill, maintain nothing-by-mouth status. Insert a gastric tube, as ordered, and connect to suction. Auscultate bowel sounds every 8 hours.
8. Additional individualized interventions: ____________

____

NURSING DIAGNOSIS: *Knowledge deficit related to complex disease and therapy*
Interventions
1. See the "Knowledge Deficit" care plan, page 45.
2. When the patient's condition allows, determine learning needs.
3. When the patient's condition allows, begin a teaching program.
4. Document learning needs and teaching. When the patient is leaves the intensive care unit (ICU), arrange for teaching plan to continue.
5. Additional individualized interventions: ____________

____

PATIENT-FAMILY TEACHING CHECKLIST
___ cause and implications of diabetes mellitus
___ precipitators of diabetic ketoacidosis, including signs and symptoms and appropriate responses
___ significance of insulin
___ signs, symptoms, and interventions for hyperglycemia and hypoglycemia
___ dietary management
___ exercise plan
___ blood and urine testing
___ plan for completing unmet learning needs

DOCUMENTATION CHECKLIST
___ clinical status on admission
___ significant changes in status
___ pertinent laboratory and diagnostic test findings
___ I.V. fluid therapy
___ pharmacologic intervention
___ oxygen administration
___ patient-family teaching
___ transfer planning

ASSOCIATED CARE PLANS
Acute Renal Failure
Grieving and Dying
Hyperglycemic Hyperosmolar Nonketotic Coma
Knowledge Deficit
Sensory-Perceptual Alteration
Shock

Disseminated Intravascular Coagulation

COLLABORATIVE PROBLEM: *Potential hemorrhage related to consumption of clotting factors, increased fibrinolysis, and presence of endogenous anticoagulants*
Interventions
1. Collaborate with the doctor to identify and treat the cause of disseminated intravascular coagulation (DIC).
2. Monitor the presence and degree of hemorrhage.
3. Monitor coagulation panel, as ordered.
4. Administer heparin, as ordered. Monitor the clotting time.
5. Give transfusion therapy, as ordered.
6. Maintain a normal blood pressure by giving fluid and medications, as ordered.
7. Monitor for the development of fluid overload.
8. Additional individualized interventions: ____________

____

COLLABORATIVE PROBLEM: *Ischemia related to microcirculatory thrombosis*
1. Assess status of organ systems at least every 4 hours, including:
• neurologic function
• cardiovascular function
• gastrointestinal function.
2. Monitor renal function closely. Document hourly urine output.
3. Implement measures to treat the underlying cause(s) of tissue ischemia, as ordered (for example, fluid administration).
4. Additional individualized interventions: ____________

____

COLLABORATIVE PROBLEM: *Potential hypoxemia related to increased pulmonary shunting, anemia, and acidosis*
Interventions
1. Monitor arterial blood gas levels, as ordered.
2. Assess physical indicators of pulmonary status at least every 4 hours.
3. Administer supplemental oxygen, positive end-expiratory pressure, or mechanical ventilation, as ordered.
4. Additional individualized interventions: ____________

____

NURSING DIAGNOSIS: *Impaired skin integrity related to capillary fragility*
Interventions
1. Avoid puncturing patient's skin with needles whenever possible. If necessary, use the smallest needle gauge possible and apply pressure afterward.
2. Handle the patient very gently.
3. Use cushioning and pressure-relieving devices.
4. Provide gentle mouth care.
5. Additional individualized interventions: ____________

____

NURSING DIAGNOSIS: *Pain related to tissue ischemia, hematomas, or bleeding into organ or joint capsules*
Interventions
1. Assess for pain frequently. Consult the "Acute Pain" care plan, page 10, for details.
2. Administer pain medications I.V.
3. Additional individualized interventions: ____________

____

PATIENT-FAMILY TEACHING CHECKLIST
__ basic pathophysiology and implications of DIC
__ rationale for therapy
__ pain-relief measures

DOCUMENTATION CHECKLIST
__ clinical status on admission
__ significant changes in status
__ pertinent laboratory and diagnostic test findings
__ bleeding episodes
__ transfusion and fluid replacement therapy
__ pain-relief measures
__ patient-family teaching
__ transfer planning

ASSOCIATED CARE PLANS
Acute Heart Failure
Acute Pain
Acute Renal Failure
Adult Respiratory Distress Syndrome
Cardiac Surgery
Impaired Physical Mobility
Ineffective Coping
Liver Failure
Major Burns
Mechanical Ventilation
Multiple Trauma
Nutritional Deficit
Shock

Gastrointestinal Hemorrhage

COLLABORATIVE PROBLEM: *Potential hypovolemic shock related to blood loss*
Interventions
1. See the "Shock" care plan, page 173.
2. Assess the amount of blood loss by:
• maintaining accurate intake and output records and documenting guaiac testing of all vomitus and stools
• evaluating orthostatic vital signs every 4 hours, unless the patient is syncopal, frankly hypotensive, or severely tachycardic when supine
• evaluating vital signs, hemodynamic pressures, and EKG findings
• obtaining appropriate laboratory studies, as ordered, including complete blood count, blood urea nitrogen, and creatinine level
• assessing the patient frequently for clinical signs of hypovolemia
• inserting and maintaining a gastric tube, as ordered, and checking drainage for blood.

3. Replace blood loss by:
• establishing and maintaining I.V. access with a large-bore cannula
• administering packed red blood cells, fresh frozen plasma, or other blood components or volume expanders, as ordered.
4. Initiate measures to stop bleeding, as ordered, by:
• ensuring strict bed rest
• starting gastric lavage—usually with room temperature normal saline solution, with or without norepinephrine (Levophed) added to solution; question orders for iced lavage
• administering vasopressin (Pitressin) I.V.
• instilling topical thrombin through the gastric tube
• inserting Sengstaken-Blakemore or other compression tubes
• administering vitamin K_1 (AquaMEPHYTON) I.M.
• preparing for surgery if bleeding remains uncontrolled for more than 24 hours, requires more than 6 units of blood, or results in severe hypovolemia, or if the hematocrit does not increase in response to administered blood products.
5. Administer medications, as ordered, to control gastric acidity, monitoring gastric aspirate pH and adjusting dosage to maintain a pH >5.0:
• histamine (H_2) blockers, such as cimetidine (Tagamet) or ranitidine (Zantac)
• antacids.
6. Prepare for diagnostic procedures, such as endoscopic examination, angiography, or other studies, as ordered.
7. Additional individualized interventions: ____________

____

NURSING DIAGNOSIS: *Potential for injury: complications related to undetected bleeding, inadequate organ perfusion, accumulation of toxins, electrolyte imbalance, release of procoagulants, or perforation of ulcer*
Interventions
1. Continue to test all gastric contents and stools for occult blood at least daily, even after the patient's condition stabilizes.
2. Immediately report and thoroughly investigate any chest pain complaint.
3. Monitor parameters of renal and hepatic functions. Note daily serum electrolyte values.
4. Observe for bleeding from other sites.
5. Immediately alert doctor to any complaint of sudden, severe abdominal pain or rigidity, and prepare for surgery.
6. Additional individualized interventions: ____________

____

NURSING DIAGNOSIS: *Fear related to sight of blood and distressing physical symptoms*
Interventions
1. Provide care promptly. Remain calm and avoid displaying alarm at the sight of bleeding. Acknowledge the patient's feelings of fear.
2. After bleeding is controlled, encourage patient to verbalize feelings. See the "Ineffective Coping" care plan, page 26.
3. Accept expressions of anxiety related to possible dying. See the "Grieving and Dying" care plan, page 15.
4. Additional individualized interventions: ____________

____

NURSING DIAGNOSIS: *Knowledge deficit related to potential recurrent bleeding*
Interventions
1. See the "Knowledge Deficit" care plan, page 45.
2. Defer detailed teaching until patient is alert and physiologically stable; then, as permitted by condition, discuss:
• precipitating or contributing factors of bleeding episode
• signs and symptoms indicating possible recurrence
• other causes of dark stools
• dietary recommendations.
3. Additional individualized interventions: ____________

____

PATIENT-FAMILY TEACHING CHECKLIST
__ cause and site of bleeding
__ precipitating or contributing factors
__ signs and symptoms indicating possible recurrence of bleeding
__ dietary recommendations, if any

DOCUMENTATION CHECKLIST
__ clinical status on admission
__ significant changes in status
__ pertinent laboratory and diagnostic test findings
__ bleeding episodes
__ fluid and blood replacement measures
__ intake and output measurements
__ emotional response
__ pharmacologic interventions
__ procedures to stop bleeding
__ patient-family teaching
__ transfer planning

ASSOCIATED CARE PLANS
Acute Renal Failure
Disseminated Intravascular Coagulation
Grieving and Dying
Impaired Physical Mobility
Ineffective Coping
Knowledge Deficit
Liver Failure
Nutritional Deficit
Pancreatitis
Shock

Impaired Physical Mobility

NURSING DIAGNOSIS: *Potential ineffective airway clearance related to reduced diaphragmatic and costal excursion, stasis of secretions, decreased ciliary activity, weakness, and underlying disease process*
Interventions
1. Assess pulmonary capabilities at least every 2 hours.
2. Evaluate for risk factors that affect pulmonary status.
3. Monitor vital signs, intake and output, hemodynamic pressures, and EKG findings.

4. Obtain and monitor arterial blood gas (ABG) levels, as ordered.
5. Initiate measures to promote effective breathing:
• Assist patient to Fowler's or semi-Fowler's position. Change position every 1 to 2 hours.
• Encourage deep breathing at least every hour. Assist with incentive spirometry.
• Splint incisions.
• Reduce abdominal distention.
6. Initiate measures to promote airway clearance:
• deep breathing (check with the doctor about including coughing)
• humidification
• adequate fluid intake
• suction
• chest physiotherapy every 4 hours while awake, or more frequently.
7. Monitor for pulmonary complications:
• pneumonia
• atelectasis
• pulmonary embolus.
8. Additional individualized interventions: ____________

____

COLLABORATIVE PROBLEM: *Potential thromboembolic phenomena related to venous pooling, loss of vasomotor tone, lack of skeletal muscle contraction, and increased blood viscosity*
Interventions
1. Evaluate for thromboembolism risk factors.
2. Initiate measures to promote venous return or decrease venous pooling:
• Help patient exercise legs every 1 to 2 hours while awake.
• Avoid raising knee gatch, crossing legs, and placing pillows directly under the popliteal area.
• Apply graded antiembolism stockings. Discuss using pneumatic devices with doctor.
• Increase patient activity as soon as condition permits.
3. Administer prophylactic anticoagulants, if ordered for high-risk patients (typically, low-dose heparin or warfarin sodium). Monitor clotting studies.
4. Monitor for thromboembolic complications, such as pulmonary embolus and thrombophlebitis.
5. Additional individualized interventions: ____________

____

NURSING DIAGNOSIS: *Potential impaired skin integrity related to impeded capillary flow, possible altered sensation, and venous stasis*
Interventions
1. On admission to the unit, and at least daily thereafter, inspect the patient's skin carefully.
2. Evaluate skin breakdown risk factors.
3. Initiate measures to prevent skin breakdown:
• turn and reposition patient every 1 to 2 hours
• use careful turning technique
• use skin lotion judiciously, avoid harsh soaps, and wash the skin gently
• provide pressure relieving devices
• ensure adequate nutrition.
4. Watch for impending skin breakdown.
5. If a pressure sore develops, begin therapeutic regimen immediately.
6. Additional individualized interventions: ____________

____

NURSING DIAGNOSIS: *Potential altered urinary elimination pattern related to diuresis, stasis of urine, positioning, and bone demineralization*
Interventions
1. Assess the patient's normal urinary elimination pattern, if possible.
2. Evaluate for urinary complication risk factors.
3. Initiate these measures to promote normal urinary elimination:
• bedside commode or upright urination, if condition permits
• adequate fluid intake
• as much activity as condition permits
• privacy during attempts to void
• measures to promote bladder emptying
• urinary catheterization only as needed.
4. Measure urine output hourly and report values that remain <60 ml/hour for 2 hours. Assess for bladder distention every 8 hours. Measure urine pH every 8 hours and report values >6.
5. Monitor for signs of urinary tract complications, such as infection and calculi.
6. If signs of urinary tract complications appear, notify the doctor promptly and collaborate in treatment.
7. Additional individualized interventions: ____________

____

NURSING DIAGNOSIS: *Potential altered bowel elimination related to lack of contraction of abdominal muscles, weakness, loss of defecation reflex, slowed peristalsis, altered nutritional intake, and psychological inhibition*
Interventions
1. Assess the patient's normal bowel elimination pattern, if possible.
2. Evaluate for constipation risk factors.
3. Initiate these measures to promote normal bowel elimination:
• bedside commode or toilet, if condition permits
• contracting abdominal muscles, while exhaling, during defecation attempts
• exercises to maintain or strengthen abdominal musculature
• adequate fluid intake
• high-fiber diet and foods that stimulate bowel activity, such as stewed prunes, as permitted
• privacy during elimination.
4. Assess for constipation indicators.
5. As necessary, collaborate with the doctor to select appropriate elimination aids, such as laxatives.
6. Additional individualized interventions: ____________

____

COLLABORATIVE PROBLEM: *Potential muscle atrophy or joint contractures related to disuse, nonfunctional positioning, or reduced muscle tone*
Interventions
1. Evaluate for factors that increase the risk of significant muscle, bone, or joint-related complications.

2. Initiate measures to preserve motor function and strength:
• permit weight bearing as condition permits
• encourage active exercise, as condition permits
• perform complete range-of-motion exercises with all joints at least four times daily
• position carefully to maintain functional alignment.
3. Additional individualized interventions: ___________

____

NURSING DIAGNOSIS: *Disturbed self-concept: body image, role performance related to dependent patient role*
Interventions
1. Assess the effects of reduced mobility on self-concept.
2. Encourage patient participation in self-care and decision making, as permitted by condition.
3. Anticipate such behaviors as regression, withdrawal, aggression, apathy, and crying. Try to help the patient interpret these normal responses to loss.
4. See the "Sensory-Perceptual Alteration" care plan, page 60.
5. See the "Ineffective Coping" care plan, page 26.
6. Additional individualized interventions: ___________

____

PATIENT-FAMILY TEACHING CHECKLIST
___ activity recommendations, restrictions, and limitations
___ measures to avert orthostatic hypotension and activity intolerance
___ indicators of clinically significant activity intolerance
___ signs of complications related to impaired mobility
___ use of any aids to mobility

DOCUMENTATION CHECKLIST
___ clinical status on admission
___ significant changes in status
___ pertinent laboratory and diagnostic test findings
___ response to resumed activity
___ complications of immobility, if any
___ protective and prophylactic measures initiated
___ patient-family teaching
___ transfer planning

ASSOCIATED CARE PLANS
Ineffective Coping
Nutritional Deficit
Acute Pain
Sensory-Perceptual Alteration

Increased Intracranial Pressure

COLLABORATIVE PROBLEM: *Potential cerebral ischemia related to fluctuations in arterial blood pressure, stressful events, nursing activities, hypoxemia, or hypercapnia*
Interventions
1. Assess the patient's level of consciousness (LOC), behavior, motor and sensory function, pupillary reactions, and respiratory patterns every 1 to 2 hours and as necessary.
2. Monitor intracranial pressure (ICP), if an ICP monitoring device is in place, and mean arterial pressure (MAP) continuously. Calculate cerebral perfusion pressure (CPP) as changes occur.
3. Maintain MAP at a level that will result in a CPP of at least 60 mm Hg:
• Administer dopamine hydrochloride (Intropin) or other vasopressors, as ordered.
• If patient has systemic hypertension, titrate fluid restriction, vasodilator administration, or other therapies according to CPP, as ordered.
4. Monitor arterial blood gas (ABG) values as ordered. Maintain ABG values within prescribed parameters.
5. Observe ICP levels (recorded by the ICP monitoring device) during activities that precipitate sustained increases in ICP.
6. Instruct the alert patient to avoid extreme hip flexion as well as straining at stool, coughing, blowing his nose, and moving or turning in bed while holding his breath.
7. Tell the alert patient to avoid pushing the feet against footboard or pushing the arms against the bed.
8. Administer medications, as ordered, for shivering and abnormal posturing.
9. Structure the environment to reduce unpleasant stimuli.
10. Assess the patient's comfort level and administer medications as needed.
11. Use restraints only when necessary and as ordered.
12. Space activities when possible.
13. Maintain venous drainage from the brain by proper alignment and positioning. Keep the head of the bed elevated 15 to 60 degrees at all times, or as ordered.
14. Implement therapeutic measures, as ordered, including:
• corticosteroids
• diuretics
• CSF drainage
• barbiturate coma.
15. When noninvasive therapeutic interventions fail to control ICP, prepare the patient and family for surgical intervention.
16. Additional individualized interventions: ___________

____

NURSING DIAGNOSIS: *Potential for infection related to invasive techniques, immunosuppression, or surgical or other trauma*
Interventions
1. Maintain strict sterile or aseptic technique.
2. Change dressings as ordered.
3. Maintain ICP and hemodynamic monitoring devices as closed systems.
4. Assess periodically for infection.
5. Administer antibiotics, as ordered.
6. Additional individualized interventions: ___________

____

COLLABORATIVE PROBLEM: *Potential for increased cerebral metabolism related to temperature elevations caused by infection and hypothalamic injury*
Interventions
1. Monitor temperature every 4 hours and as needed.
2. Administer antipyretics, as ordered.

3. Apply a cooling (hypothermia) blanket, as ordered.
4. Maintain appropriate precautions while the patient uses the hypothermia blanket.
• Cover the hypothermia blanket with a sheet or bath blanket.
• Check rectal temperature every 30 minutes (or use a rectal probe).
• Turn off blanket when rectal temperature reaches 99.8° F. (37.7 C.).
• Control shivering by administering medication, as ordered.
5. Remove excess bed clothes, and allow for adequate ventilation.
6. Additional individualized interventions: ____________

____

COLLABORATIVE PROBLEM: *Potential for respiratory failure related to increased ICP, cerebral dysfunction, obstructed airway, absence of spontaneous respirations and gag or cough reflex, aspiration, atelectasis, ventilation and perfusion abnormalities, alteration in LOC, or neurogenic pulmonary edema*

Interventions

1. Assess the respiratory rate, depth, and pattern every 15 to 60 minutes. Assist with intubation if the patient cannot maintain adequate airway, respiratory depth, or respiratory pattern.
2. Auscultate breath sounds every 2 hours and as needed.
3. Assess respiratory secretions for color, amount, and consistency.
4. Monitor ABG values, as ordered. Obtain chest X-rays, as ordered.
5. Position the patient with the head of bed elevated to the prescribed height.
6. Reposition the patient every 2 hours, if ICP levels allow.
7. Suction as needed.
8. Implement care related to mechanical ventilation, if used.
9. Additional individualized interventions: ____________

____

NURSING DIAGNOSIS: *Potential for fluid volume deficit related to diuretic therapy, fluid restriction, diabetes insipidus (DI), hyperthermia, or gastrointestinal suction*

Interventions

1. See Appendix C, Fluid-Electrolyte Imbalances, page 317.
2. Monitor and correlate intake and output measurements hourly and cumulatively. Measure urine specific gravity. Report:
• output >200 ml/hour for 2 hours, with urine specific gravity 1.001 to 1.005
• output <30 ml/hour for 2 hours, with urine specific gravity >1.030.
3. Monitor laboratory values, as ordered.
4. Monitor the EKG and hemodynamic pressures continually.
5. Administer replacement therapy, as ordered.
6. Additional individualized interventions: ____________

____

NURSING DIAGNOSIS: *Potential fluid volume excess related to stress, steroid therapy, or syndrome of inappropriate secretion of antidiuretic hormone (SIADH)*

Interventions

1. See Appendix C, Fluid-Electrolyte Imbalances, page 317.
2. Monitor intake and output measurements hourly.
3. Monitor electrolyte, blood urea nitrogen, creatinine, osmolality, and hematocrit values daily or as ordered.
4. Monitor the EKG and hemodynamic pressures continually.
5. Institute therapy, as ordered:
• fluid restriction
• diuretics.
6. Additional individualized interventions: ____________

____

NURSING DIAGNOSIS: *Potential for injury related to decreased level of consciousness, seizure activity, and drug therapy*

Interventions

1. Observe the patient closely at all times. Keep side rails up.
2. Assess for seizure activity. Implement seizure precautions.
3. Assess for gastric bleeding. Administer medications, as ordered, usually antacids or cimetidine (Tagamet).
4. Assess for an absent corneal reflex and apply artificial tears or eye patches, as needed.
5. Additional individualized interventions: ____________

____

PATIENT-FAMILY TEACHING CHECKLIST

__ increased ICP causes
__ extent of neurologic deficits, if any
__ continued family support needed
__ requirements for rehabilitation program, if known

DOCUMENTATION CHECKLIST

__ clinical status on admission
__ significant changes in status
__ pertinent laboratory and diagnostic test findings
__ fluid intake and output levels
__ neurologic status
__ neurologic deficits, if any
__ gastrointestinal bleeding, if any
__ seizure activity, if any

ASSOCIATED CARE PLANS

Acute Pain
Impaired Physical Mobility
Ineffective Coping
Knowledge Deficit
Nutritional Deficit
Sensory-Perceptual Alteration

Ineffective Coping

NURSING DIAGNOSIS: *Ineffective coping related to overwhelming threat*

Interventions

1. Establish rapport. Introduce yourself to the patient and family and explain your role clearly. Emphasize the staff's availability. Try to provide consistency in staffing.
2. Use nonverbal communication to reinforce verbal exchanges.
3. Provide orientation to the health care unit.
4. Identify unfamiliar stimuli, such as sounds, that may contribute to the patient's tension or anxiety.
5. Repeat explanations, as necessary.
6. Encourage verbal expression of feelings.
7. Recognize patient's and family's need to share or repeat details of events leading to hospitalization. Provide positive feedback when possible.
8. Help patient and family list components of threat, encouraging them to separate and prioritize problems. Focus discussion on modifiable factors, emphasizing and allowing choices whenever possible.
9. Additional individualized interventions: ____________

____

NURSING DIAGNOSIS: *Ineffective coping related to inadequate resources*

Interventions

1. Assess previous health history. Ask patient and family how they handled previous problems.
2. Share specific observations of positive family interactions or personal strengths.
3. Assess patient's and family's external resource base. Arrange appropriate referrals as indicated.
4. Explore with the patient and family new ways of looking at identified problems.
5. Consider organizing an ongoing family support group. Without a formally organized group, facilitate supportive interactions among families when possible.
6. Encourage family members to participate in patient care.
7. Additional individualized interventions: ____________

____

NURSING DIAGNOSIS: *Ineffective coping related to inability to mobilize existing resources*

Interventions

1. Allow time for adaptation. Avoid forcing issues. Be especially alert to avoided topics and nonverbal cues.
2. Rule out organic causes for behavioral changes.
3. Whenever possible, reduce or eliminate environmental barriers that interfere with coping ability. Establish routines.
4. If the patient exhibits maladaptive behavior, examine your own biases and values in relation to the behavior. Attempt to understand behavior in terms of the threat to the individual; try to show acceptance.
5. Teach patient and family effective relaxation techniques.
6. Help the patient and family develop plans for dealing with each identified problem.
7. Assess suicide potential by asking direct questions; intervene as indicated. See the "Grieving and Dying" care plan, page 15, for details.
8. As much as possible, prepare patient and family for eventual, possibly abrupt, transfer from the critical care unit.
9. Additional individualized interventions: ____________

____

PATIENT-FAMILY TEACHING CHECKLIST

__ diagnosis, treatment plan, and prognosis
__ expected psychological responses
__ resources available for help
__ effective coping strategies

DOCUMENTATION CHECKLIST

__ clinical status on admission
__ significant stress-related physiologic responses
__ patient's and family's subjective perception of threat
__ identified problems
__ response to staff members
__ patient-family support and interaction
__ coping history
__ pain control measures
__ sleep patterns
__ nutritional intake
__ relaxation techniques
__ other interventions to increase coping ability
__ suicide assessment
__ referrals made
__ teaching

ASSOCIATED CARE PLANS

Acute Pain
Grieving and Dying
Knowledge Deficit
Sensory-Perceptual Alteration

Liver Failure

COLLABORATIVE PROBLEM: *Deteriorating neurologic status related to hepatic encephalopathy syndrome*

Interventions

1. Assess neurologic status hourly.
2. Assess for asterixis.
3. Auscultate the chest and assess respiratory rate hourly. Administer oxygen by nasal prongs, as ordered.
4. Stop dietary protein intake. Also stop administering all nitrogen-containing drugs, as ordered.
5. Administer neomycin by nasogastric tube, if ordered.
6. Administer lactulose by nasogastric tube, if ordered. Monitor for diarrhea.
7. Stop any diuretic therapy, as ordered.
8. Administer enema solutions, as ordered.
9. Avoid all sedatives primarily metabolized by the liver.
10. Provide patient and family teaching associated with above interventions, as appropriate.
11. Additional individualized interventions: ____________

____

COLLABORATIVE PROBLEM: *Potential for fever related to liver disease or infection.*

Interventions

1. Take patient's temperature every 4 hours.
2. Observe for cloudy, concentrated urine.

3. Auscultate lung fields at least every 2 hours.
4. Auscultate bowel sounds at least every 4 hours.
5. If infection is diagnosed, assist with treatment, as ordered. If fever from liver failure is diagnosed, provide appropriate care.
6. Additional individualized interventions: ___________

____

COLLABORATIVE PROBLEM: *Fluid and electrolyte imbalance related to ascites*
Interventions
1. Monitor fluid and electrolyte status closely.
2. Percuss and palpate the abdomen every 4 hours.
3. Maintain strict bed rest.
4. Implement dietary restrictions, as ordered.
5. Provide patient and family teaching related to above measures, as appropriate.
6. Additional individualized interventions: ___________

____

COLLABORATIVE PROBLEM: *Potential gastrointestinal hemorrhage related to esophageal varices*
Interventions
1. Observe for and report signs of esophageal bleeding. See the "Gastrointestinal Hemorrhage" care plan, page 191.
2. Additional individualized interventions: ___________

____

NURSING DIAGNOSIS: *Nutritional deficit related to catabolism from liver disease*
Interventions
1. Implement dietary prescriptions, as ordered.
2. If the patient has encephalopathy, do not administer protein. Once encephalopathy has subsided, begin protein intake at 20 g/day increments.
3. Emphasize to the patient and family the importance of dietary control.
4. Additional individualized interventions: ___________

____

NURSING DIAGNOSIS: *Potential for impaired skin integrity related to jaundice, increased bleeding tendencies, malnutrition, and ascites*
Interventions
1. Monitor skin condition.
2. Monitor prothrombin time, as ordered.
3. Reposition the patient and apply lotion to bony prominences at least every 2 hours. Implement the additional measures in the "Impaired Physical Mobility" care plan, page 33, as appropriate.
4. Provide palliative care for pruritus, as necessary.
5. Additional individualized interventions: ___________

____

PATIENT-FAMILY TEACHING CHECKLIST
__ relationship between alcohol consumption and exacerbation of liver disease
__ causes of neurologic status changes and relationship to liver disease
__ effects of ascites and treatment methods
__ importance of diet in liver disease

DOCUMENTATION CHECKLIST
__ clinical status on admission
__ significant changes in status
__ pertinent laboratory and diagnostic test findings
__ weight
__ intake and output measurements
__ fluctuations in fever and associated symptoms
__ skin integrity
__ signs of gastrointestinal bleeding
__ patient-family teaching
__ transfer planning

ASSOCIATED CARE PLANS
Gastrointestinal Hemorrhage
Impaired Physical Mobility
Nutritional Deficit
Sensory-Perceptual Alteration

Mechanical Ventilation

COLLABORATIVE PROBLEM: *Ineffective alveolar ventilation related to failure to maintain prescribed ventilator settings*
Interventions
1. Confirm orders for mechanical ventilation:
• type of ventilator (pressure or volume cycled)
• inspiratory mode—control, assist-control, intermittent mandatory ventilation (IMV)
• expiratory maneuvers—positive end-expiratory pressure, continuous positive airway pressure (CPAP), expiratory retard.
2. Collaborate with the respiratory therapist to monitor prescribed settings:
• rate
• tidal volume
• minute ventilation (MV)
• inspiratory flow rate
• inspiratory-expiratory ratio
• airway pressure
• pressure limit
• sensitivity
• sigh.
3. In collaboration with the respiratory therapist, monitor compliance every 8 hours.
4. Evaluate pulmonary status at least every 2 hours.
5. Additional individualized interventions: ___________

____

COLLABORATIVE PROBLEM: *Potential hypoxemia related to insufficient oxygen delivery or inadequate level of positive end-expiratory pressure (PEEP)*
Interventions
1. Compare delivered oxygen percentage with desired percentage.
2. Note fraction of inspired oxygen (FIO_2). If 50% or greater:
• Consider, with the doctor, the oxygen toxicity risk in relation to the oxygen therapy need.
• If the oxygen dose cannot be lowered, observe for signs and symptoms of oxygen toxicity.
3. Note PEEP.
• Visually monitor the PEEP level.
• Assist with titration of PEEP.

4. Additional individualized interventions: ____________

____

NURSING DIAGNOSIS: *Ineffective airway clearance related to endotracheal tube, increased secretions, and underlying pathology*

Interventions

1. Provide artificial airway care, including:
• supporting the ventilator tubing
• measuring cuff pressures and volumes every 8 hours
• using minimal occluding volume or minimal leak technique.
2. Monitor endotracheal tube position.
3. Keep a manual self-inflating bag and mask at the bedside. If accidental extubation occurs, open the airway and ventilate with the bag and mask and 100% oxygen. Summon medical assistance.
4. Reposition the patient every 1 to 2 hours. Provide chest physiotherapy as indicated.
5. Suction when needed. Observe these guidelines:
• If the patient's PaO_2 is normal or low, oxygenate before and after with 100% oxygen.
• If the patient is receiving PEEP, use a manual self-inflating bag with a PEEP valve.
• Monitor blood pressure (BP), heart rate, and EKG pattern.
• While suctioning, observe for paroxysmal coughing without deep breaths; remove the catheter if it occurs.
• If the patient reacts adversely to traditional suctioning, consult with the doctor.
6. Additional individualized interventions: ____________

____

COLLABORATIVE PROBLEM: *Potential for injury: complications related to patient deterioration, mechanical breakdown, increased intrathoracic pressure, or bypassed defense mechanisms*

Interventions

ABRUPT RESPIRATORY DISTRESS

1. Keep ventilator alarms turned on at all times.
2. Familiarize yourself with troubleshooting techniques in advance of need.
3. Continually assess patient's breathing in synchrony with the ventilator. If the patient develops sudden respiratory distress or if the ventilator fails abruptly:
• Immediately disconnect the ventilator, open the airway, and ventilate the patient using a manual self-inflating bag and 100% oxygen.
• After establishing ventilation, reassess the patient. If distress subsides, check the ventilator settings. Obtain arterial blood gas (ABG) studies immediately or evaluate oximetric monitoring data.
• If the distress continues, perform a rapid assessment, suction if indicated, and obtain medical assistance.
• Assess for signs of tension pneumothorax. If present, anticipate needle thoracentesis or chest tube insertion.
• If a problem remains unidentified and you suspect patient panic, bag-ventilate to gain control of respiratory rate. Then reconnect the ventilator, coaching the patient to breathe in synchrony with the ventilator.
• If the problem persists, implement changes in ventilator settings, sedate the patient (usually with morphine sulfate), or paralyze the patient as ordered. If paralysis is prescribed, be sure that prescription includes an amnesic agent.
4. Monitor patients on PEEP for barotrauma, decreased cardiac output, water retention, and increased intracranial pressure.
5. Additional individualized interventions: ____________

____

DECREASED CARDIAC OUTPUT

1. Monitor the patient for signs of decreased cardiac output. Administer I.V. fluid or vasopressors, as ordered.
2. Read pulmonary artery and wedge pressures at end-expiration.
3. If the patient is on PEEP, consult the doctor about the specific technique for reading wedge pressures. Monitor the trend of values.
4. Additional individualized interventions: ____________

____

PULMONARY INFECTION

1. Monitor the humidifier's water level and temperature.
2. Drain "rained out" fluid in the ventilator tubing into a basin.
3. Observe for pulmonary infection signs.
4. If patient has pulmonary infection signs, consult the doctor.
5. Additional individualized interventions: ____________

____

GASTROINTESTINAL BLEEDING

1. Insert a nasogastric tube, as ordered.
2. Administer antacids, ranitidine, or cimetidine, as ordered.
3. Additional individualized interventions: ____________

____

FLUID RETENTION

1. Monitor for fluid retention signs. If present, consult with the doctor.
2. Additional individualized interventions: ____________

____

NURSING DIAGNOSIS: *Fear related to inability to speak and dependence on a machine for life support*

Interventions

1. Implement the general measures in the "Ineffective Coping" care plan, page 26, as appropriate.
2. Establish a communication method.
3. Reduce the patient's need for communication. Emphasize that a nurse is available immediately if needed.
4. Explain the reason for mechanical ventilation. Stress the temporary nature of ventilation, if true.
5. Additional individualized interventions: ____________

____

COLLABORATIVE PROBLEM: *Potential ineffective weaning related to lack of physiologic or psychological readiness*

Interventions

1. Anticipate weaning when the patient meets weaning criteria.

2. Make sure the patient is rested, well nourished, oriented, able to follow commands, and receiving no respiratory depressants.
3. Explain the weaning process to the patient and family.
4. Obtain baseline vital signs, ABG values, and pulmonary function measurements. Suction the airway.
5. Implement the weaning method ordered: CPAP, IMV, or T-piece.
6. Monitor the BP, heart rate, EKG rhythm, respiratory rate, ease of breathing, level of consciousness, and level of fatigue constantly for the first 20 to 30 minutes and every 5 minutes thereafter until weaning is complete.
7. With the doctor, terminate weaning if adverse reactions occur.
8. If weaning continues, measure the tidal volume, MV, and ABG values after 20 to 30 minutes.
9. If physiologic parameters indicate weaning is feasible, but the patient resists, assess the possibility of psychological dependence on the ventilator. Consult with the doctor, pulmonary nurse specialist, or psychiatric nurse clinician, as appropriate.
10. Assist with extubation, when ordered.
11. Additional individualized interventions: ______

______

PATIENT-FAMILY TEACHING CHECKLIST
__ reason for mechanical ventilation
__ communication measures
__ alarms
__ weaning process

DOCUMENTATION CHECKLIST
__ clinical status on admission
__ significant changes in status
__ pertinent laboratory and diagnostic test findings
__ ventilator and patient checks
__ ventilator alarm status
__ airway care
__ measures to prevent or detect and treat complications
__ communication measures
__ emotional support
__ sedative or paralyzing pharmacologic agents, if used
__ weaning process
__ patient-family teaching
__ transfer planning

ASSOCIATED CARE PLANS
Adult Respiratory Distress Syndrome
Impaired Physical Mobility
Ineffective Coping
Nutritional Deficit
Sensory-Perceptual Alteration

Nutritional Deficit

NURSING DIAGNOSIS: *Nutritional deficit related to difficulty chewing or swallowing, sore throat after endotracheal extubation, or dry mouth*
Interventions
1. Assess and document causes. Initiate referrals as appropriate.
2. Assess level of consciousness, ability to chew and swallow, and gag reflex.
3. With the dietitian, and as ordered, provide a diet appropriate to the patient's abilities, for example, liquids, soft foods, or food requiring little cutting.
4. If the patient has a sore mouth or throat, obtain an order for viscous lidocaine.
5. Assist the patient to an upright sitting position (with the head flexed forward) for meals, unless contraindicated.
6. Suction food, fluids, or accumulated saliva as needed.
7. Provide assistance, as needed.
8. Document feeding technique and food intake.
9. Additional individualized interventions: ______

______

NURSING DIAGNOSIS: *Nutritional deficit related to anorexia*
Interventions
1. Assess possible causes of anorexia.
2. Provide as pleasant an eating environment as possible.
3. Before meals, provide rest; administer analgesics or antiemetics, as ordered; avoid painful procedures; and provide oral hygiene.
4. Emphasize the importance of eating.
5. Provide social interaction during meals.
6. Offer small, frequent feedings of highly nutritious foods.
7. Limit fluid intake at mealtimes.
8. If the person begins to feel nauseated, encourage slow deep breathing. If vomiting occurs, document the amount and type of emesis. Provide oral hygiene.
9. Praise the patient for signs of increased appetite.
10. Additional individualized interventions: ______

______

COLLABORATIVE PROBLEM: *Nutritional deficit related to inability to digest nutrients or to hypermetabolic state*
Interventions
1. Anticipate patient's increased nutrient needs. Also observe for signs of inability to absorb nutrients.
2. Obtain a comprehensive nutritional assessment.
3. Assess and document bowel sounds and abdominal distention every 4 hours.
4. Collaborate with nutritional experts to establish nutrient requirements.
5. Provide appropriate nutritional replacements, as ordered:
• enteral feeding
—nutrient supplements
—meal replacements
—defined-formula diets
• parenteral nutrition
—peripheral venous nutrition
—central venous nutrition, also known as total parenteral nutrition (TPN) or hyperalimentation.
6. If the patient is receiving tube feedings:
• Check tube placement before each feeding.
• Keep the head of the bed elevated during feedings, and after feedings for 1 hour.
• Begin with small amounts of dilute solution. Increase the amount and concentration as tolerated.
• Use a continuous infusion pump, if possible.

7. If the patient is receiving TPN, ensure delivery of prescribed solutions and monitor for complications.
8. Additional individualized interventions: ____________

____

PATIENT-FAMILY TEACHING CHECKLIST

__ nutrition's importance in recovery
__ rationale for selecting specific nutritional support method

DOCUMENTATION CHECKLIST

__ clinical status on admission
__ significant changes in status
__ pertinent laboratory and diagnostic test findings
__ specific nutritional support method
__ tolerance of method
__ complications, if any
__ daily nutritional intake
__ medications administered, if any
__ attitude toward eating
__ patient-family teaching
__ transfer planning

ASSOCIATED CARE PLANS

Refer to care plan for specific underlying condition.

Seizures

NURSING DIAGNOSIS: *Ineffective airway clearance related to loss of consciousness, apnea, excessive secretions, jaw clenching, and/or airway occlusion by tongue or foreign body*

Interventions

1. If patient reports an aura or warning phase, clear the mouth of foreign bodies and insert a soft cloth or gauze pad at the mouth's corners. Without warning, do not try to force the jaw open or insert oral airways. Maintain an open airway.
2. Suction the oropharynx, as needed. Provide supplemental oxygen by nasal cannula.
3. If seizure activity persists or recurs frequently, despite drug therapy, notify the doctor immediately. Anticipate required endotracheal intubation and mechanical ventilation.
4. Insert a nasogastric tube and connect it to low suction, as ordered.
5. Additional individualized interventions: ____________

____

COLLABORATIVE PROBLEM: *Potential status epilepticus related to inadequate pharmacologic control or misidentification of underlying cause*

Interventions

1. Administer I.V. anticonvulsant medication, as ordered:
• diazepam (Valium)
• phenobarbital sodium (Luminal) and other barbiturate anticonvulsants
• phenytoin sodium (Dilantin).
2. Consider possible underlying causes, such as:
• head trauma
• electrolyte imbalance
• hypoxia
• hypoglycemia or hyperglycemia
• brain tumors
• infections
• cerebral hemorrhage
• toxins.
3. If seizure activity is refractory to drug therapy, anticipate possible neuromuscular blockage or general anesthesia, combined with mechanical ventilation.
4. Additional individualized interventions: ____________

____

NURSING DIAGNOSIS: *Potential for injury: trauma or myoglobinuria related to excessive uncontrolled muscle activity*

Interventions

1. At the seizure's onset, ensure safe patient positioning. Place pillows around the patient and pad the side rails. Do not restrain extremities.
2. Stay with the patient during seizure.
3. After motor activity stops, perform a neurologic evaluation and inspect the oropharynx, tongue, and teeth.
4. Prevent excessive environmental stimulation during the postictal period.
5. If seizure activity was prolonged, monitor urine output for possible myoglobin content.
6. Additional individualized interventions: ____________

____

PATIENT-FAMILY TEACHING CHECKLIST

__ cause and implications of seizure activity
__ treatment modalities instituted
__ signs of possible recurrence
__ safety precautions

DOCUMENTATION CHECKLIST

__ clinical status on admission
__ significant changes in status
__ pertinent laboratory and diagnostic test findings
__ episodes of seizure activity
__ safety precautions instituted
__ pharmacologic interventions
__ patient-family teaching
__ transfer planning

ASSOCIATED CARE PLANS

Craniotomy
Diabetes Mellitus
Drug Overdose
Hyperglycemic Hyperosmolar Nonketosis
Increased Intracranial Pressure
Mechanical Ventilation
Multiple Trauma
Sensory-Perceptual Alteration

Shock

COLLABORATIVE PROBLEM: *Potential hypovolemic shock related to blood loss, diuresis, dehydration, or third-space fluid shift*

Interventions

1. Observe for fluid loss signs and symptoms.

2. For active external bleeding, apply direct, continuous pressure and elevate the area, if possible.
3. Except for patients with active head and neck bleeding, suspected increased intracranial pressure, or suspected cardiogenic shock, elevate the legs above heart level.
4. Obtain initial and serial diagnostic tests.
5. Insert and maintain as ordered:
• two or more large-bore I.V. lines
• urinary catheter
• central venous pressure (CVP) catheter
6. Depending on which lines are inserted, monitor urine output and CVP every 15 minutes to 1 hour.
7. Monitor arterial blood pressure and mean arterial pressure (MAP).
• Assist with insertion of an arterial line, if ordered. Monitor blood pressure (BP) continually and measure MAP electronically.
• With no arterial line in place, measure cuff BP every 5 to 15 minutes until stable and then hourly. Calculate MAP.
• Maintain MAP within the desired range.
8. Administer crystalloid or colloid I.V. solutions, as ordered.
9. Administer a fluid challenge, if ordered.
10. During all fluid administration, monitor hemodynamic measurement trends and urinary output. Observe for fluid overload signs.
11. Additional individualized interventions: ___________

____

COLLABORATIVE PROBLEM: *Potential cardiogenic shock related to decreased myocardial contractility, dysrhythmias, or excessive vasoconstriction*
Interventions
1. Observe for signs and symptoms of poor arterial perfusion.
2. Observe for signs and symptoms of venous congestion.
3. Monitor the EKG continually.
4. Assist with insertion of a thermodilution catheter. Measure cardiac output (CO), as ordered—typically, every hour until patient stabilizes and then every 2 to 4 hours. Calculate cardiac index. Note trend of values.
5. Monitor right atrial pressure, pulmonary artery pressure, and pulmonary capillary wedge pressure, as ordered, typically every hour and as needed.
6. Calculate systemic vascular resistance. Monitor trend of readings.
7. Construct a ventricular function curve, if used in your unit.
8. Administer I.V. solutions, as ordered.
9. Administer I.V. medications to improve CO, as ordered:
• positive inotropic agents
• vasodilators.
10. Provide nursing care related to the intraaortic balloon pump, if used.
11. Additional individualized interventions: ___________

____

COLLABORATIVE PROBLEM: *Potential vasogenic shock related to loss of vasomotor tone or release of vasodilating substances*
Interventions
1. Observe for general signs and symptoms of vasogenic shock.
2. Observe for evidence of specific types of vasogenic shock:
• neurogenic
• anaphylactic
• septic: early stage (hyperdynamic, or "warm") or late stage (hypodynamic, or "cold").
3. Administer I.V. fluids, as ordered.
4. Administer pharmacologic agents, as ordered.
5. Additional individualized interventions: ___________

____

COLLABORATIVE PROBLEM: *Hypoxemia related to ventilation-perfusion imbalance and diffusion defect*
Interventions
1. Provide standard nursing care related to impaired gas exchange:
• airway
• suction
• supplemental oxygen
• intubation and mechanical ventilation, if indicated.
2. Monitor arterial blood gas values, as ordered—typically every 4 hours.
3. Administer sodium bicarbonate I.V., as ordered.
4. Additional individualized interventions: ___________

____

NURSING DIAGNOSIS: *Potential for injury: complications related to ischemia*
Interventions
1. Prevent paralytic ileus and stress ulcers. Maintain nothing by mouth (NPO) status; insert nasogastric tube, as ordered; administer cimetadine (Tagamet), ranitidine (Zantac), or antacids, as ordered. Monitor bowel sounds.
2. Observe for adult respiratory distress syndrome signs and symptoms. If present, alert the doctor and document. (See the "Adult Respiratory Distress Syndrome" care plan, page 101.)
3. Observe for acute myocardial infarction signs and symptoms. See the "Acute Myocardial Infarction" care plan, page 150.
4. Observe for heart failure signs and symptoms. Consult the "Acute Heart Failure" care plan, page 140.
5. Observe for disseminated intravascular coagulation signs and symptoms. See the "Disseminated Intravascular Coagulation" care plan.
6. Observe for acute renal failure signs and symptoms. Implement measures in the "Acute Renal Failure" care plan, page 227, as appropriate.
7. Observe for liver failure signs and symptoms. Consult the "Liver Failure" care plan, page 199.
8. Additional individualized interventions: ___________

____

NURSING DIAGNOSIS: *Fear related to life-threatening condition*
Interventions
1. Implement measures in the "Ineffective Coping" and "Grieving and Dying" care plans, pages 26 and 15, respectively, as appropriate.
2. Additional individualized interventions: ___________

____

PATIENT-FAMILY TEACHING CHECKLIST

__ cause and significance of shock
__ expectations for recovery
__ purpose of monitoring devices
__ rationales for therapeutic interventions

DOCUMENTATION CHECKLIST

__ clinical status on admission
__ significant changes in status
__ pertinent laboratory and diagnostic test findings
__ care related to invasive monitoring lines
__ fluid administration
__ inotropes, vasodilators, or other pharmacologic agents
__ intraaortic balloon pump, if used
__ ventilation and oxygenation support measures
__ emotional support
__ patient-family teaching
__ transfer planning

ASSOCIATED CARE PLANS

Acute Heart Failure
Acute Myocardial Infarction
Acute Renal Failure
Adult Respiratory Distress Syndrome
Disseminated Intravascular Coagulation
Grieving and Dying
Impaired Physical Mobility
Ineffective Coping
Liver Failure
Major Burns
Mechanical Ventilation
Multiple Trauma
Pulmonary Embolus

Appendices

Appendix A: Monitoring Standards

Monitoring of clinical signs and symptoms, laboratory tests, and diagnostic procedures is presented within specific care plans in this text. This appendix outlines generally accepted standards for implementing selected hemodynamic monitoring techniques for critically ill patients. It should be individualized according to a specific patient's needs and unit protocol. For all monitoring techniques, remember that the trend of values is more significant than isolated readings.

EKG monitoring

- Monitor EKG continuously. Observe for dysrhythmias, ST-segment changes, and T-wave abnormalities.
- Monitor in MCL_1 or MCL_6 whenever possible, because they best differentiate ectopy from aberrancy.
- Keep rate alarms on at all times.
- Mount rhythm printouts in the patient's record routinely every 4 to 8 hours and as needed for significant dysrhythmias.
- Evaluate and document atrial and ventricular rate, rhythm, PR interval, QRS duration, and appearance of P waves, QRS complex, ST segment and T waves at least once every 8 hours and as needed for significant changes.

Vital sign monitoring

- Monitor apical pulse, blood pressure, and respiratory rate every 15 minutes until stable, then every hour.
- Monitor temperature at least every 8 hours.

Intake and output (I&O) monitoring

- Monitor hourly and 8-hour or 24-hour cumulative intake and output levels.
- Besides standard nursing I&O measures (for example, including Jell-O in intake total), record the amount of all I.V. flush solutions administered.
- Measure specific gravity hourly.
- Measure glucose and acetone levels every 4 to 6 hours in diabetic patients, patients on total parenteral nutrition, postoperative cardiac surgery patients, and others, as indicated.

Arterial pressure monitoring

- Monitor arterial pressure continuously in patients with arterial lines.
- Keep pressure alarms on at all times.
- Keep all connections in constant view; the patient can exsanguinate in a matter of minutes if a disconnection occurs.
- Balance and calibrate the transducer according to the manufacturer's directions at least every 8 hours to negate the influence of atmospheric pressure on readings and to confirm the measuring accuracy.
- Use a constant low-flow closed heparinized flush solution to maintain patency.
- Periodically observe for the characteristic arterial waveform on the oscilloscope; investigate damping or abnormal appearance promptly.
- Compare to sphygmomanometer pressure every 8 hours; investigate significant discrepancies between the two.
- Check pulse, skin temperature, and skin color distal to insertion site at least every 8 hours.

Central venous pressure (CVP) monitoring

- Measure CVP every hour and as needed.
- Before measuring CVP, level the zero point on the manometer with the phlebostatic axis (fourth intercostal space in the midaxillary line).
- Before measuring CVP, confirm catheter patency by observing the manometer fluid level for the characteristic fall and fluctuations with respiration.

Monitoring Standards *(continued)*

Pulmonary artery (PA) monitoring	• Measure systolic, diastolic, and mean pressures every hour and as needed. • Use consistent baseline position for obtaining readings. • Level the transducer's air-fluid interface with the phlebostatic axis. • Follow unit protocol for removing patients from ventilators to record readings. If recording pressures while the patient is on the ventilator, read pressures at end-expiration to minimize respiratory influences on hemodynamic values. Document whether pressures are recorded when the patient is on or off the ventilator. • Balance and calibrate the transducer according to the manufacturer's directions at least every 8 hours to negate the influence of atmospheric pressure on readings and to confirm accuracy of measurement. • Use a constant low-flow closed heparinized flush solution to maintain patency. • Before readings, confirm patency by observing the oscilloscope for characteristic PA waveforms. • Usually, when the above standards are followed, regard a change in values of >5 mm Hg as clinically significant.
Pulmonary capillary wedge pressure (PCWP) monitoring	• Measure PCWP every hour and as needed. • To read PCWP, inflate the balloon with no more than the specified amount of air for that size balloon, until the characteristic PCWP waveform appears. After reading the pressure, be sure the balloon is deflated by removing the syringe used for inflation, releasing the lever if used to lock air in the balloon for the reading, and confirming on the oscilloscope the return to the usual PA waveform. • To avoid frequent wedging, which damages the balloon, and to monitor left ventricular filling pressure constantly, consider continuous monitoring of PA diastolic pressure. Verify correlation with PCWP every 4 to 8 hours by confirming that the pressures are within 5 mm Hg of each other.
Cardiac output (CO) monitoring	• Measure CO every hour and as needed. • Obtain at least three readings at a time. Discard any readings that deviate significantly from each other and average the remaining readings. • Use injectate ordinarily at room temperature. Use iced injectate if room temperature injectate readings consistently deviate >15% from each other. • Monitor cardiac index by dividing CO by the patient's body surface area, obtainable from a DuBois nomogram. • Monitor systemic vascular resistance by dividing CO into mean arterial pressure (MAP) minus mean right atrial pressure.
Intracranial pressure (ICP) monitoring	• Monitor ICP continuously in patients with ICP monitoring catheters. • Use a consistent baseline position for obtaining readings, usually a 20- to 30-degree elevation of the head of the bed. • Level the air-fluid interface of the transducer with the reference point for the foramen of Monro, usually considered to be the outer corner of the eye, top of the ear, or the external auditory meatus. • Verify patency of the line by observing the characteristic waveform on the oscilloscope. • Do not read pressures while the patient is moving, coughing, or has head turned to one side or the other; all will falsely elevate pressures. • Never aspirate an ICP line; doing so may draw brain tissue into the catheter or screw. • Do not flush an ICP line unless specifically ordered to do so by the patient's doctor. • Monitor cerebral perfusion pressure by subtracting ICP from MAP. • Balance and calibrate the transducer at least every 8 hours.

REFERENCES

Daily, E., and Schroeder, J. *Techniques in Bedside Hemodynamic Monitoring,* 3rd ed. St. Louis: C.V. Mosby Co., 1985.

Holloway, N., and Gawlinski, A. "Hemodynamic Monitoring," in *Nursing the Critically Ill Adult,* 3rd ed. Edited by Holloway, N. Menlo Park, Calif.: Addison-Wesley Publishing Co., 1988.

Nemens E., and Woods, S. "Normal Fluctuations in Pulmonary Artery and Pulmonary Capillary Wedge Pressures in Acutely Ill Patients," *Heart & Lung* 11:393-98, 1982.

Shellock, F., and Riedinger, M. "Reproducibility and Accuracy of Using Room Temperature vs. Ice-Temperature Injectate for Thermodilution Cardiac Output Determination," *Heart & Lung* 12:175-76, 1983.

Appendix B: Acid-Base Imbalances

Disorder	ABG results	Physiologic basis	Potential causes	Signs and symptoms	Compensatory mechanisms
Respiratory acidosis	↓ pH ↑ $PaCO_2$ Compensatory: ↑ HCO_3^-	Decreased alveolar ventilation, resulting in carbon dioxide retention	Depression of medullary respiratory center from drugs, injury, or disease Pulmonary diseases Inadequate tidal volume (TV) or respiratory rate on ventilator	Decreased mentation, restlessness, combativeness, headache, diaphoresis, anxiety, tachycardia	Renal compensation by HCO_3^- retention, acid elimination, and increased ammonia production
Respiratory alkalosis	↑ pH ↓ $PaCO_2$ Compensatory: ↓ HCO_3^-	Increased alveolar ventilation, resulting in carbon dioxide loss	Hyperventilation from anxiety, pain, excessive TV or respiratory rate on ventilator Respiratory-center stimulation by drugs, injury, or disease Fever or high ambient temperature Sepsis	Increased rate and depth of respirations, "tingling" or numb feeling, light-headedness or syncope, anxiety	Renal compensation by HCO_3^- elimination, acid retention, and decreased ammonia production
Metabolic acidosis	↓ pH ↓ HCO_3^- Compensatory: ↓ $PaCO_2$	HCO_3^- loss, ↑ acid formation	Diarrhea, diabetes, shock, renal failure, azotemia, small-bowel fistulas	Increased rate and depth of respirations, fatigue/lethargy, acetone odor to breath, unconsciousness	Rapid pulmonary compensation by hyperventilation, renal metabolic compensation (except in renal failure) by HCO_3^- retention, acid elimination, increased ammonia production
Metabolic alkalosis	↑ pH ↑ HCO_3^- Compensatory: ↑ $PaCO_2$	↑ HCO_3^-, and acids or potassium loss	Vomiting, gastric suctioning, prolonged use of diuretics, excessive HCO_3^- ingestion	Decreased rate and depth of respirations, hypertonicity, twitching to tetanus, convulsions, irritability, restlessness/combativeness, unconsciousness	Rapid pulmonary compensation by hypoventilation, renal metabolic compensation by HCO_3^- elimination, acid retention, decreased ammonia production

From: Strange, J. *Shock Trauma Care Plans.* Springhouse, Pa.: Springhouse Corp., 1987, pp 372-73.

Appendix C: Fluid and Electrolyte Imbalances

Causes	Signs and symptoms and Laboratory results	Treatment
Hypovolemia		
Hemorrhage, diabetes insipidus (DI), renal disease, vagal stimulation, drug reactions, hyperglycemic hyperosmolar nonketotic coma	Tachycardia, weak pulse, hypotension, oliguria, ↓ central venous pressure (CVP), ↓ level of consciousness (LOC), pallor, ↓ hematocrit/hemoglobin	Correct the cause; administer appropriate I.V. fluids.
Hypervolemia		
Excessive I.V. fluid administration	Hypertension, edema, bounding pulse, ↑ CVP, pulmonary edema, venous distention, ↓ hemoglobin/hematocrit, ↓ blood urea nitrogen (BUN)	Treat with diuretics, dialysis phlebotomy; no treatment may be needed; prevention is the best treatment.
Intravascular/interstitial shift		
Hemorrhage, ↓ water intake, concentrated tube feedings, vomiting/diarrhea, burns, prolonged gastric suctioning, soft-tissue injury, intestinal obstruction, fever	Shock state, tachycardia, weak pulse, oliguria, ↓ LOC, dry mucous membranes, ↑ hemoglobin/hematocrit, ↑ BUN, hypotension	Correct the cause; administer appropriate I.V. fluids.
Interstitial/intravascular shift		
Burns, soft-tissue injury, excessive colloid or hypertonic I.V. administration	Hypertension, bounding pulse, venous distention, ↑ CVP, weakness, ↓ hemoglobin/hematocrit, ↓ BUN, hyponatremia	No treatment is usually needed except in patients with abnormal heart, liver, or kidney function; they are usually treated with diuretics.
Hyponatremia		
Excessive sweating or water intake, ↓ salt intake, congestive heart failure (CHF), renal failure, diuretic therapy, freshwater near drowning, vomiting, diarrhea, burns	Confusion, headache, abdominal cramps, apathy, hypotension, weakness, hyperactive reflexes, convulsions, oliguria, ↓ serum sodium, ↓ chloride, ↓ urine specific gravity	Decrease water intake or increase sodium intake.
Hypernatremia		
↓ water intake, ↓ sodium intake, prolonged watery diarrhea, prolonged hyperventilation, saltwater near drowning, diabetes insipidus	Dehydration; thirst; dry mucous membranes; weakness; fever; warm, flushed skin; muscle pain; ↑ serum sodium level; ↑ serum chloride level; ↑ urine specific gravity	Correct the cause, if possible; restrict sodium intake; increase fluid intake.
Hypokalemia		
↓ potassium intake, diuretics, vomiting or diarrhea, burns, CHF, fistulas, colitis, steroids	Diminished reflexes, irregular pulse, thirst, hypotension, EKG changes, muscular weakness or irritability, ↓ serum potassium level, ↓ serum chloride level	Increase dietary potassium intake; administer P.O. or I.V. potassium supplements.
Hyperkalemia		
↑ potassium intake, burns, soft tissue injury, advanced kidney disease, adrenal insufficiency, hemorrhagic shock, excessive I.V. administration	Irritability, nausea, diarrhea, confusion, flaccid muscles, EKG changes, hypotension, abdominal cramping, ↑ serum potassium level	Decrease intake; treat with dialysis; give a sodium polystyrene sulfonate enema; give sodium bicarbonate, glucose, and insulin together I.V.

(continued)

Fluid and Electrolyte Imbalances *(continued)*

Causes	Signs and symptoms and laboratory results	Treatment
Hypocalcemia		
Diarrhea, burns, renal failure, draining wounds, citrated blood administration, acidosis overcorrection, vitamin D deficiency	Carpopedal spasms; tetany; convulsions; tingling in fingers, toes, lips; muscle cramps; EKG changes; ↓ serum calcium level	Administer calcium P.O. or I.V.
Hypercalcemia		
Vitamin D overdose, renal disease, excessive antacid use, excessive calcium intake	Pathologic fractures, deep-bone or flank pain, lethargy, nausea, vomiting, EKG changes, osteoporosis, kidney stones, kidney infections, ↑ serum calcium level	Correct the cause; administer disodium phosphate, sodium sulfate, diuretics.
Hypomagnesemia		
Alcohol abuse, vomiting, ↓ intake, malnutrition, diuretics, prolonged GI suctioning, diarrhea, pancreatitis, kidney disease	Tetany, lethargy, nausea, vomiting, tachydysrhythmias, hypotension, confusion, hyperactive reflexes, ↓ serum magnesium level	Increase dietary intake, administer I.V. magnesium.
Hypermagnesemia		
Excessive intake, kidney disease, severe dehydration, repeated magnesium-containing enemas, magnesium antacids in renal failure	Lethargy, flushing, depressed respirations, hypotension, flaccid muscles or paralysis, dysrhythmias, ↑ serum magnesium level	Decrease intake; administer I.V. 10% calcium gluconate; treat renal-failure patients with dialysis.

From: Strange, J. *Shock Trauma Care Plans.* Springhouse, Pa.: Springhouse Corp., 1987, pp 374-75.

Appendix D: Organ Donation

Organ donation offers the families of dying or deceased patients an opportunity to turn their tragedy into a "gift of life" for another person. Organ donation can help families find meaning in what otherwise seems a senseless, premature death. Approximately 75% of organ donors are trauma victims. As many as 80% to 85% of families who are approached about organ donation agree to it. The nurse should be alert for potential donors and learn the individual institution's procedure; organ donor programs and criteria for donation may vary slightly among states.

Considerations in identifying donors

Age. Most donor programs seek donors between age 5 and 65; some organs, such as eyes, may be harvested at any age.

Underlying systemic conditions. Patients who have acquired immunodeficiency syndrome, hepatitis, syphilis, tuberculosis, kidney disease, chronic hypertension, sepsis, cancer, or any active, transmittable disease will not be suitable organ donors in most cases. Diabetic patients may or may not be suitable donors, depending on individual status.

Underlying conditions of donor organs:
- heart and lungs—no history of cardiovascular disease or tracheostomy
- kidney—no renal disease
- liver—no history of alcoholism or hepatobiliary disease
- cornea—no history of eye surgery or corneal disease
- pancreas—no history of diabetes in either donor or first-generation relative, and no history of alcoholism.

Patient preference. Many people now carry Uniform Anatomical Gift cards, have a "donor" notation on their state driver's license, or have expressed their wishes regarding this issue to family members.

Cultural-religious background. Some cultures and religions may find organ donation unacceptable.

Brain death criteria. All donors must meet specific brain death criteria. These may vary slightly by law among states but include cerebral and brain stem unresponsiveness, as manifested by the following:
- unresponsiveness to sensory input
- absence of decerebrate or decorticate posturing
- absence of pupillary, gag, and corneal reflexes
- absence of eye movement in response to oculocephalic or oculovestibular testing
- absence of spontaneous respiratory effort even after $Paco_2$ reaches 60 mm Hg
- cause of coma identified as other than drug intoxication, hypothermia, shock, hypoxia, or other potentially reversible conditions. All these criteria must be present and must persist for a prescribed length of time, as follows:
  —at least 6 hours with a confirmatory isoelectric EEG
  —at least 12 or 24 hours without an isoelectric EEG, depending on the cause of brain death

(continued)

Organ Donation *(continued)*

Family counseling

The family of the potential donor should be given ample opportunity for discussion, grieving, and questions in an unhurried atmosphere. The following concerns should be addressed:

- meaning of "brain death"
- absence of pain for the donor because brain stem function has ceased
- donor's appearance unchanged for funeral purposes
- expected length of procedure (varies with organs)
- no effect on funeral arrangements
- no cost to donor or donor's family
- transportation for organ arranged by involved institutions
- confidentiality: although confidentiality is maintained, the family may later learn the general identity of the recipient, for example, "Your brother's kidney was successfully transplanted into a 12-year-old girl with kidney disease."

Donor maintenance until transplantation

Careful assessment and corrective intervention, as needed, are essential until the transplant team arrives. This must include frequent assessments of vital signs and hemodynamic parameters; optimally administered mechanical ventilation; maintenance of cardiac output, peripheral perfusion, and fluid balance; maintenance of normothermia; and prevention of infection, skin breakdown, or other complications. Large volumes of dilute urine may indicate development of diabetes insipidus, a common condition in donors because of the failure of the hypothalamus to produce or the pituitary gland to release antidiuretic hormone.

REFERENCES

American Association of Critical Care Nurses. Position Statement: Required Request and Routine Inquiry: Methods to Improve the Organ and Tissue Donation Process. *Focus on Critical Care* 14(2):79, 1987.

Cox, J. "Organ Donation: The Challenge for Emergency Nursing," *Journal of Emergency Nursing* 12(4):199-204, 1986.

Diggs, C. "Recognition and Nursing Care of Organ Donors," *Journal of Emergency Nursing* 12(4):205-9, 1986.

Goldsmith, J., and Montefusco, C. "Nursing Care of the Potential Organ Donor," *Critical Care Nurse* 5(6):22-9, 1985.

Hart, D. "Helping the Family of the Potential Organ Donor: Crisis Intervention and Decision Making," *Journal of Emergency Nursing* 12(4):210-12, 1986.

Holler, D., and Groves, M. "Organ Donation," in *Shock Trauma Care Plans.* Edited by Strange, J. Springhouse, Pa.: Springhouse Corp., 1987.

Johnson, L. "A Case for Organ Donation," *Journal of Emergency Nursing* 12(4):196-98, 1986.

Tooke, M., et al. "Corneal Transplantation," *American Journal of Nursing* 86(6):685-87, June 1986.

Appendix E: Pediatric Considerations

Care of the critically ill child involves a working knowledge of normal growth and development and an awareness of specific principles that can guide interventions. Although care for a particular disorder is similar for patients of any age, remember that children are not merely small adults.

This appendix reviews major considerations in the care of children; consult current pediatric nursing texts for further details.

Pediatric concerns in the CCU

Age and developmental level. Do the patient's overall behavior, weight, height, intellectual ability, and motor coordination fall within normal range for the patient's age group?

Nonverbal behavior. Because children may be unable to articulate their symptoms or needs as an adult would, close observation for nonverbal cues is essential. For example, abdominal pain in children may be evidenced by doubling or curling up, hesitancy to move, or facial grimacing. Because parents are usually the best sources of information regarding the child's normal behavior and response to illness, it is wise to rely heavily on their observations regarding the child's condition.

Physical examination. Although a head-to-toe technique may be most appropriate for adults, some clinicians recommend a different approach in children. Beginning with extremities usually is less threatening to the child and may produce less crying and agitation, which can interfere with the examination.

Vital signs. Normal vital signs vary considerably with age, as shown by the table below. Body temperature in children is usually considered within a range of normal limits. Partly because of their higher metabolic rate, children commonly display elevated temperature even in the absence of significant abnormalities. As in adults, however, any persistent elevation, particularly if accompanied by other symptoms or in the presence of underlying illness, should be investigated promptly.

Pediatric Glasgow Coma Scale (GCS). An age-referenced adaptation of the GCS is used for children, as shown in the table on page 322.

Interventions

Fluid status. Infants and young children are more susceptible to fluid imbalances than adults because a greater proportion of their body weight is water. Also, children's total blood volume (TBV), approximately 75 to 80 ml/kg, is much less than that of adults. The premature newborn may have a TBV of only 100 to 200 ml. After age 1, TBV is usually 735 to 860 ml, and by age 13, TBV begins to approach that of most adults. All children's I.V. infusions should be administered via an infusion control pump in the CCU. If this equipment is not immediately available, use a volume control chamber to minimize the possibility of inadvertent fluid overload.

A guide for maintenance I.V. fluid in children follows:
- first 10 kg body weight: 100 ml/kg/24 hours
- next 10 kg body weight: 50 ml/kg/24 hours
- for each kg over 20 kg body weight: 20 ml/kg/24 hours.

Fluid selection. Dextrose 5% with ¼, ⅓, or ½ normal saline solution is generally preferred for a maintenance solution in children. Dextrose 5% in water is typically avoided to minimize possible hyponatremia. Ringer's lactate solution or blood is commonly used in trauma or shock situations when rapid volume infusion is desired.

Nutritional needs. Children have a higher basal metabolic rate, and thus greater obligatory energy needs in relation to their body size than adults. Also, children have less stored nutritional energy reserves. The newborn, for example, requires 110 to 120 kcal/kg/day for basal metabolic, energy, and growth needs, compared to the approximately 2,500 kcal needed by a 132 lb (60 kg) adult male (41 to 42 kcal/kg/day). This means that nutritional depletion can occur much more rapidly in children, particularly if fever or other conditions that increase metabolic rate are present.

(continued)

Pediatric Considerations *(continued)*

Interventions *(continued)*

Medication dosages. Because children vary widely in size, medication dosages must be calculated in dose per kilogram of body weight or, alternatively, according to body surface area, using appropriate nomograms. The nurse also must verify that the dose per kilogram ordered does not exceed the 24-hour dose recommendations, regardless of the appropriateness of the individual dose. Keeping drug cards or charts with commonly used emergency medication dosages precalculated for weight ranges in kilograms can save time and reduce the possibility of error.

REFERENCES

Aoki, B. *Principles in the Stabilization and Transport of Critically Ill Children.* Oakland, Calif: Children's Hospital Medical Center of Northern California, 1982.

Strange, J. "General Pediatric Care Considerations," in *Shock Trauma Care Plans.* Springhouse, Pa.: Springhouse Corp., 1987.

Normal pediatric vital signs

Normal heart rates by age	Newborn: 120 to 160 beats/minute preschool: 120 to 140 beats/minute School age: 100 to 120 beats/minute	**Normal respiratory rates by age**	1 week: 30 breaths/minute 3 years: 22 breaths/minute 5 years: 20 breaths/minute 8 years: 18 breaths/minute 12 years: 16 breaths/minute
Age-related calculation of normal systolic blood pressure	(age × 2) + 80 = normal systolic pressure	**Normal lung volumes in children**	Tidal volume: 6 to 7 ml/kg Vital capacity: 50 to 70 ml/kg

Pediatric coma scale*

Response	Score	Over 1 year	Less than 1 year	
Eyes opening	4	Spontaneously	Spontaneously	
	3	To verbal command	To shout	
	2	To pain	To pain	
	1	No response	No response	
Response		**Over 1 year**	**Less than 1 year**	
Best motor	6	Obeys		
	5	Localizes pain	Localizes pain	
	4	Flexion withdrawal	Flexion withdrawal	
	3	Flexion—abnormal (decorticate rigidity)	Flexion—abnormal (decorticate rigidity)	
	2	Extension (decerebrate rigidity)	Extension (decerebrate rigidity)	
	1	No response	No response	
Response		**Over 5 years**	**2–5 years**	**0–23 months**
Best verbal	5	Oriented and converses	Appropriate words and phrases	Smiles, coos, cries appropriately
	4	Disoriented and converses	Inappropriate words	Cries
	3	Inappropriate words	Cries and/or screams	Inappropriate crying and/or screaming
	2	Incomprehensible sounds	Grunts	Grunts
	1	No response	No response	No response
Total	3–15			

*Modification of Glasgow Coma Scale: A sum of seven or less is an objective measure of coma. The lower the score, the deeper the coma.

Appendix F: Preventing Postoperative Complications

Complications	Preventive nursing measures
Respiratory arrest	• Maintain airway. • Monitor respiratory parameters continuously. • Maintain I.V. infusion.
Shock	• Monitor hemodynamic parameters. • Measure intake and output levels. • Monitor neurologic status. • Report excessive postoperative bleeding. • Monitor hemoglobin and hematocrit values.
Pulmonary infection	• Supervise incentive spirometry every 2 hours. • Coach coughing or deep breathing. • Encourage position changes at least every 2 hours. • Maintain hydration. • Encourage activity to tolerance. • Assess and report lung sounds.
Wound infection	• Practice conscientious hand washing. • Monitor vital signs and report fever, tachycardia, or tachypnea. • Report redness, swelling, purulent exudate. • Provide aseptic wound care.
Urinary retention	• Promote early spontaneous voiding, using relaxation and positioning measures. • Maintain hydration. • Obtain order to catheterize if patient cannot void for 8 hours after surgery or shows marked distention or discomfort.
Paralytic ileus	• Encourage early activity, as permitted. • Assess bowel sounds. • Withhold food and fluid until peristalsis returns. • Insert gastric tube, as ordered. • Administer rectal tube or return-flow enema, as ordered. • Administer laxatives or suppositories, as ordered.
Thromboembolism	• Remind patient about hourly leg exercises. • Apply antiembolic stockings, as ordered. • Avoid knee gatch. • Report evidence of phlebitis or thrombosis. • Have patient begin weight bearing as soon as possible postoperatively.
Pain	• Provide analgesic medication, as ordered, and positioning or relaxation measures; see the "Acute Pain" care plan, page 10. • Prevent GI distention. • Control or remove noxious stimuli. • Administer antiemetics, as ordered. • Coach in use of relaxation techniques.
Dehiscence	• Leave original dressing undisturbed, unless otherwise recommended. • Reinforce dressing as needed. • Provide gentle wound care. • Minimize pull on incision.

For further details on postoperative care, see: Moir, E. "Surgical Intervention," in *Medical-Surgical Care Plans*. Edited by Holloway, N. Springhouse, Pa.: Springhouse Corp., 1988.

Appendix G: Nursing Diagnosis Grouped According to Functional Health Patterns

Health perception–health management pattern
Airway clearance, ineffective
Breathing pattern, ineffective
Gas exchange, impaired

Cardiac output, decreased†
Tissue perfusion, altered†: renal, cerebral, cardiopulmonary, gastrointestinal, peripheral

Tissue integrity, impaired†
Skin integrity, impaired

Injury, potential for: poisoning, suffocation, trauma
Infection, potential for

Adjustment, impaired
Growth and development, altered
Health maintenance, altered
Noncompliance (specify)

Nutritional-metabolic pattern
Fluid volume deficit
Fluid volume excess

Body temperature, altered: potential
Hypothermia
Hyperthermia
Thermoregulation, ineffective

Oral mucous membrane, alteration in
Nutrition, altered: less than body requirements
Nutrition, altered: more than body requirements
Swallowing, impaired

Elimination pattern
Bowel elimination, altered: constipation
Bowel elimination, altered: diarrhea
Bowel elimination, altered: incontinence

Incontinence, functional
Incontinence, reflex
Incontinence, stress
Incontinence, urge
Incontinence, total
Urinary elimination, altered patterns
Urinary retention

Activity-exercise pattern
Activity intolerance
Diversional activity deficit
Home maintenance management, impaired
Mobility, impaired physical
Self-care deficit: feeding, bathing/hygiene, dressing/grooming, toileting

Sleep-rest pattern
Sleep pattern disturbance

Cognitive-perceptual pattern
Comfort, altered: chronic pain
Comfort, altered: pain

Knowledge deficit (specify)
Thought processes, altered

Sensory-perceptual alterations: visual, auditory, kinesthetic, gustatory, tactile, olfactory
Unilateral neglect

Self-perception–self-concept pattern
Hopelessness
Powerlessness
Self-concept, disturbance in: body image
Self-concept, disturbance in: self-esteem
Self-concept, disturbance in: personal identity

Role-relationship pattern
Communication, impaired verbal
Family processes, alteration in
Parenting, altered
Social interaction, impaired
Social isolation
Violence, potential for
Role performance, altered

Sexuality-reproductive pattern
Sexuality, altered patterns
Sexual dysfunction
Rape-trauma syndrome

Coping–stress tolerance pattern
Coping, ineffective individual
Coping, ineffective family: compromised
Coping, ineffective family: disabling
Coping, family: potential for growth
Anxiety
Fear
Grieving, anticipatory
Grieving, dysfunctional
Post-trauma response

Value-belief pattern
Spiritual distress

*The functional health patterns are from Gordon, M. *Nursing Diagnosis: Process and Application,* 2nd ed. New York: McGraw-Hill Book Co., 1987. The nursing diagnoses are modified from McLane, A. *Classification of Nursing Diagnoses: Proceedings of the Seventh Conference.* St. Louis: C.V. Mosby Co., 1987.

†The editor believes that these diagnoses represent renaming of commonly accepted medical terms and recommends that they not be used for nursing diagnoses guiding independent nursing care. Interdependent nursing care related to these problems is included in the list of collaborative problems and labeled with the already familiar terms (shock, ischemia, and so forth) in this book.

Appendix H: Transfer Criteria Guidelines

Although the decision to transfer a patient is a medical one, the critical care nurse often has input in the decision. The following presents general criteria for transfer from a critical care unit to a "stepdown" or medical-surgical unit. Additional disease-specific criteria are presented within the appropriate care plans in this text. These transfer criteria guidelines should be individualized according to the patient's needs and unit protocol.

If desired, this list could be developed into a checklist of criteria that must be met before transfer to another unit. The nurse could check off each item accomplished and then use the list as the standard for communicating information during the transfer report.

General considerations

- No longer requires constant surveillance
- Discharge planning initiated, with assessments made of patient's living arrangements before admission, discharge prognosis, anticipated length of stay, ability to perform activities of daily living, educational goals, family or friend's ability and willingness to assist the patient after discharge, and referrals initiated to appropriate ancillary services
- Resuscitation status specified in medical order

Neurologic system

- Improved or unchanged level of consciousness and other neurologic vital signs for 12 hours
- Absence of intracranial pressure monitoring line

Pulmonary system

- Pulmonary status stable for 12 hours
- If still requires mechanical ventilation, transfer to caregivers experienced with this therapy
- PaO_2 >50 mm Hg
- $PaCO_2$ <10 mm Hg above patient's normal value

Cardiovascular system

- No longer needs I.V. pharmacologic therapy requiring continuous cardiac monitoring
- Blood pressure within 30 mm Hg of patient's normal value (or otherwise acceptable value) for 12 hours, without I.V. drugs, such as inotropes, vasodilators, or vasoconstrictors; or mechanical assist devices, such as intraaortic balloon pump
- Absent arterial line and pulmonary artery catheter

Renal system

- Urinary output ≥1 ml/kg/hour, except in chronic renal failure
- If receiving concentrated potassium infusion >20 mEq/hour, transfer to monitored bed

Index

A

B

C

D

Page numbers with a "t" indicate tables

Page numbers with a "t" indicate tables

Page numbers with a "t" indicate tables

U

V

W

Z

Page numbers with a "t" indicate tables

Notes

Notes

Notes

Notes

Notes

Notes